1993

Pocket Book of Infectious Disease Therapy

Pocket Book of Infectious Disease Therapy

John G. Bartlett, M.D.

Chief, Division of Infectious Diseases
The Johns Hopkins University School of Medicine
and The Johns Hopkins Hospital
Baltimore, Maryland

WILLIAMS & WILKINS
BALTIMORE • HONG KONG • LONDON • MUNICH
PHILADELPHIA • SYDNEY • TOKYO

Editor: Jonathan Pine
Associate Editor: Molly Mullen
Copy Editor: Susan S. Vaupel
Designer: Wilma Rosenberger
Illustration Planner: Ray Lowman
Production Coordinator: Kim Nawrozki

Accurate indications, adverse reactions, and dosage schedules for drugs are provided in
this book, but it is possible that they may change. The reader is urged to review the package
information data of the manufacturers of the medications mentioned.

Printed in the United States of America

First Edition 1990
ISBN 0-683-00443-3

93 94 95 96
1 2 3 4 5 6 7 8 9 10

■ PREFACE

The *1993 Pocket Book of Infectious Disease Therapy* is intended for physicians and other care providers who manage adult patients with infectious diseases. These include internists, generalists, surgeons, obstetricians, gynecologists, medical subspecialists and surgical subspecialists.

This book has the same lofty goals as the first three books: to provide standards of care with particular emphasis on antimicrobial agents, their selection and dosing regimens. As with prior editions there is extensive use of recommendations from various authoritative sources such as the Centers for Disease Control (CDC), the *Medical Letter on Drugs and Therapeutics,* the American Hospital Formulary Service, AMA Drug Evaluations and learned societies such as official statements of the American Heart Association (AHA), the American Thoracic Society and the Infectious Diseases Society of America (IDSA).

This book has extensive changes in terms of additions, deletions and revisions. Nearly all the tabular material has been updated to account for newly approved antibiotics, newly detected microbes and new recommendations for management. Extensive revisions have been made in the sections dealing with drug interactions, vaccinations, treatment of viral infection, tuberculosis, meningitis, hepatitis and urinary tract infections and HIV infection. New sections include the sepsis syndrome and a guide to the use of corticosteroids in infectious diseases and telephone numbers. New antibiotics included in tabular data include azithromycin, cefpodoxime, cefprozil, clarithromycin, dideoxycytidine (ddC), dideoxyinosine (ddI), itraconazole, ofloxacin, lomefloxacin, loracarbef, oxamniquine and teicoplanin.

The reader is encouraged to notify the author [Ross Research Building, Room 1159, The Johns Hopkins University School of Medicine, Baltimore, MD 21205; (410) 955-3150] if there are errors, differences of opinion or suggested additions.

■ CONTENTS

PREPARATIONS AND RECOMMENDED DOSING REGIMENS FOR ANTIMICROBIAL AGENTS (ADAPTED FROM DRUG INFORMATION 92, AMERICAN HOSPITAL FORMULARY SERVICE, 1992 pp 33-481)

Agent	Trade Names	Dosage Form	Usual Adult Regimen: Daily Dose, Route & Dose Interval
Acyclovir	Zovirax	5% ointment 3 & 15 gm tubes 200 mg caps 800 mg tabs 200 mg/5 ml susp 500;1000 mg vials (IV)	Topical q3h 200 mg po; x3-5/day 800 mg po; x5/day 200-800 mg po; x3-5/day 15-36 mg/kg/day IV over 1hr q8h
Amantadine	Symmetrel	100 mg cap & tabs 50 mg/5 ml syrup	100-200 mg/day po q12-24h
Amdinocillin	Coactin	0.5; 1 gm vial	40-60 mg/kg/day IM or IV q4-6h
Amikacin	Amikin	0.1;0.5;1 gm vials	15 mg/kg/day IV q8-12h
Aminosalicylic acid	PAS	0.5 gm tabs	150 mg/kg/day po q6-12h
Amoxicillin	Amoxil, Polymox, Trimox, Utimox, Wymox, Larotid	250;500 mg caps 125;250 mg/5 ml syrup	.75-2 gm/day po q6-8h
Amoxicillin + K clavulanate	Augmentin	125/31 mg/5 ml susp 250/62 mg/5 ml susp 125/31 mg tabs 250/125 mg tabs 500/125 mg tabs	.75-1.5 gm/day (amoxicillin) po q8h
Amphotericin B	Fungizone	50 mg vial	0.3-1 mg/kg/day IV over 4-8 hr q 1-2 days
Ampicillin	Omnipen, Amcill, Penamp, Polycillin, Principen, Totacillin	250;500 mg caps 125;250;500 mg/5 ml susp 3.5 gm + probenecid, 1 gm (for GC)	1-2 gm/day po q6h
Ampicillin sodium	Omnipen-N, Polycillin-N, Totacillin-N	0.125;0.25;0.5; 1; 2; 10 gm vials	2-8 gm/day IV q4-6h
Ampicillin + sulbactam	Unasyn	1:0.5 gm + 2:1.0 gm vials (Amp:sulbactam)	4-8 gm ampicillin/ day IV or IM q6h

(continued)

Agent	Trade Names	Dosage Form	Usual Adult Regimen: Daily Dose, Route & Dose Interval
Atovaquone	Mepron	250 mg tabs	750 mg po 3x/day w/food
Azithromycin	Zithromax	250 mg tabs	500 mg po first day, then 250 mg q24h x 5
Azlocillin	Azlin	2; 3; 4 gm vials	8-24 gm/day IV q6-8h
AZT	(see zidovudine)		
Aztreonam	Azactam	0.5; 1; 2 gm vials	1.5-6 gm/day IV or IM q6-8h
Bacampicillin	Spectrobid	400 mg tabs (equivalent to 280 mg ampicillin) 125 mg/5 ml syrup (equiv to 87 mg amp)	.8-1.6 gm/day po q12h
Bacitracin	Baci-IM	50,000 unit vials	10,000-25,000 units IM q6h; 25,000 units po q6h
Capreomycin	Capastat	1 gm vial	1 gm/day IM
Carbenicillin indanyl sodium	Geocillin	382 mg tabs	382-764 mg po q6h
Cefaclor	Ceclor	250;500 mg caps 125;187;250 & 375 mg/5 ml susp	1-2 gm/day po q8h
Cefadroxil	Duricef, Ultracef	500 mg caps; 1 gm tab; 125; 250; 500 mg/5 ml susp	1-2 gm/day po 1-2 x/day
Cefamandole nafate	Mandol	0.5;1;2;10 gm vials	2-18 gm/day IM or IV q4-6h
Cefazolin	Ancef, Kefzol, Zolicef	0.25;0.5;1;5;10;20 gm vials	2-6 gm/day IV or IM q8h
Cefixime	Suprax	200;400 mg tabs; 100 mg/5 ml susp	400 mg/day po, 1-2 x/day
Cefmetazole	Zefazone	1;2 gm vials	4-8 gm/day IV q6-12h
Cefonicid	Monocid	0.5;1;10 gm vials	1-2 gm/day IV or IM in 1 dose/day
Cefoperazone	Cefobid	1;2;10 gm vials	2-8 gm/day IM or IV q8-12h
Ceforanide lysine	Precef	0.5;1 gm vials	1-3 gm/day IV or IM q12h (continued)

2

Agent	Trade Names	Dosage Form	Usual Adult Regimen: Daily Dose, Route & Dose Interval
Cefotaxime sodium	Claforan	0.5;1;2;10 gm vials	2-12 gm/day IV or IM q6h
Cefotetan	Cefotan	1;2;10 gm vials	2-4 gm/day IV or IM q12h
Cefoxitin sodium	Mefoxin	1;2;10 gm vials	2-18 gm/day IV or IM q4-6h
Cefpodoxime proxetil	Vantin	100;200 mg tabs 50 mg/5 ml; 100 mg/5 ml susp	200-800 mg/day po, q12h
Cefprozil	Cefzil	250;500 mg tabs 125;250 mg/5 ml susp	0.5-2 gm/day po, q12-24h usually 500 mg qd or bid
Ceftazidime	Fortaz, Tazidime, Tazicef, Ceptaz	0.5;1;2;6 gm vials	3-6 gm/day IV or IM q8-12h
Ceftizoxime sodium	Cefizox	1;2;10 gm vials	2-12 gm/day IV or IM q6-8h
Ceftriaxone	Rocephin	0.25;0.5;1;2;10 gm vial	1-2 gm IV or IM q12-24h
Cefuroxime	Zinacef	0.75;1.5 gm vial	2.25-4.5 gm/day IV or IM q6-8h
Cefuroxime axetil	Ceftin	0.125;0.25;0.5 gm tabs	0.5-1.0 gm/day po q12h
Cephalexin monohydrate	Keflex, Keftab, Cefanex, Keflet	0.25;0.5 gm caps 0.25;0.5 gm tabs 125;250 mg/5 ml susp	1-2 gm/day po q6h
Cephalothin sodium	Keflin	1;2;20 gm vials	2-12 gm/day IV q4-6h
Cephapirin sodium	Cefadyl	0.5;1;2;4 gm vials	2-4 gm/day IV q6h
Cephradine	Anspor	250;500 mg caps 125;250 mg/5 ml susp	1-2 gm/day po q6h
	Velosef	0.25;0.5;1;2 gm vials	2-8 gm/day IV or IM q6h
Chloramphenicol	Chloromycetin	250 mg caps	1-2 gm/day po q6h

(continued)

Agent	Trade Names	Dosage Form	Usual Adult Regimen: Daily Dose, Route & Dose Interval
Chloramphenicol palmitate	Chloromycetin	150 mg/5 ml syrup	1-2 gm/day po q6h
Chloramphenicol Na succinate	Chloromycetin sodium succinate	1 gm vial	2-4 gm/day IV q6h
Chloroquine HCl	Aralen HCl	250 mg amp (150 mg base)	200-250 mg base q6h IM or IV
Chloroquine PO₄	Aralen PO₄	500 mg tabs (300 mg base) 250 mg tabs (150 mg base)	300-600 mg (base) qd - q week
Chloroquine hydroxy	Plaquenil	200 mg tabs (155 mg base)	10 mg/kg/day po q24h
Cinoxacin	Cinobac	250;500 mg cap	1 gm/day po q6-12h
Ciprofloxacin	Cipro Cipro IV	250;500;750 mg tabs 200;400 mg vials	0.5-1.5 gm/day po q12h 800 mg/day IV q12h
Clarithromycin	Biaxin	250;500 mg tabs	500 mg/day po q12h
Clindamycin HCl	Cleocin HCl	75;150;300 mg cap	0.6-1.8 gm/day po q6-8h
Clindamycin PO₄	Cleocin PO₄	150 mg/ml in vials (2,4,6 ml)	1.8-2.7 gm/day IV q6-8h
Clindamycin palmitate HCl	Cleocin pediatric	75 mg/5 ml solution	0.6-1.8 gm/day po q6-8h
Clindamycin vaginal cream	Cleocin VC	2% 40 gm tube	Topical: 1/day x 7 days
Clofazimine	Lamprene	50;100 mg caps	50-300 mg/day po q8-24h
Cloxacillin	Tegopen Cloxapen	250;500 mg caps 125 mg/5 ml solution	1-2 gm/day po q6h
Colistin	Coly-Mycin S Coly-Mycin M	25 mg/5 ml susp 150 mg vial (IV)	2.5-5.0 mg/kg/day IV q6-12h
Cyclacillin	Cyclapen-W	250;500 mg cap 125;250 mg/5 ml susp	1-2 gm/day po q6h
Cycloserine	Seromycin	250 mg caps	0.5-1 gm/day po in 2 doses
Dapsone		25;100 mg tabs	25-100 mg/day po q24h

(continued)

4

Agent	Trade Names	Dosage Form	Usual Adult Regimen: Daily Dose, Route & Dose Interval
Demeclocycline	Declomycin	150;300 mg caps	600 mg/day po q6-12h
Dicloxacillin	Dycill, Dynapen Pathocil	125;250;500 mg cap 62.5 mg/5 ml susp	1-2 gm/day po q6h
Didanosine (Dideoxyinosine) (ddI)	Videx	25;50;100;150 mg tabs and 100;167;250;375 mg packets	>60 kg:200 mg (tabs) bid <60 kg:125 mg (tabs) bid
Dideoxycytidine (ddC)	HIVID	0.375;0.75 mg tabs	0.75 mg po tid
Diethylcarba-mazine	Hetrazan	50 mg tabs	6-13 mg/kg/day, 1-3 doses
Diloxanide	Furamide		500 mg po q8h
Doxycycline	Vibramycin Doxy caps, Doxy tabs Vibra-tabs Doxy-100,200	50 mg/5 ml susp 100 mg tabs 50;100 mg caps 100;200 mg vial	100-200 mg/day po q12-24h 200 mg/day IV q12h
Eflornithine	Ornidyl		400 mg/kg/day IV; 100 mg/kg po q8h
Emetine HCl		65 mg/ml (1 ml vial)	1-1.5 mg/kg/day up to 90 mg/day; IM or deep SC injection
Enoxacin	Penetrex	200;400 mg tabs	400-800 mg/day po q12h
Erythromycin	E-mycin;ERYC; Ery-Tab; E-Base Erythromycin Base Ilotycin, PCE, RP-Mycin, Robimycin	250 mg caps 250;333;500 mg tabs 2% topical	1-2 gm/day po q6h (topical for acne)
Erythromycin estolate	Ilosone	250 mg caps, 500 mg tabs 125;250 mg/5 ml susp	1-2 gm/day po q6h
Erythromycin ethylsuccinate	E.E.S. EryPed	200;400 mg tabs 200;400 mg/5 ml susp	1.6-3.2 gm/day po q6h
Erythromycin gluceptate	Ilotycin gluceptate	1 gm vial	2-4 gm/day IV q6h
Erythromycin lactobionate	Erythrocin lactobionate	0.5;1 gm vial	1-4 gm/day IV q6h

(continued)

Agent	Trade Names	Dosage Form	Usual Adult Regimen: Daily Dose, Route & Dose Interval
Erythromycin stearate	Eramycin Erypar; Erythrocin stearate; Ethril; Wyamycin S SK-erythromycin	250;500 mg tabs	1-2 gm/day po q6h
Ethambutol	Myambutol	100;400 mg tabs	15 mg/kg/day po q24h
Ethionamide	Trecator-SC	250 mg tabs	0.5-1 gm/day po in 1-3 daily doses
Fluconazole	Diflucan	50;100;200 mg tabs 100;200 mg vials	100-200 mg/day po or IV q24h
Flucytosine	Ancobon	250;500 mg cap	50-150 mg/kg/day po q6h
Foscarnet	Foscavir	24 mg/ml, 500 ml	90-180 mg/kg/day IV qd or tid
Furazolidone	Furoxone	100 mg tabs 50 mg/15 ml susp	100 mg po q6h
Ganciclovir	Cytovene	0.5 gm vial	5 mg/kg IV bid (induction) or qd (maintenance)
Gentamicin	Garamycin Gentamicin SO₄ Injection Isotonic (NaCl) Gentamicin SO₄ ADD-Vantage Gentamicin SO₄ in 5% dextrose piggyback	40;60;70;80;90; 100;120 mg vials 2 mg/ml for intrathecal use	3-5 mg/kg/day IV or IM q8h
Griseofulvin	Grisactin Fulvicin Grifulvin V Gris-PEG Grisactin Ultra Fulvicin P/G	microsize: 250 caps, 250;500 mg tabs 125 mg/5 ml susp ultramicrosize: 125; 165;250;330 mg tabs	500 mg - 1 gm po/day

330-750 mg po/day |
| Imipenem/ Cilastatin | Primaxin | 0.25;0.5;0.75 gm vials (Imipenem: cilastatin is 1:1) | 1-4 gm/day IV q6h |
| Interferon Alfa 2a | Roferon-A | 3,18,36 mil unit vials | 3 mil units 3x/wk (HCV) 30-35 mil units/wk (HBV) 30 mil units/m2 3x/wk (Kaposi Sarcoma) 1 mil units intralesion (condylomata) |

(continued)

Agent	Trade Names	Dosage Form	Usual Adult Regimen: Daily Dose, Route & Dose Interval
Interferon (continued) Alfa 2b	Intron A	3,5,10,25,50 mil unit vials	As above
Iodoquinol	Yodoxin Diquinol Yodoquinol	210 mg tabs 650 mg tabs	650 mg/day po q8h
Isoniazid	Laniazid Tubizid	50;100;300 mg tabs 50 mg/5 ml (oral solu)	300 mg/day po q24h
	Nydrazid	1 gm vial (IM)	300 mg/day IM q12-24h
Itraconazole	Sporanox	100 mg caps	200-400 mg/day po q12-24h
Kanamycin	Kantrex Klebcil	.075;0.5; 1 gm vial 500 mg caps	15 mg/kg/day IV q8h
Ketoconazole	Nizoral	200 mg tabs	200-400 mg/day po q12-24h up to 1.6 gm/day
Lincomycin	Lincocin	250;500 mg caps 300 mg/ml (2,10 ml)	1.5-2.0 gm/d po q6-8h 1.8-8 gm/d IV q8-12h
Loracarbef	Lorabid	200 mg parvule	400-800 mg/day po q12h
Lomefloxacin	Maxaquin	400 mg caps	400 mg/day po q24h
Mefloquine	Lariam	250 mg tabs	1250 mg po x 1 (treatment); 250 mg po q wk (prophylaxis)
Mebendazole	Vermox	100 mg tabs	100 mg po x 1-2 up to 2 gm/day
Methacycline	Rondomycin	150;300 mg caps	600 mg/d po
Methenamine hippurate	Hiprex	1 gm tabs	1-2 gm/day po q12h
Methenamine mandelate	Mandelamine	0.35;0.5;1 gm tabs 250;500 mg/5 ml syrup 0.5; 1 gm granules	1-4 gm/day po q6h
Methicillin	Staphcillin	1;4;6;10 gm vial	4-12 gm/day IV or IM q6h
Metronidazole	Flagyl, Metryl Metizol, Protostat	250;500 mg tabs	0.75-2 gm/day po q12h
	Metric 21, Satric	500 mg vial	0.75-2 gm/day IV q6-12h

(continued)

7

Agent	Trade Names	Dosage Form	Usual Adult Regimen: Daily Dose, Route & Dose Interval
Mezlocillin Na	Mezlin	1;2;3;4 gm vial	6-24 gm/day IV q 4-6h
Miconazole	Monistat	200 mg amp 200 mg vaginal supp	0.6-3.6 gm/day IV q8h qd x 3
Minocycline	Minocin	50;100 mg caps & tabs 50 mg/5 ml syrup 100 mg vial	200 mg/day po q6-12h 200 mg/day IV q6-12h
Moxalactam	Moxam	1 gm vial	2-8 gm/day IV q6-8h
Nafcillin	Unipen	250 mg caps; 500 mg tabs	1-2 gm/day po q6h
	Nafcil, Nallpen, Unipen	0.5;1;2;10 gm vial	2-12 gm/day IV or IM q4-6h
Nalidixic acid	NegGram	0.25;0.5;1 gm tabs 250 mg/5 ml susp	4 gm/day po q6h
Neomycin	Mycifradin	500 mg tabs 125 mg/5 ml solu	3-12 gm po/day
Netilmicin	Netromycin	100 mg/ml vials	4-6.5 mg/kg/day IV or IM q8h
Niclosamide	Niclocide	500 mg tabs	2 gm (single dose)

Nitrofurantoin	Macrodantin
	Furadantin
	Furaton
	Furalan
	Faran
		macrocrystals:
		25;50;100 mg caps
		microcrystals:
		50;100 caps/tabs
		25 mg/5 ml susp
			50-100 mg po q6h
			  Suppressive treatment:
			  50-100 mg qd

Norfloxacin	Noroxin	400 mg tabs	400 mg po bid
Novobiocin	Albamycin	250 mg caps	1-2 gm/day po q6-12h
Nystatin	Mycostatin Nystex Nilstat	100,000 units/ml 500,000 unit tab 0.05;0.15;0.25;0.5;1;2; 5;10 billion units powder	5 ml swish, swallow or 5-10 ml po 3-5 x daily
Ofloxacin	Floxin	200;300;400 mg tabs	200-400 mg po q12h
Oxacillin	Bactocill, Prostaphlin	250; 500 mg caps 250 mg/5 ml solu 0.25;0.5;1;2;4;10 gm vials	2-4 gm/day po q12h 2-12 gm/day IV or IM q4-6h

(continued)

8

Agent	Trade Names	Dosage Form	Usual Adult Regimen: Daily Dose, Route & Dose Interval
Oxamniquine	Vansil	250 mg caps	12-15 mg/kg x 1 15 mg/kg q12h x 4
Paromomycin	Humatin	250 mg caps	2-4 gm/day po q6-12h
Penicillin G and V Crystalline G potassium	Pentids	(1 unit = 0.6 mcg) 0.2;0.25;0.4;0.8 million unit tabs 0.4 million units/5ml	1-2 gm po/day q6h
	Penicillin G for injection Pfizerpen	1;2;3;5;10;20 million unit vials	2-20 million units/day IV q4-6h
Crystalline G sodium	Penicillin G sodium for injection	5 million unit vial	2-20 million units IV/day q4-6h
Benzathine	Bicillin Bicillin L-A Permapen	200,000 unit tabs 3 million unit vial; 600,000 units/ml vial (1,2,4,10 ml vials)	Not recommended po 1.2-2.4 mil units IM
Benzathine+ procaine	Bicillin C-R	Benzathine: procaine/ml 150,000:150,000 units (10 ml) 300,000:150,000 (1,2,4 ml) 450,000:150,000 units (2 ml)	1.2-2.4 mil units IM
Procaine	Crysticillin Pfizerpen Wycillin	300,000 units (10 ml) 500,000 units (12 ml) 600,000 units (1,2,4 ml syringe)	0.6-4.8 mil units/day IM q6-12h
Phenoxyethyl penicillin (V)	Beepen VK, Betapen VK, Pen-Vee K, V-Cillin K, Veetids, Ledercillin VK, Robicillin VK	125;250;500 mg tabs 125;250 ml/5 ml susp	1-2 gm/day po q6h
Pentamidine	Pentam 300 NebuPent	300 mg vial 300 mg aerosol	4 mg/kg/day IV qd 300 mg/day/mo (prophylaxis)
Piperacillin	Pipracil	2;3;4;40 gm vials	6-24 gm/day IV q4-6h
Piperazine		250 mg tabs 500 mg/5 ml	3.5-5 gm/day

(continued)

9

Agent	Trade Names	Dosage Form	Usual Adult Regimen: Daily Dose, Route & Dose Interval
Polymyxin B	Aerosporin	500,000 unit vials 1 mg = 1,000 units 200,000 units + 40 mg neomycin	1.5-2.5 mg/kg/day IM or IV q4-6h
Praziquantel	Biltricide	600 mg tabs	20-75 mg/kg/day po in 3 doses
Primaquine		15 mg (base) tabs	15 mg po qd
Pyrantel	Antiminth	50 mg/ml susp	11 mg/kg x 1
Pyrazinamide		500 mg tabs	15-30 mg/kg/day po in 6-8 doses
Pyrimethamine	Daraprim	25 mg tabs	25 mg po q wk or daily up to 200 mg/day
Pyrimethamine + sulfadoxine	Fansidar	Sulfa-500 mg plus pyrimeth-25 mg	1 tab/wk 3 tabs (1 dose)
Quinacrine	Atabrine	100 mg	300-800 mg po/day
Quinine	Legatrin Quine 200,300 Quin-260 etc	130;200;300;325 mg caps 260;325 mg tabs	325 mg bid 650 mg q8h po
Quinine dihydrochloride		IV available from CDC	600 mg IV q8h
Rifabutin	Mycobutin	150 mg caps	600 mg/day po
Rifampin	Rifadin Rifamate	150;300 mg caps 300 mg cap with 150 mg INH 600 mg vials	600 mg/day po (TB) 600-1200 mg/day po (other indications) 600 mg/day IV
Spectinomycin	Trobicin	2;4 gm vials	2 gm IM x 1
Streptomycin		1 & 5 gm vial	1-2 gm IM/day
Sulfonamides Trisulfa- pyrimidines	Triple sulfa Neotrizine Terfonyl	Sulfadiazine, Sulfamerazine & Sulfamethazine, 167 mg (each) tabs and 167 mg (each) 5 ml susp	2-4 gm/day po q4-8h
Sulfadiazine	Microsulfon	0.5 gm tabs	2-4 gm/day po q4-8h

(continued)

Agent	Trade Names	Dosage Form	Usual Adult Regimen: Daily Dose, Route & Dose Interval
Sulfamethox-azole	Gantanol	0.5; 1 gm tabs	2-4 gm/day po q8-12h
Sulfapyridine		0.5 gm tabs	1-4 gm/day po q6h
Sulfasalazine	Azulfidine	0.5 gm tabs 0.25 mg/5 ml susp	3-4 gm/day po q6h
Sulfisoxazole	Gantrisin	0.5 gm tabs	4-8 gm/day po q4-6h
Teicoplanin	Targocid	400 mg vials	6-12 mg/kg/day IV q24h
Tetracyclines			
Demeclocycline	Declomycin	150 mg cap 150;300 mg tab	600 mg/day po q6-12h
Doxycycline	Vibramycin	50;100 mg tabs 50;100 mg caps 50 mg/5 ml susp 100 mg vials	100-200 mg/day po q12-24h 200 mg/day IV q12-24h
Minocycline	Minocin	50;100 mg caps 50;100 mg tabs 100 mg vials	200 mg/day po or IV q12h
Oxytetracycline	Terramycin Uri-Tet	250 mg cap 50;125 mg/ml with lidocaine (IM)	1-2 gm/day po q6h 0.5-1 gm/day IM q12h
Tetracycline	Achromycin; Tetralan Brodspec; Panmycin Robitet; Sumycin, etc.	100;250;500 mg caps 250;500 mg tabs 125 mg/5 ml susp	1-2 gm/day po q6h
Thiabendazole	Mintezol	500 mg tabs 500 mg/5 ml susp	1-3 gm po/day
Ticarcillin	Ticar	1;3;6;20;30 gm vials	4-24 gm/day IV q4-6h
Ticarcillin + clavulanic acid	Timentin	3 gm ticarcillin + 100 mg CA vials	4-24 gm/day (ticarcillin) IV q4-6h
Tobramycin	Nebcin	20;60;80 & 1200 mg vials	3-5 mg/kg/day IV or IM q8h
Trimethoprim	Proloprim; Trimpex	100;200 mg tabs	200 mg/day po q12-24h

(continued)

11

Agent	Trade Names	Dosage Form	Usual Adult Regimen: Daily Dose, Route & Dose Interval
Trimethoprim-sulfamethoxazole	Bactrim, Septra Cotrim	Trimethoprim:sulfa 40 mg:200 mg/5 ml susp 80 mg:400 mg tabs 160 mg:800 mg DS tabs 16 mg:80 mg/ml (IV) (5,10,20 ml vials)	2-20 mg/kg/day (trimethoprim) po or IV q6-8h
Vancomycin	Vancocin pulvules Vancocin HCl (oral solu) Vancocin HCl IV Lyphocin	125;250 mg caps 1;10 gm vials 0.5;1 gm vials (IV)	0.5-2 gm/day po q6h 1-2 gm/day IV q6-12h
Vidarabine	Vira-A, Ara-A	200 mg/ml	15 mg/kg/day IV
Zidovudine	Retrovir, AZT	100 mg caps; 50 mg/ 5 ml syrup 240 ml Infusion - 10 mg/ml (20 ml)	500-600 mg/day po q4-8h 1-2 mg/kg IV q4h

COST OF ANTIMICROBIAL AGENTS

Acyclovir	200 mg cap	$ 0.82		Chloroquine	500 mg tab	$ 2.40
	800 mg cap	$ 3.32		Plaquenil	200 mg tab	$ 0.95
	500 mg vial**	$ 44.02		Ciprofloxacin	750 mg tab	$ 4.97
Amantadine	100 mg tab	$ 0.72			400 mg vial**	$ 28.80
Amikacin	1 gm vial**	$119.42		Clarithromycin	250 mg tab	$ 2.50
Amoxicillin	250 mg cap	$ 0.82			500 mg tab	$ 2.50
Amoxil	250 mg cap	$ 0.21		Clindamycin	300 mg vial**	$ 7.04
Amoxicillin +				Cleocin	300 mg cap	$ 2.14
clavulanate	250 mg cap	$ 1.70		Clofazimine	100 mg cap	$ 0.20
Amphotericin B	50 mg vial**	$ 38.60		Clotrimazole	10 mg tab	$ 0.68
Ampicillin	250 mg cap	$ 0.07		Cloxacillin	500 mg tab	$ 0.38
Omnipen	250 mg cap	$ 0.62		Cycloserine	250 mg pulv	$ 3.14
Ampicillin	2 gm vial**	$ 12.64		Dapsone	100 mg tab	$ 0.18
Ampicillin +				ddC	0.75 mg	$ 2.13
sulbactam	1.5 gm vial**	$ 5.80		ddI	100 mg	$ 1.43
Atovaquone	250 mg tab	$ 2.13		Dicloxacillin	500 mg cap	$ 0.11
Azithromycin	250 mg tab	$ 8.12		Vibramycin	100 mg tab	$ 3.15
Aztreonam	1 gm vial**	$ 14.54			100 mg vial**	$ 16.15
Azulfidine	500 mg tab	$ 0.18		Erythromycin	250 mg cap	$ 0.11
Bacitracin	50,000 unit vial	$ 8.51		E-mycin	250 mg tab	$ 0.24
Bicillin	2.4 mil units**	$ 20.97		Erythromycin	1 gm vial**	$ 21.50
Cefaclor	250 mg pulv	$ 1.83		Erythropoietin	3000 unit vial	$ 36.00
Cefadroxil	500 mg cap	$ 2.70		Ethambutol	400 mg tab	$ 1.18
Cefamandole	2 mg vial**	$ 18.80		Fluconazole	50 mg	$ 4.37
Cefazolin	500 mg cap	$ 3.00			100 mg tab	$ 6.87
Cefixime	200 mg tab	$ 2.56			200 mg vial**	$119.00
Cefmetazole	2 gm vial**	$ 14.33		Flucytosine	500 mg cap	$ 1.66
Cefonicid	1 gm vial**	$ 27.11		Foscarnet	6 gm vial**	$ 73.25
Cefoperazone	2 gm vial**	$ 31.69		Gamimmune	250 ml vial**	$714.00
Ceforanide	1 gm vial**	$ 12.54		Ganciclovir	0.5 gam vial**	$ 34.80
Cefotaxime	2 gm vial**	$ 21.00		G-CSF	300 mcg vial**	$135.00
Cefotetan	1 gm vial**	$ 10.84		GM-CSF	350 mcg vial**	$135.00
Cefoxitin	2 gm vial**	$ 17.71		Gentamicin	80 mg vial**	$ 1.04
Cefprozil	250 mg tab	$ 2.63		Garamycin	80 mg vial**	$ 3.44
Ceftazidime	1 gm vial**	$ 14.60		Griseofulvin	500 mg tab	$ 0.93
	2 gm vial**	$ 20.73		ultramicro	250 mg tab	$ 0.68
Ceftriaxone	250 mg vial**	$ 10.24		Imipenem	500 mg vial**	$ 23.59
	1 gm vial**	$ 30.46		Interferon alpha	3 MU vial**	$ 26.96
Cefuroxime	750 mg vial**	$ 7.10		Isoniazid	300 mg tab	$ 0.02
Cefuroxime axeil	250 mg tab	$ 2.79		Itraconazole	100 mg cap	$ 4.10
Cephalexin	500 mg tab	$ 0.28		Ketoconazole	200 mg tab	$ 2.32
Keflex	500 mg tab	$ 2.30		Leukovorin	5 mg tab	$ 2.71
Cephalothin				Lomefloxin	400 mg	$ 4.47
Keflin	2 gm vial**	$ 6.55		Methenamine	1 gm tab	$ 0.33
Cephapirin	1 gm vial**	$ 3.98		Metronidazole	500 mg tab	$ 0.07
Cephradine	500 mg cap	$ 1.62		Flagyl	500 mg tab	$ 2.09
	500 mg vial**	$ 4.13			500 mg vial**	$ 7.81
	500 mg vial**	$ 5.20		Flagyl	500 mg vial**	$ 15.53
Chloramphenicol	1 gm vial**	$ 5.20		Mezlocillin	3 gm vial**	$ 11.90
Chloromycetin	250 mg cap	$ 1.05				

(continued)

13

Miconazole	200 mg vial**	$ 38.05	Rifampin	300 mg cap	$ 1.97
vag supp	200 mg	$ 7.05	Streptomycin	1 gm vial**	$ 3.95
2% creme	30 mg	$ 18.00	Sulfamethoxazole	500 mg tab	$ 0.06
Minocycline	100 mg cap	$ 1.90	Gantanol	500 mg tab	$ 0.47
Nafcillin	250 mg tab	$ 0.87	Sulfisoxazole	500 mg tab	$ 0.03
	2 gm vial**	$ 16.00	Gantrisin	500 mg tab	$ 0.21
Nalidixic acid	500 mg tab	$ 0.97	Tetracycline	500 mg tab	$ 0.05
Netilmicin	100 mg vial**	$ 10.11	Acromycin	500 mg tab	$ 0.06
Nitrofurantoin	50 mg tab	$ 0.60	Ticarcillin	3 gm vial**	$ 9.30
Macrodantin	50 mg tab	$ 0.59	Ticarcillin +		
Norfloxacin	400 mg tab	$ 2.25	clavulanate	3 gm vial**	$ 12.85
Nystatin tab	100,000 units	$ 0.15	Tobramycin	80 mg vial**	$ 7.88
Mycostatin tab	100,000 units	$ 0.90	Trimethoprim	100 mg tab	$ 0.14
susp 100,000			Trimethoprim-	DS tab	$ 0.07
units/ml	60 ml	$ 6.00	sulfamethoxazole	160 mg vial**	$ 5.80
Ofloxacin	400 mg tab	$ 3.38	Bactrim	DS tab	$ 1.05
	200 mg tab	$ 2.70	Septra	DS tab	$ 0.99
Oxacillin	500 mg caps	$ 1.30	Vancomycin	1 gm vial**	$ 37.00
	2 gm vial**	$ 21.74		125 mg parv	$ 4.73
Penicillin G	1 million unit vial**	$ 1.30	Vivonex TEN	1 packet	$ 5.39
	20 million unit vial**	$ 10.11	Zidovudine (AZT)	100 mg	$ 1.44
	500 mg tab	$ 0.07			
Penicillin V	250 mg tab	$ 0.04			
Pen-Vee-K	500 mg tab	$ 0.12			
Pentamidine	300 mg vial**	$ 98.75			
Piperacillin	3 gm vial**	$ 16.75			
Podofilox	3.5 ml bottle	$ 48.00			
Praziquantel	600 mg tab	$ 9.48			
Pyrazinamide	500 mg tab	$ 1.01			
Pyrimethamine	25 mg tab	$ 0.33			
Pyrimethamine +					
sulfadoxine	25/500 mg tab	$ 3.04			
Quinacrine	100 mg tab	$ 0.32			
Quinine	325 mg pulv	$ 0.38			

---

*   Approximate wholesale prices; price to consumer will be higher. Prices are provided by generic name alphabetically; prices for both trade and generic name are provided for some products.

**   Indicates preparation for parenteral administration.

PREFERRED ANTIMICROBIAL AGENTS FOR SPECIFIC PATHOGENS
(Adapted in part from The Medical Letter on Drugs and Therapeutics 34:49, 1992)

Organism	Usual Disease	Preferred Agent	Alternatives
Achromobacter xylosoxidans	Meningitis, septicemia	Antipseudomonad penicillin (2) Imipenem	Cephalosporins - 3rd gen (5) Sulfa-trimethoprim Imipenem Ticarcillin + clavulanic acid
Acinetobacter calcoaceticus var antitratum (Herellea vaginicola; var lwoffi (Mima polymorpha)	Sepsis (esp line sepsis) Pneumonia	Imipenem Aminoglycoside (tobramycin or amikacin) + ceftazidime or antipseudomonad penicillin (2)	Fluoroquinolone (6) Cephalosporin - 3rd gen (5) Tetracycline (4) Antipseudomonad penicillin (2)
Actinobacillus actinomycetemcomitans	Actinomycosis	Penicillin	Clindamycin Tetracycline (4) Erythromycin Cephalosporins (5)
	Endocarditis	Penicillin + aminoglycoside (1)	Cephalosporin (5) + aminoglycoside (1)
Actinomyces israelii (also A. naeslundii, A. viscosus, A. odontolyticus and Arachnia proprionica)	Actinomycosis	Penicillin G	Clindamycin Tetracycline (4) Erythromycin
Aeromonas hydrophila	Diarrhea	Fluoroquinolone (6) Sulfa-trimethoprim	Tetracycline (4)
	Bacteremia	Cephalosporin (3rd gen)	Sulfa-trimethoprim Aminoglycoside (1)

(continued)

15

Organism	Usual Disease	Preferred Agent	Alternatives
Aeromonas hydrophila (cont.)	Cellulitis/myositis/ osteomyelitis	Fluoroquinolone (6) Sulfa-trimethoprim	Aminoglycoside (1) Imipenem
Afipia felis	Cat scratch disease	Fluoroquinolone (6) (usually not treated)	Sulfa-trimethoprim Gentamicin Amoxicillin-clavulanate
Bacillus anthracis	Anthrax	Penicillin G Penicillin + streptomycin (meningitis or inhalation anthrax)	Erythromycin Tetracycline (4) Chloramphenicol
Bacillus cereus	Food poisoning Invasive disease	Not treated Clindamycin, erythromycin, vancomycin	
Bacillus species	Septicemia (comp host)	Vancomycin	Imipenem Aminoglycosides (1) Fluoroquinolones (6)
Bacteroides bivius	Female genital tract infections	Metronidazole Clindamycin Cefoxitin Cefotetan	Chloramphenicol Antipseudomonad penicillin (2) Imipenem Betalactam-betalactamase inhibitor (7)
"B. fragilis group"	Abscesses Bacteremia Intra-abdominal sepsis	Metronidazole Clindamycin Cefoxitin	Chloramphenicol Antipseudomonad penicillin (2) Imipenem Betalactam-betalactamase inhibitor (7) Cefmetazole
"B. melaninogenicus group"	Oral-dental & pulmonary infections Female genital tract infections	Metronidazole Clindamycin Cefoxitin	Chloramphenicol Betalactam-betalactamase inhibitor (7) Imipenem Cefotetan Cefmetazole

(continued)

16

Organism	Usual Disease	Preferred Agent	Alternatives
Bartonella bacilliformis	Bartonellosis	Chloramphenicol Penicillin	Tetracycline + streptomycin
Bordetella pertussis	Pertussis	Erythromycin	Sulfa-trimethoprim Ampicillin
Borrelia burgdorferi	Lyme disease	Tetracycline (4) (early disease) Ceftriaxone (late complications)	Penicillin G po or IV Amoxicillin Cefuroxime axetil Erythromycin/Azithromycin(?) Cefotaxime
Borrelia recurrentis	Relapsing fever	Tetracycline (4)	Penicillin G Erythromycin Chloramphenicol
Brucella	Brucellosis	Doxycycline + rifampin Doxycycline + gentamicin or streptomycin	Chloramphenicol ± streptomycin Sulfa-trimethoprim Rifampin + cephalosporin (3rd gen) (5) (CNS involvement)
Calymmatobacterium granulomatis	Granuloma inguinale	Tetracycline (4)	Sulfa-trimethoprim Erythromycin (pregnancy)
Campylobacter fetus	Septicemia, vascular infections, meningitis	Gentamicin Imipenem	Chloramphenicol Erythromycin Clindamycin Tetracycline (4)
Campylobacter jejuni	Diarrhea	Erythromycin Fluoroquinolone (6)	Tetracycline (4) Furazolidine Gentamicin
Capnocytophaga ochracea	Periodontal disease Bacteremia in neutropenic host Tonsillitis (?)	Clindamycin Erythromycin	Amoxicillin–clavulanic acid Imipenem Cefoxitin Cephalosporins (3rd gen) (5) Fluoroquinolone (6) Tetracycline (continued)

Organism	Usual Disease	Preferred Agent	Alternatives
Capnocytophaga canimorus (DF$_2$)	Dog and cat bites Bacteremia meningitis (asplenia)	Penicillin Clindamycin	Cephalosporins (3rd gen) (5) Imipenem Vancomycin Fluoroquinolones (6)
Cardiobacterium	Bacteremia Endocarditis	Penicillin + aminoglycoside	Cephalosporin (5) ± aminoglycoside (1)
Cat scratch disease, agent of	Cat scratch disease with lymphadenitis	Fluoroquinolone (6)	Gentamicin Amoxicillin–clavulanate Trimethoprim-sulfamethoxazole
Chlamydia pneumoniae (TWAR agent)	Pneumonia	Tetracycline (4) Erythromycin	Clarithromycin Azithromycin
Chlamydia psittaci	Psittacosis	Tetracycline (4)	Chloramphenicol
Chlamydia trachomatis	Urethritis Endocervicitis PID Epididymitis Urethral syndrome	Tetracycline (4) Azithromycin	Erythromycin Ofloxacin Sulfisoxazole
	Trachoma	Tetracycline (4) (topical + oral)	Sulfonamide (topical + oral)
	Lymphogranuloma venereum	Tetracycline (4)	Erythromycin
	Inclusion conjunctivitis	Erythromycin (topical or oral)	Sulfonamide
Citrobacter diversus	Urinary tract infections, pneumonia	Aminoglycoside (1) Cephalosporin (2nd & 3rd gen) (5) Sulfa-trimethoprim	Tetracycline (4) Fluoroquinolone (6) Imipenem Piperacillin

(continued)

18

Organism	Usual Disease	Preferred Agent	Alternatives
Citrobacter freundii	Urinary tract infection, wound infection, septicemia, pneumonia	Imipenem Fluoroquinolone (6) Sulfa-trimethoprim Aminoglycoside (1)	Tetracycline (4) Cephalosporin (3rd gen) (5)
Clostridium difficile	Antibiotic-associated colitis	Vancomycin (oral) Metronidazole (oral)	Bacitracin (oral) Cholestyramine Lactobacilli Vancomycin + rifampin
Clostridium sp.	Gas gangrene Sepsis Tetanus Botulism Crepitant cellulitis	Penicillin G Tetanus immune globulin or IGIV Trivalent equine antitoxin (CDC)*	Chloramphenicol Metronidazole Antipseudomonad penicillin (2) Clindamycin Imipenem
Corynebacterium diphtheriae	Diphtheria	Penicillin or erythromycin + antitoxin (CDC)*	
Corynebacterium JK strain	Septicemia	Vancomycin	Penicillin G + gentamicin Fluoroquinolone (6)
Corynebacterium minutissimum	Erythrasma	Erythromycin	
Corynebacterium ulcerans	Pharyngitis	Erythromycin	
Coxiella burnetii	Q fever	Tetracycline (4)	Chloramphenicol Ciprofloxacin (6) Rifampin (7)
Dysgonic fermenter type 2 (DF₂)	See Capnocytophaga canimoris		

(continued)

19

Organism	Usual Disease	Preferred Agent	Alternatives
Edwardsiella tarda	Gastroenteritis (usually not treated) Wound infection Bacteremia, liver abscesses	Ampicillin	Cephalosporin (5) Aminoglycoside (1) Chloramphenicol Tetracycline (4)
Ehrlichia canis	Ehrlichiosis	Tetracycline (4)	Chloramphenicol (?)
Eikenella corrodens	Oral infections, bite wounds	Ampicillin/amoxicillin Penicillin G	Tetracycline (4) Amoxicillin-clavulanic acid Cephalosporin (5) Imipenem
Enterobacter aerogenes, E. cloacae	Sepsis, pneumonia, wound infections	Aminoglycoside (1) Sulfa-trimethoprim Fluoroquinolone (6)	Aztreonam Imipenem Antipseudomonad penicillin (2) Cephalosporin-3rd gen (5)
	Urinary tract infection	Sulfa-trimethoprim Cephalosporin-3rd gen (5)	Antipseudomonad penicillin (2) Aminoglycoside Fluoroquinolone (6) Imipenem
Enterococcus (E. faecalis and E. faecium)	Urinary tract infections	Ampicillin/amoxicillin	Penicillin + aminoglycoside (1) Vancomycin Nitrofurantoin Fluoroquinolone (6)
	Wound infections, intra-abdominal sepsis	Ampicillin	Vancomycin Penicillin + aminoglycoside (1) Imipenem (E. faecalis)
	Endocarditis	Penicillin G/ampicillin + gentamicin, streptomycin or amikacin	Vancomycin + gentamicin or streptomycin

(continued)

20

Organism	Usual Disease	Preferred Agent	Alternatives
Enterococcus (Vancomycin-resistant)		Moderate resistance: high dose penicillin + vancomycin ± aminoglycoside(MIC ≤ 32 μg/ml) High resistance + deep infection: ciprofloxacin ± rifampin and gentamicin	Teicoplanin (many strains resistant)
Erwinia agglomerans	Urinary tract infections Bacteremia Pneumonia	Aminoglycosides (1)	Fluoroquinolone (6) Chloramphenicol Cephalosporins (5)
Erysipelothrix rhusiopathiae	Localized cutaneous	Penicillin	Erythromycin
	Endocarditis/ disseminated	Penicillin	Cephalosporins (5)
E. coli	Septicemia Intra-abdominal sepsis Wound infection	Cephalosporin (3rd gen) (5) Ampicillin (if sensitive)	Aminoglycoside (1) Sulfa-trimethoprim Imipenem Fluoroquinolone (6) Cephalosporin (1st or 2nd gen) (5) Aztreonam Antipseudomonad penicillin (2)
	Urinary tract infection	Ampicillin (if sensitive) Tetracycline (4) Sulfa-trimethoprim Aminoglycoside (1) Cephalosporin (5) Antipseudomonad penicillin (2)	Imipenem Aztreonam Fluoroquinolone (6) Sulfonamide
Flavobacterium meningosepticum	Sepsis	Vancomycin	Sulfa-trimethoprim Erythromycin Clindamycin Imipenem Fluoroquinolone (6)

(continued)

21

Organism	Usual Disease	Preferred Agent	Alternatives
Francisella tularensis	Tularemia	Streptomycin or gentamicin	Tetracycline (4) Chloramphenicol (7)
Fusobacterium	Oral/dental/pulmonary infection; liver abscess	Penicillin G Metronidazole	Cefoxitin/cefotetan Chloramphenicol Imipenem Clindamycin
Gardnerella vaginalis	Vaginitis	Metronidazole	Clindamycin (po or topical)
Haemophilus aphrophilus	Sepsis, endocarditis	Penicillin G + aminoglycoside (1)	Cephalosporin-3rd gen (5) + aminoglycoside (1)
H. ducreyi	Chancroid	Ceftriaxone Erythromycin	Sulfa-trimethoprim Amoxicillin + clavulanic acid Fluoroquinolone (6)
H. influenzae	Meningitis	Cefotaxime, ceftriaxone Chloramphenicol	
	Epiglottitis Pneumonia Arthritis Cellulitis	Cephalosporin - 3rd gen (5) Sulfa-trimethoprim Cefamandole/cefuroxime Ampicillin (if sensitive)	Chloramphenicol ± ampicillin Betalactam-betalactamase inhibitor (7)
	Otitis Sinusitis Bronchitis	Sulfa-trimethoprim Ampicillin/amoxicillin (if sens)	Erythromycin - sulfonamide Cephalosporin - 2nd or 3rd gen (5) Tetracycline (4) Betalactam-betalactamase inhibitor (7) Fluoroquinolone (6)
Hafnia alvei	Pneumonia, wound infection, urinary tract infection	Aminoglycosides (1)	Ciprofloxacin (6) Chloramphenicol Antipseudomonad penicillin (2)

(continued)

22

Organism	Usual Disease	Preferred Agent	Alternatives
Helicobacter pylori (Campylobacter pylori)	Gastritis Recurrent duodenal ulcer disease	Bismuth subcitrate plus metronidazole plus tetracycline	Bismuth plus metronidazole plus amoxicillin Omeprazole plus amoxicillin
Kingella sp.	Endocarditis Septic arthritis	Penicillin + aminoglycoside	Cephalosporin (5) + aminoglycoside (1)
Klebsiella pneumoniae, K. oxytoca	Septicemia Pneumonia Intra-abdominal sepsis	Cephalosporin (3rd gen) (5)	Aminoglycoside (1) Sulfa-trimethoprim Piperacillin/mezlocillin Imipenem Betalactam-betalactamase inhibitor (7) Aztreonam Fluoroquinolone (6)
Klebsiella sp.	Urinary tract infection	Sulfa-trimethoprim Cephalosporin (5) Tetracycline (4)	Aminoglycoside (1) Betalactam-betalactamase inhibitor (7) Fluoroquinolone (6) Piperacillin/mezlocillin Imipenem
Legionella sp.	Legionnaires' disease	Erythromycin ± rifampin	Sulfa-trimethoprim + rifampin Fluoroquinolone (6) + rifampin Clarithromycin (7) Azithromycin (7)
Leptospira	Leptospirosis	Penicillin G or ampicillin	Tetracycline (4)
Leptotrichia buccalis	Orodental infections "Vincent's infection"	Penicillin G	Tetracycline (4) Clindamycin Erythromycin Metronidazole

(continued)

23

Organism	Usual Disease	Preferred Agent	Alternatives
Listeria monocytogenes	Meningitis Septicemia	Ampicillin or penicillin ± gentamicin	Sulfa-trimethoprim
Moraxella	Ocular infections Bacteremia	Aminoglycoside (1) Penicillins	Cephalosporin - 3rd gen (5) Imipenem Fluoroquinolone (6) Antipseudomonad penicillin (2)
Moraxella catarrhalis (Branhamella catarrhalis)	Otitis, sinusitis, pneumonitis	Sulfa-trimethoprim	Amoxicillin-clavulanic acid Erythromycin Clarithromycin/azithromycin Tetracycline (4) Cephalosporin (5) Fluoroquinolone (6)
Morganella morganii	Bacteremia Urinary tract infection Pneumonia Wound infection	Aminoglycoside Fluoroquinolone (6) Imipenem Cephalosporin (3rd gen) (5)	Sulfa-trimethoprim Aztreonam Antipseudomonad penicillin (2) Betalactam-betalactamase inhibitor (7) Tetracycline (4)
Mycobacterium tuberculosis (See page 126)	Tuberculosis	INH + rifampin pyrazinamide, ± ethambutol	Streptomycin, Capreomycin or Kanamycin Ciprofloxacin or Ofloxacin Ethionamide PAS Cycloserine
M. kansasii (See page 133)	Pulmonary infection	INH + rifampin + ethambutol ± streptomycin	Ethionamide Cycloserine

(continued)

24

Organism	Usual Disease	Preferred Agent	Alternatives
M. avium-intracellulare (See page 133)	Pulmonary infection	INH + rifampin + ethambutol + streptomycin	Clofazimine (extrapul dis) Clarithromycin Ethionamide Amikacin Cycloserine Ciprofloxacin/Ofloxacin
	Disseminated infection (AIDS)	Clarithromycin + ethambutol or clofazimine ± ciprofloxacin (6) 3-5 of the following: rifampin, ethambutol, amikacin, kanamycin, clofazimine, clarithromycin, ciprofloxacin	Rifampin or rifabutin Eithionamide Cycloserine Pyrazinamide Imipenem Amikacin
M. chelonae (See page 134)	Skin and soft tissue	Amikacin and/or cefoxitin, clofazimine or clarithromycin, then sulfonamide, rifampin, doxycycline or erythromycin	
M. fortuitum (See page 133)	Soft tissue and wound infections	Amikacin, ciprofloxacin + sulfonamide	Clofazimine Clarithromycin Cefoxitin Doxycycline Imipenem
M. marinum (See page 133)	Soft tissue infections	Rifampin + ethambutol or Sulfa-trimethoprim or Minocycline (doxycycline)	Ciprofloxacin (6)
M. ulcerans	Pulmonary	INH, rifampin + ethambutal	
M. leprae	Leprosy	Sulfone sensitive strains: Dapsone + rifampin Sulfone resistant strains: Clofazimine ± rifampin	Ethionamide (Protionamide) Minocycline Ofloxacin

(continued)

25

Organism	Usual Disease	Preferred Agent	Alternatives
Mycoplasma fermentans	Genital tract infections	Doxycycline	
Mycoplasma pneumoniae	Pneumonia	Erythromycin Tetracycline (4)	Clarithromycin (?) Azithromycin (?) Fluoroquinolone (?)
Neisseria gonorrhoeae	Urethritis Salpingitis Cervicitis Arthritis-dermatitis	Ceftriaxone Cefixime Fluoroquinolone (6)	Spectinomycin Sulfa-trimethoprim Cefotaxime, Cefoxitin Ceftizoxime Cefuroxime axetil
N. meningitidis	Meningitis Bacteremia Pericarditis Pneumonia	Penicillin G	Ampicillin Chloramphenicol Sulfa-trimethoprim Cephalosporin-cefotaxime, ceftizoxime, ceftriaxone
	Prophylaxis	Rifampin Fluoroquinolone (6)	
Nocardia asteroides	Nocardiosis: pulmonary infection, abscesses - skin, lung, brain	Sulfonamide (usually sulfadiazine) Sulfa-trimethoprim (sulfa level maintained at 10-20 mg/dl)	Sulfasoxazole Imipenem ± amikacin Minocycline ± sulfa Amikacin ± sulfa Cycloserine
Pasteurella multocida	Animal bite wound	Penicillin G	Tetracycline (4) Ciprofloxacin (6) Amoxicillin-clavulanic acid
	Septicemia Septic arthritis/ osteomyelitis	Penicillin G	Cephalosporins (5) Betalactam-betalactamase inhibitor (7) Chloramphenicol

(continued)

Organism	Usual Disease	Preferred Agent	Alternatives
Peptostreptococcus	Oral/dental/pulmonary infection; intra-abdominal sepsis; gynecologic infection	Penicillin G Ampicillin/amoxicillin	Clindamycin Metronidazole Cephalosporin (5) Chloramphenicol Erythromycin Vancomycin Imipenem
Plesiomonas shigelloides	Diarrhea (usually not treated)	Sulfa-trimethoprim Tetracycline (4) Fluoroquinolone (6)	Chloramphenicol Aminoglycosides (1)
	Extra-intestinal infection	Cephalosporin-3rd gen (3) Aminoglycoside (1)	Aztreonam Sulfa-trimethoprim Imipenem Fluoroquinolone (6)
Propionibacterium acnes	Acne	Tetracycline (4)	Clindamycin (topical)
	Systemic infection	Penicillin	Clindamycin
Proteus mirabilis	Septicemia Urinary tract infection Intra-abdominal sepsis Wound infection	Ampicillin	Aminoglycosides (1) Cephalosporins (5) Sulfa-trimethoprim Antipseudomonad penicillin Aztreonam Imipenem Fluoroquinolone (6)
Proteus indole positive	Septicemia Urinary tract infection	Cephalosporin-3rd gen (5)	Aminoglycoside (1) Sulfa-trimethoprim Antipseudomonad penicillin (2) Aztreonam Imipenem Betalactam-betalactamase inhibitor (7) Fluoroquinolone (6)

(continued)

Organism	Usual Disease	Preferred Agent	Alternatives
Providencia rettgeri	Septicemia Urinary tract infection	Cephalosporin-3rd gen (5)	Aminoglycoside (1) Antipseudomonad penicillin (2) Imipenem Aztreonam Sulfa-trimethoprim Fluoroquinolone (6)
Providencia stuartii	Septicemia Urinary tract infection	Cephalosporin-3rd gen (5)	Aminoglycoside (1) Antipseudomonad penicillin (2) Sulfa-trimethoprim Imipenem Aztreonam Fluoroquinolone (6) Betalactam-betalactamase inhibitor (7)
Pseudomonas aeruginosa	Septicemia, pneumonia Intra-abdominal sepsis	Aminoglycoside (tobramycin) ± antipseudomonad penicillin (2)	Aminoglycoside (1) ± cefoperazone, imipenem or ceftazidime Aztreonam Ciprofloxacin (6)
	Urinary tract infections	Aminoglycoside (1) Antipseudomonad penicillin (2) Fluoroquinolone (6)	Imipenem Ceftazidime Cefoperazone Aztreonam
Ps. cepacia	Septicemia Pneumonia	Sulfa-trimethoprim	Betalactam-betalactamase inhibitor (7) Ceftazidime Fluoroquinolone (6)
Ps. mallei	Glanders	Streptomycin + tetracycline	Chloramphenicol + streptomycin
Ps. maltophilia (Xanthomonas maltophilia)	Septicemia	Sulfa-trimethoprim	Ticarcillin–clavulanic acid

(continued)

28

Organism	Usual Disease	Preferred Agent	Alternatives
Ps. pseudomallei	Melioidosis	Ceftazidime ± sulfa-trimethoprim	Sulfa-trimethoprim Tetracycline (4) + chloramphenicol Imipenem Cefotaxime Amoxicillin + clavulanate
Ps. putida	Septicemia, pneumonia, urinary tract infections	Aminoglycosides (1) Fluoroquinolone (6)	
Rhodococcus equi	Pneumonia, pulmonary abscess, bacteremia	Vancomycin ± ciprofloxacin, imipenem or amikacin	Imipenem Erythromycin Ciprofloxacin (6) Amikacin
Rickettsia	Rocky Mountain spotted fever, Q fever, tick bite fever, murine typhus, scrub typhus, typhus, trench fever	Tetracycline (4)	Chloramphenicol Fluoroquinolone (6)
Rochalimaea henselae	(See Afipia felix)		
Rochalimaea quintana	Bacillary angiomatosis	Erythromycin	Aminoglucosides Aztreonam Sulfa-trimethoprim Tetracycline (4)
Salmonella typhi	Typhoid fever	Ceftriaxone	Chloramphenicol Sulfa-trimethoprim Ampicillin/amoxicillin Fluoroquinolones (6) Cefotaxime/cefoperazone/ ceftriaxone

(continued)

29

Organism	Usual Disease	Preferred Agent	Alternatives
Salmonella sp. (other)	Enteric fever Mycotic aneurysm	Cefotaxime/cefoperazone/ ceftriaxone	Ampicillin/amoxicillin Sulfa-trimethoprim Chloramphenicol Fluoroquinolone (6)
Serratia marcescens	Septicemia Urinary tract infection Pneumonia	Cephalosporin-3rd gen (5)	Gentamicin or amikacin ± antipseudomonad penicillin or cephalosporin-3rd gen (5) Cephalosporins-3rd gen (5) Sulfa-trimethoprim Antipseudomonad penicillin (2) Imipenem Fluoroquinolone (6) Aztreonam
Shigella	Colitis	Sulfa-trimethoprim	Ampicillin Tetracycline (4) Ciprofloxacin/nalidixic acid (6)
Spirillum minus	Rat bite fever	Penicillin G	Tetracycline (4) Streptomycin
Staphylococcus aureus Methicillin-sensitive	Septicemia Pneumonia Wound infection	Penicillinase resistant penicillin (3) ± rifampin or gentamicin Cephalosporins-1st gen (5) Cefuroxime/cefamandole	Erythromycin/clindamycin Vancomycin Betalactam-betalactamase inhibitor (7) Imipenem Fluoroquinolone (6) Clindamycin
Methicillin-resistant		Vancomycin ± rifampin or gentamicin	Sulfa-trimethoprim Fluoroquinolones (6) Minocycline Teicoplanin (investigational)

(continued)

Organism	Usual Disease	Preferred Agent	Alternatives
Staph. saprophyticus	Urinary tract infections	Sulfa-trimethoprim Ampicillin/amoxicillin Fluoroquinolone (6)	Cephalosporins (5) Tetracycline (4)
Staph. epidermidis	Septicemia Infected prosthetic devices	Vancomycin	Sulfa-trimethoprim Penicillinase resistant penicillin (3) Cephalosporin (5) Fluoroquinolone (6) Imipenem
Streptococcus, Group A,B, C,G; bovis, milleri, pneumoniae, viridans, anaerobic	Pharyngitis Soft tissue infection Pneumonia Abscesses	Penicillin G or V	Cephalosporin (5) Clindamycin Vancomycin Erythromycin Clarithromycin
	Endocarditis	Penicillin G ± streptomycin or gentamicin	Cephalosporin (5) Vancomycin
	Meningitis	Penicillin G	Chloramphenicol Cephalosporin-3rd gen (5)
S. pneumoniae (resistant strains)		Vancomycin ± rifampin (for meningitis) Erythromycin	Chloramphenicol Sulfa-trimethoprim Tetracycline
Streptobacillus moniliformis	Rat bite fever Haverhill fever	Penicillin G	Tetracycline (4) Streptomycin
Treponema carateum	Pinta	Penicillin G	Tetracycline
Treponema pallidum	Syphilis	Penicillin G	Tetracycline (4) Erythromycin Ceftriaxone
Treponema pallidum ss. endemicum	Bejel	Penicillin G	

(continued)

Organism	Usual Disease	Preferred Agent	Alternatives
Treponema pallidum ss pertenue	Yaws	Penicillin G	Tetracycline (4)
Ureaplasma urealyticum	Urethritis Endocervicitis PID (?)	Erythromycin	Tetracycline (4)
Vibrio cholerae	Cholera	Tetracycline (4)	Erythromycin Sulfa-trimethoprim Furazolidone (6) Fluoroquinolone (6)
Vibrio vulnificus	Septicemia Wound infection	Tetracycline (4)	Cefotaxime
Xanthomonas maltophilia	Septicemia UTI Pneumonia	Sulfa-trimethoprim	Ceftazidine Fluoroquinolone (6)
Yersinia enterocolitica	Enterocolitis (usually not treated) Mesenteric adenitis (usually not treated)	Sulfa-trimethoprim	Cephalosporin-3rd gen (5) Ciprofloxacin (6) Tetracycline (4)
	Septicemia	Aminoglycoside (gentamicin)	Chloramphenicol Cephalosporins-3rd gen (5)
Yersinia pestis	Plague	Streptomycin	Chloramphenicol Tetracycline (4) Gentamicin
Yersinia pseudotuberculosis	Mesenteric adenitis (usually not treated) Septicemia	Aminoglycoside (1) Ampicillin	Sulfa-trimethoprim Tetracycline (4)

(continued)

32

* Available from CDC 404-639-3670

1. Aminoglycosides = Gentamicin, tobramycin, amikacin, netilmicin
2. Antipseudomonad penicillin = Ticarcillin, piperacillin, mezlocillin; carbenicillin and azocillin are no longer available
3. Penicillinase resistant penicillins: Nafcillin, oxacillin, methicillin, cloxacillin, dicloxacillin
4. Tetracycline = Tetracycline, doxycycline, minocycline
5. Cephalosporins
   1st generation: Cefadroxil, cefprozil, cefazolin, cephalexin, cephalothin, cephapirin, cephradine
   2nd generation: Cefaclor, cefamandole, cefonicid, ceforanide, cefotetan, cefoxitin, cefuroxime, cefmetazole
   3rd generation: Cefotaxime, ceftizoxime, ceftazidime, cefoperazone, ceftriaxone, moxalactam, cefixime, cefpodoxime, ceftibutin,
   Carbacefems: Loracarbef, cefprozil
6. Fluoroquinolones: Norfloxacin, ciprofloxacin, ofloxacin and lomefloxacin. Systemic infections are usually treated with ciprofloxacin. With regard to spectrum: Ps. aeruginosa
   — ciprofloxacin or ofloxacin; all may be used for urinary tract infections. With regard to spectrum: Ps. aeruginosa
   exoxacin, lomefloxacin or ofloxacin; Mycobacteria — ciprofloxacin or ofloxacin; C. trachomatis — ofloxacin
   — ciprofloxacin; S. pneumoniae — ofloxacin; Mycobacteria — ciprofloxacin or ofloxacin
7. Betalactam-betalactamase inhibitor: Amoxicillin + clavulanate, ticarcillin + clavulanate and ampicillin + sulbactam

33

ANTIMICROBIAL DOSING REGIMENS IN RENAL FAILURE

A. **General Principles**

1. The initial dose is not modified.
2. Adjustments in subsequent doses for renally excreted drugs may be accomplished by **a)** giving the usual maintenance dose at extended intervals, usually 3 half lives (extended interval method); **b)** giving reduced doses at the usual intervals (dose reduction method); or **c)** a combination of each.
3. Adjustments in dose are usually based on creatinine clearance that may be estimated as follows:

   a. Formula: Males: $\dfrac{\text{weight (kg) x (140-age in yrs)}}{72 \text{ x serum creatinine (mg/dl)}}$

   Females: above value x 0.85

   b. Nomogram (Kampmann J et al. Acta Med Scand 196:617,1974).

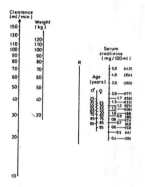

Use a straight edge to connect the patient's weight (2nd line on the left) and the patient's age (4th line). Mark intercept on R (3rd line) and swing straight edge to serum creatinine (5th line). Intercept on first line provides creatinine clearance

   c. Pitfalls and notations with calculations
      (1) Elderly patient: Serum creatinine may be deceptively low with danger of overdosing) due to reduced muscle mass.
      (2) Pregnancy and volume expansion: GFR may be increased (with danger of underdosing) in third trimester of pregnancy and patients with normal renal function who receive massive parenteral fluids.
      (3) Obese patients: Use lean body weight.
      (4) Renal failure: Formulas assume stable renal function; for patients with anuria or oliguria assume CCr of 5-8 ml/min.

B. Aminoglycoside Dosing

1. Guidelines of Johns Hopkins Hospital Clinical Pharmacology Department

Agent	Loading dose (regardless of renal function)	Susequent doses (prior to level measurements)		Therapeutic levels (1 hr after infusion over 20-30 min)
		CCr>70 ml/mm	CCr<70 ml/mm	
Gentamicin	2 mg/kg	1.7-2 mg/kg/8h	0.3 x CCr=mg/kg/8h	5-10 mcg/ml
Tobramycin	2 mg/kg	1.7-2 mg/kg/8h	0.3 x CCr=mg/kg/8h	5-10 mg/ml
Netilmicin	2.2 mg/kg	2-2.2 mg/kg/8h	0.3 x CCr=mg/kg/8h	5-10 mg/ml
Amikacin	8 mg/kg	7.5-8 mg/kg/8h	.12 x CCr=mg/kg/8h	20-40 mg/ml
Kanamycin	8 mg/kg	7.5-8 mg/kg/8h	.12 x CCr=mg/kg/8h	20-40 mg/ml

Note:
1. CCr = creatinine clearance.
2. Doses for gentamicin, tobramycin and netilmicin should be written in multiples of 5 mg; doses of amikacin and kanamycin should be written in multiples of 25 mg.
3. For obese patients use calculated lean body weight plus 40% of excess adipose tissue.
4. For patients who are oliguric or anuric use CCr of 5-8 ml/min.

Mayo Clinic guidelines (Van Scoy RE and Wilson WR, Mayo Clin Proc 62:1142, 1987)
a. Initial dose: Gentamicin, tobramycin, netilmicin: 1.5-2 mg/kg
Amikacin, kanamycin, streptomycin: 5.0-7.5 mg/kg
b. Maintenance dose: Usual daily dose x CCr/100

Reduced dose nomogram developed for tobramycin

Weight		Usual dose (q8h)	
lbs	kg	1 mg/kg	1.7 mg/kg
264	120	120	200
242	110	110	185
220	100	100	165
198	90	90	150
176	80	80	135
154	70	70	115
132	60	60	100
110	50	50	85
88	40	40	65

Source: Package insert of Tobramycin.

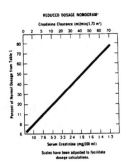

REDUCED DOSAGE NOMOGRAM*

Creatinine Clearance (ml/min/1.73 m²)

Percent of Normal Dosage from Table I

Serum Creatinine (mg/100 ml)

Scales have been adjusted to facilitate dosage calculations.

4. **Guidelines for AMA Drug Evaluations, American Medical Assoc., Chicago, Vol. II 6:3, 1990 and Drug Information 92, American Hospital Formulary Service, pg 57, 1992**

   a. Loading dose based on estimated ideal body weight

Agent	Dose (mg/kg ideal wt)	Peak conc. (mcg/ml)
Tobramycin	1.5-2 mg/kg	4-10
Gentamicin	1.5-2 mg/kg	4-10
Netilmicin	1.3-3.25 mg/kg	4-12
Amikacin	5-7.5 mg/kg	15-30
Kanamycin	5-7.5 mg/kg	15-30

   b. Maintenance dose as % of loading dose according to desired dosing interval and the corrected creatinine clearance CCr*

$$CCr \ (male) = \frac{(140 - age)}{serum \ creatinine}$$

   CCr (female) = 0.85 x CCr male

CCr (ml/min)	Half life (hrs)**	Dosing 8	Interval 12	(hr) 24
90	3.1	84%	-	-
80	3.4	80%	91%	-
70	3.9	76%	88%	-
60	4.5	71%	84%	-
50	5.3	65%	79%	-
40	6.5	57%	72%	92%
30	8.4	48%	63%	86%
25	9.9	43%	57%	81%
20	11.9	37%	50%	75%
17	13.6	33%	46%	70%
15	15.1	31%	42%	67%
12	17.9	27%	37%	61%
10***	20.4	24%	34%	56%
7	25.9	19%	28%	47%
5	31.5	16%	23%	41%
2	46.8	11%	16%	30%
0	69.3	8%	11%	21%

* From: Sarubbi FA Jr, Hull JH. Ann Intern Med, 89:612, 1978.
** Maintenance dose may be one half the loading dose at an interval approximately the estimated half life.
*** Serum concentrations should be measured to assist dose selection when the CCr is < 10 ml/min.

C. DRUG THERAPY DOSING GUIDELINES

(Adapted from Bennett WM, et al Ann Intern Med 93:62,1980, AMA Drug Evaluations, 1990, section 13, pp 1:1-8,35 and Drug Information 92, American Formulary Service, 1990, pp 33-481, 1992)

Drug	Major excretory route	Half life (hr) Normal	Half life (hr) Anuria	Usual regimen Oral	Usual regimen Parenteral	Maintenance regimen renal failure* Glomerular filtration rate in mL/min 50-80	10-50	<10
Acyclovir	Renal	2-2.5	20	200 mg 2-5x/day 800 mg 5x/day --	-- -- 5-12 mg/kg q8h	Usual Usual Usual	Usual 800 mg q8h 5-12 mg/kg q12-24h	200 mg q12h 800 mg q12h 2.5-6 mg/kg q24h
Amantidine	Renal	15-20	170	100 mg bid	--	100-150 mg q day	100-200 mg 2-3 x/wk	100-200 mg q wk
Amdinocillin	Renal	1	3.3	--	10 mg/kg q4-6h	Usual	10 mg/kg q6h	10 mg/kg q8h
Amikacin	Renal	2	30	--	7.5 mg/kg	See pages 35, 36	See pages 35, 36	↓ ↓ ↓ ↓
Amoxicillin	Renal	1	15-20	250-500 mg q8h	--	.25-.5 gm q12h	.25-.5 gm q12-24h	.25-.5 gm q12-24h
Amoxicillin-clavulanic acid	Renal	1	8-16	250-500 mg q8h	--	Usual	0.25-0.5 gm q12h	0.25-0.5 gm q20-36h
Amphotericin B	Nonrenal	15 days	15 days	--	0.3-1.4 mg/kg/day	Usual	Usual	Usual
Ampicillin	Renal	1	8-12	.25-0.5 gm q6h	1-3 gm q4-6h	Usual	Usual 1-2 gm IV q8h	Usual 1-2 gm IV q12h

(continued)

37

Drug	Major excretory route	Half life (hr)		Usual regimen		Maintenance regimen renal failure* Glomerular filtration rate in mL/min		
		Normal	Anuria	Oral	Parenteral	50-80	10-50	<10
Ampicillin-sulbactam	Renal	1	8-12	--	1-2 gm q6h	1-2 gm IV q8h	1-2 gm IV q8h	1-2 gm IV q12h
Atovaquone	Gut	69.6	69.6	750 mg tid w/food	--	Usual	Usual	Unknown
Azlocillin	Renal	1	5	--	2-4 gm q4-6h	Usual	1.5-2 gm q8h	1.5-3 gm q12h
Azithromycin	Hepatic	68	68	250 mg/d	--	Usual	No data -- "use caution"	No data -- "use caution"
Aztreonam	Renal	1.7-2	6-9	--	1-2 gm q6h	1-2 gm q8-12h	1-2 gm q12-18h	1-2 gm q24h
Bacampicillin	Renal	1	8-12	0.4-0.8 gm q12h	--	Usual	Usual	Usual
Capreomycin	Renal	4-6	50-100	1 gm q day-2x/wk	--	Usual	7.5 mg/kg q 1-2 days	7.5 mg/kg 2x/wk
Carbenicillin	Renal	1	13-16	.5-1 gm	5-6 gm IV q4h	Usual Usual	Usual 2-3 gm q6h	Avoid 2 gm q12h
Cefaclor	Renal	0.75	2.8	.25-0.5 gm q8h	--	Usual	Usual	Usual
Cefadroxil	Renal	1.4	20-25	.5-1 gm q12-24h	--	Usual	.5 gm q12-24h	.5 gm q36h
Cefamandole	Renal	0.5-2.1	10	--	0.5-2 gm q4-8h	.5-2 gm q6h	1-2 gm q8h	0.5-1 gm q12h
Cefazolin	Renal	1.8	18-36	--	0.5-2 gm	0.5-1.5 gm q8h	.5-1 gm q8-12h	0.25-0.75 gm q18-24h

(continued)

38

Drug	Major excretory route	Half life (hr)		Usual regimen		Maintenance regimen renal failure* Glomerular filtration rate in mL/min		
		Normal	Anuria	Oral	Parenteral	50-80	10-50	<10
Cefixime	Renal	3-4	12	200 mg q12h	--	Usual	300 mg/d	200 mg/d
Cefmetazole	Renal	1.2		--	2 gm q6-12h	1-2 gm q12h	1-2 gm q16-24h	1-2 gm q 48h
Cefonicid	Renal	4-5	50-60	--	.5-2 gm q24h	8-25 mg/kg q24h	4-15 mg/kg q24-48h	3-15 mg/kg q3-5d
Cefoperazone	Gut	1.9-2.5	2-2.5	--	1-2 gm q 6-12h	Usual	Usual	Usual
Ceforanide	Renal	3	20-40	--	0.5-1 gm q12h	Usual	0.5-1 gm q24h	0.5-1 gm q48-72h
Cefotaxime	Renal	1.1	3	--	1-2 gm q8-12h	Usual	1-2 gm q12-24h	1-2 gm q24h
Cefotetan	Renal	3-4	12-30	--	1-2 gm q12h	Usual	1-2 gm q24h	1-2 gm q48h
Cefoxitin	Renal	0.7	13-22	--	1-2 gm q6-8h	1-2 gm q8-12h	1-2 gm q12-24h	0.5-1 gm q12-48h
Cefprozil	Renal	1.3	5-6	0.25-0.5 gm q12h	--	Usual	0.25-0.5 gm q24h	0.25 gm q12-24h
Ceftazidime	Renal	0.9-1.7	15-25	--	1-2 gm q8-12h	Usual	1 gm q12-24h	0.5 gm q24-48h
Ceftizoxime	Renal	1.4-1.8	25-35	--	1-3 gm q6-8h	0.5-1.5 q8h	.25-1 gm q12h	.25 gm q24h

(continued)

39

Drug	Major excretory route	Half life (hr) Normal	Half life (hr) Anuria	Usual regimen Oral	Usual regimen Parenteral	Maintenance regimen renal failure* Glomerular filtration rate in mL/min 50-80	10-50	<10
Ceftriaxone	Renal & gut	6-9	12-15	--	0.5-1 gm q12-24h	Usual	Usual	Usual
Cefuroxime	Renal	1.3-1.7	20	--	.75-1.5 gm q8h	Usual	0.75-1.5 gm q8-12h	0.75 gm q24h
Cefuroxime axetil	Renal	1.2	20	250 mg q12h	--	Usual	Usual	250 mg q24h
Cephalexin	Renal	0.9	5-30	0.25-1.0 gm q6h	--	Usual	0.25-1.0 gm q8-12h	0.25-1 gm q24-48h
Cephalothin	Renal	0.5-0.9	3-8	--	.5-2 gm q4-6h	Usual	1.0-1.5 gm q6h	.5 gm q8h
Cephapirin	Renal	0.6-0.9	2.4	--	0.5-2 gm q4-6h	0.5-2 gm q6h	0.5-2 gm q8h	0.5-2 gm q12h
Cephradine	Renal	.7-1	8-15	0.25-1.0 gm q6h --	0.5-2 gm q4-6h	0.5-1 gm q6h	0.5 gm q6h / 0.5-1 gm q6-24h	0.25 gm q12h / 0.5-1 gm q24-72h
Chloramphenicol	Hepatic	2.5	3-7	0.25-0.75 gm q6h	.25-1 gm q6h	Usual	Usual	Usual
Chloroquine	Renal & metabolized	48-120	?	300-600 mg po qd	--	Usual	Usual	150-300 mg po qd

(continued)

Drug	Major excretory route	Half life (hr) Normal	Half life (hr) Anuria	Usual regimen Oral	Usual regimen Parenteral	Maintenance regimen renal failure* Glomerular filtration rate in ml/min 50-80	10-50	<10
Cinoxacin	Renal	1.5	8.5	.25-.5 gm q12h	--	.25 gm q8h	.25 gm q12h	.25 gm q24h
Ciprofloxacin	Renal & hepatic metabolism	4	5-10	.25-.75 gm q12h	400 mg q12h	Usual	.25-.5 gm q12h / .4 gm q18h	.25-.5 gm q18h / .4 gm q24h
Clarithromycin	Hepatic metabolism & renal	4	slight↑	250-500 mg q12h	--	Usual	Usual	250-500 mg q24h
Clindamycin	Hepatic	2-2.5	2-3.5	150-300 mg q6h	300-900 mg q6-8h	Usual	Usual	Usual
Clofazimine	Hepatic	8 days	8 days	50 mg qd 100 mg tid	--	Usual	Usual	Usual
Cloxacillin	Renal	0.5	0.8	0.5-1.0 gm q6h	--	Usual	Usual	Usual
Colistin	Renal	3-8	10-20	--	1.5 mg/kg q6-12h day	2.5-3.8 mg/kg q24-36h	1.5-2.5 mg/kg	.6 mg/kg q24h
Cyclacillin	Renal	0.6	0.6	0.5-1.0 gm q6h	--	Usual	Usual	0.5-1.0 gm q12h
Cycloserine	Renal	8-12	?	250-500 mg bid	--	Usual	250-500 mg qd	250 mg qd
Dapsone	Hepatic metabolism	30	slight↑	50-100 mg/day	--	Usual	Usual	(No data)
Dicloxacillin	Renal	0.5-0.9	1-1.6	0.25-0.5 gm q6h	--	Usual	Usual	Usual

(continued)

41

Drug	Major excretory route	Half life (hr) Normal	Half life (hr) Anuria	Usual regimen Oral	Usual regimen Parenteral	Maintenance regimen renal failure* Glomerular filtration rate in mL/min 50-80	10-50	<10
Didecoxyinosine (ddI)	Renal & nonrenal	1.3-1.6	?	200 mg bid	--	Usual	Consider dose reduction; note Mg load -- 60 mEq/tab	
Dideoxycytidine (ddC, zalcitibine)	Renal	2	8	0.75 mg tid	--	Usual	0.75 mg bid	0.75 mg po qd
Doxycycline	Renal & gut	14-25	15-36	100 mg bid	100 mg bid	Usual	Usual	Usual
Enoxacin	Renal & hepatic metabolism	3-6	--	200-400 mg mg bid	--	Usual	½ usual dose	½ usual dose
Erythromycin	Hepatic	1.2-2.6	4-6	.25-.5 gm q6h	1 gm q6h	Usual	Usual	Usual
Ethambutol	Renal	3-4	8	15-25 mg/kg q24h	--	15 mg/ kg q24h	15 mg/kg q24-36h	15 mg/kg q48h
Ethionamide	Metabolized	4	9	.5-1 gm/day 1-3 doses	--	Usual	Usual	5 mg/kg q24h
Fluconazole	Renal	20-50	100	100-200 mg/day	100-200 mg/day	Usual	50-100 mg/day	25-50 mg/day
Flucytosine	Renal	3-6	70	37 mg/kg q6h	--	Usual	37 mg/kg q12-24h	Not recommended
Foscarnet induction maintenance	Renal	3	†	--	60 mg/kg q8h 90 mg/kg qd 120 mg/kg qd	40-50 mg/kg q8h 60-70 mg/kg qd 80-90 mg/kg qd	20-30 mg/kg q8h 50-70 mg/kg qd 60-80 mg/kg qd	Contraindicated (CrCl<20/ml) Contraindicated (CrCl<20/ml) Contraindicated (CrCl<20/ml) Contraindicated (CrCl<20/ml)

42

(continued)

Drug	Major excretory route	Half life (hr) Normal	Half life (hr) Anuria	Usual regimen Oral	Usual regimen Parenteral	Maintenance regimen renal failure* — Glomerular filtration rate in mL/min 50-80	10-50	<10
Ganciclovir - induction doses (maintenance - 1/2 dose)	Renal	1.5-3	10	--	5.0 mg/kg bid	2.5 mg/kg bid	2.5 mg/kg qd	1.25 mg/kg qd
						2.5 mg/kg/d	1.2 mg/kg/d	0.6 mg/kg/d
Gentamicin	Renal	2	48	--	1.7 mg/kg q8h	→ → → → →	See pages 35, 36	→ → → →
Griseofulvin microsize	Hepatic metabolism	24	24	.5-1 gm qd	--	Usual	Usual	Usual
ultramicrosize	(Same)	(Same)	(Same)	.33-.66 gm qd	--	Usual	Usual	Usual
Imipenem	Renal	.8-1	3.5	--	0.5-1 gm q6h	0.5 gm q6-8h	0.5 gm q8-12h	0.25-0.5 mg q12h
Isoniazid	Hepatic	0.5-4	2-10	300 mg q24h	300 mg q24h	Usual	Usual	Slow acetylators 1/2 dose
Itraconazole	Hepatic	20-60	20-60	100-200 mg/day	--	Usual	Usual	Usual
Kanamycin	Renal	2-3	27-30	--	7.5 mg/kg	→ → → → →	See pages 35, 36	→ → → → →
Ketoconazole	Hepatic metabolism	1-4	1-4	200-400 mg q12-24h	--	Usual	Usual	Usual
Lomefloxacin	Renal	8	45	400 mg q24h	--	Usual	400 mg; then 200 mg qd	400 mg; then 200 mg qd
Loracarbef	Renal	1	32	200-400 mg q12h	--	Usual	200-400 mg q24h	200-400 mg q 3-5 days
Mefloquine	Hepatic	2-4 wks	2-4 wks	1250 mg x 1 / 250 mg q wk	--	Usual	Usual	Usual

(continued)

Drug	Major excretory route	Half life (hr) Normal	Half life (hr) Anuria	Usual regimen Oral	Usual regimen Parenteral	Maintenance regimen renal failure* Glomerular filtration rate in mL/min 50-80	10-50	<10
Methenamine hippurate	Renal	3-6	?	1 gm q12h	--	Usual	Avoid	Avoid
mandelate	Renal	3-6	?	1 gm q12h	--	Usual	Avoid	Avoid
Methicillin	Renal (hepatic)	0.5	4	--	1-2 gm q4-6h	1-2 gm q6h	1-2 gm q8h	1-2 gm q12h
Metronidazole	Hepatic	6-14	8-15	.25-7.5 gm tid	.5 gm q6h	Usual	Usual	Usual
Mezlocillin	Renal	1	1.5	--	3-4 gm q4-6h	Usual	3 gm q8h	2 gm q8h
Miconazole	Hepatic	0.5-1	0.5-1	--	0.4-1.2 gm q8h	Usual	Usual	Usual
Minocycline	Hepatic & metabolized	11-26	17-30	100 mg q12h	100 mg q12h	Usual	Usual	Usual or slight decrease
Moxalactam	Renal	2	20	--	1-4 gm q8-12h	3 gm q8h	2-3 gm q12h	1 gm 12-24h
Nafcillin	Hepatic metabolism	0.5	1.2	0.5-1 gm 96h	0.5-2 gm q4-6h	Usual	Usual	Usual
Nalidixic acid	Renal & hepatic metabolism	1.5	21	1 gm q6h	--	Usual	Usual	Avoid
Netilmicin	Renal	2.5	35	--	2.0 mg/kg q8h	↑ ↑ ↑ ↑	See pages 35, 36	↓ ↓ ↓ ↓
Nitrofurantoin	Renal	0.3	1	50-100 mg q6-8h	--	Usual	Avoid	Avoid

(continued)

Drug	Major excretory route	Half life (hr) Normal	Anuria	Usual regimen Oral	Parenteral	Maintenance regimen renal failure* Glomerular filtration rate in mL/min 50-80	10-50	<10
Norfloxacin	Renal & hepatic metabolism	3.5	8	400 mg bid	--	Usual	400 mg qd	400 mg qd
Nystatin	Not absorbed	--	--	.4-1 mil units 3-5 x daily	--	Usual	Usual	Usual
Ofloxacin	Renal	6	40	200-400 mg bid	--	Usual	200-400 mg qd	100-200 mg qd
				--	200-400 mg q12h	Usual	200-400 mg q24h	100-200mg q24h
Oxacillin	Renal	0.5	1	0.5-1 gm	0.5-2 gm	Usual	Usual	Usual
Penicillin G crystalline	Renal	0.5	7-10	0.4-0.8 mil units q6h	1-4 mil units q4-6h	Usual	Usual	1/2 usual dose
procaine	Renal	24		--	0.6-1.2 mil units IM q12h	Usual	Usual	Usual
benzathine	Renal	days		--	0.6-1.2 mil units IM	Usual	Usual	Usual
V	Renal	0.5-1.0	7-10	0.4-0.8 mil units q6h	--	Usual	Usual	Usual
Pentamidine	Non-renal	6	6-8	--	4 mg/kg q24h	Usual	4 mg/kg q24-36h	4 mg/kg q48h
Piperacillin	Renal	1	3	--	3-4 gm	Usual q4-6h	3 gm q8h	3 gm q12h
Polymyxin B	Renal	6	48	--	.8-1.2 gm IV q12h	1-1.5 mg/kg qd	1-1.5 mg/kg q2-3d	1 mg/kg q5-7d

45

(continued)

Drug	Major excretory route	Half life (hr)		Usual regimen		Maintenance regimen renal failure* Glomerular filtration rate in mL/min		
		Normal	Anuria	Oral	Parenteral	50-80	10-50	<10
Praziquantel	Hepatic metabolism	0.8-1.5	?	10-25 mg/kg tid	--	Usual	Usual	Usual
Pyrazinamide	Metabolized	10-16	?	15-35 mg/kg daily	--	Usual	Usual	12-20 mg/kg/day
Pyrimethamine	Non-renal	1.5-5 days	?	25-75 mg/day	--	Usual	Usual	Usual
Quinine	Hepatic metabolism	4-5	4-5	650 mg tid	7.5-10 mg/kg q8h	Usual	Usual	Usual
Quinacrine	Renal	5 days	--	100-200 mg q6-8h	--	Usual	Usual	?
Rifampin	Hepatic	Early 2-5 Late 2	2-5	600 mg/kg/day	600 mg/day	Usual	Usual	Usual
Spectinomycin	Renal	1-3	?	--	2 gm IM/day	Usual	Usual	Usual
Streptomycin	Renal	2.5	100-110	--	500 mg q12h	7.5 mg/kg q24h	7.5 mg/kg q24-72h	7.5 mg/kg q72-96h
Sulfadiazine	Renal	8-17	22-34	0.5-1.5 gm q4-6h	30-50 mg/kg q6-8h	Usual	0.5-1.5 gm q8-12h / 30-50 mg/kg q12-18h	0.5-1.5 gm q12-24h / 30-50 mg/kg q18-24h
Sulfisoxazole	Renal	3-7	6-12	1-2 gm q6h	--	Usual	1 gm q8-12h	1 gm q12-24h
Teicoplanin	Renal	6	41	--	6-12 mg/kg/d	Usual	1/2 usual dose	1/3 usual dose

46

(continued)

Drug	Major excretory route	Half life (hr)		Usual regimen		Maintenance regimen renal failure* Glomerular filtration rate in mL/min		
		Normal	Anuria	Oral	Parenteral	50-80	10-50	<10
Tetracycline	Renal	8	50-100	.25-.5 gm q6h	.5-1 gm q12h	Usual	Use doxycycline	
Ticarcillin	Renal	1-1.5	16	--	3 gm q4h	Usual	2-3 gm q6-8h	2 gm q12h
Ticarcillin + clavulanic acid	Renal	1-1.5	16	--	3 gm q4h	Usual	2-3 gm q6-8h	2 gm q12h
Tobramycin	Renal	2.5	56	--	1.7 mg/kg q8h	↑ ↑ ↑ ↑ ↑	See pages 35, 36 ↓ ↓ ↓ ↓ ↓	↓
Trimethoprim	Renal	8-15	24	100 mg q12h q18-24h	--	Usual	100 mg	Avoid
Trimethoprim-sulfamethoxazole	Renal	T:8-15 S:7-12	T:24 S:22-50	2-4 tabs/d or 1-2 DS/day	3-5 mg/kg q6-12h	3-5 mg/ kg q 18h	3-5 mg/kg q24h	Avoid
Vancomycin	Renal	6-8	200-250	.125-.5 gm q6h	--	Usual dose 1 gm q24h	Usual dose 1 gm q3-10d	0.125 mg po 1 gm q5-10d
Vidarabine	Renal	3.5	--	--	15 mg/kg/day	Usual	Usual	10 mg/kg/day
Zidovudine AZT	Hepatic metabolism to G-AZT → renal	1	3	100 mg q4h x 5/d	--	Usual	Usual	100 mg q8h

47

D. **ANTIMICROBIAL DOSING REGIMENS DURING DIALYSIS**
(Adapted from: Norris S, Nightengale CH and Mandell GL: In: Principles and Practice
of Infectious Diseases, 3rd Ed., Churchill Livingstone, NY 1990, pp 440-457; American
Hospital Formulary Service Drug Information 92, pp 33-481, 1992, and Berns JS et al, J
Amer Soc Neph 1:1061, 1991.)

	Hemodialysis	Peritoneal dialysis
Acyclovir	2.5-5.0 mg/kg/day + dose post-dialysis	2.5 mg/kg/day
Amdinocillin	No extra dose	--
Amikacin	2.5-3.75 mg/kg post-dialysis	Loading dose predialysis 9-20 mg/L dialysate*
Amoxicillin	0.25 gm post-dialysis	Usual regimen
Amoxicillin + clavulanic acid	0.50 gm (amoxicillin) + .125 (CA) halfway through dialysis and another dose at end	Usual regimen
Amphotericin B	Usual regimen	Usual regimen
Ampicillin	Usual dose post-dialysis	Usual regimen
Ampicillin + sulbactam	2 gm ampicillin post-dialysis	Usual regimen
Atovaquone	Unknown	Unknown
Azithromycin	Usual regimen	Usual regimen
Aztreonam	One-eighth initial dose (60-250 mg) post-dialysis	Usual loading dose, then one-fourth usual dose at usual intervals
Carbenicillin	.75-2.0 gm post-dialysis	2 gm 6-12h
Cefaclor	Repeat dose post-dialysis	Usual regimen
Cefadroxil	0.5-1 gm post-dialysis	0.5 gm/day
Cefamandole	Repeat dose post-dialysis	0.5-1 gm q12h
Cefazolin	0.25-0.5 gm post-dialysis	0.5 gm q12h
Cefixime	300 mg/day	200 mg/day
Cefonicid	No extra dose	Usual regimen
Cefoperazone	Schedule dose post-dialysis	Usual regimen

(continued)

48

	Hemodialysis	Peritoneal dialysis
Cefotaxime	0.5-2 gm daily plus supplemental dose post-dialysis	1-2 gm/day
Cefotetan	One-fourth usual dose q24h on non-dialysis days and one-half dose on dialysis days	1 gm/day
Cefoxitin	1-2 gm post-dialysis	1 gm/day
Cefprozil	250-500 mg post-dialysis	0.25 gm q12-24h
Ceftazidime	1 gm loading 1 gm post-dialysis	0.5-1 gm loading then 0.5 gm/day or 250 mg in each 2 L dialysate
Ceftizoxime	Scheduled dose post-dialysis	1 gm/day
Ceftriaxone	No extra dose	Usual regimen
Cefuroxime	Repeat dose post-dialysis	15 mg/kg post-dialysis or 750 mg/day
Cephalexin	0.25-1 gm post-dialysis	250 mg po tid
Cephalothin	Supplemental dose post-dialysis	Option to add $\leq$ 6 mg/dL to dialysate
Cephapirin	7.5-15 mg/kg before dialysis and q12h after	1-2 gm q12h
Cephradine	250 mg pre-dialysis, then at 12 and 36-48 hr later	1 gm/day (IV) 250 mg bid (po)
Chloramphenicol	Schedule dose post-dialysis	Usual regimen
Ciprofloxacin	250-500 mg q24h post-dialysis	250-500 mg/day
Clindamycin	Usual regimen	Usual regimen
Cloxacillin	Usual regimen	Usual regimen

(continued)

	Hemodialysis	Peritoneal dialysis
Clofazamine	Usual regimen	Usual regimen
Dicloxacillin	Usual regimen	Usual regimen
Doxycycline	Usual regimen	Usual regimen
Erythromycin	Usual regimen	Usual regimen
Ethambutol	15 mg/kg/day post-dialysis	15 mg/kg/day
Fluconazole	Usual dose post-dialysis	½ usual dose
Flucytosine	20-37.5 mg/kg post-dialysis	0.5-1 gm/day
Ganciclovir	1.25 mg/kg q24h given post-dialysis on dialysis days	?
Gentamicin	1.0-1.7 mg/kg post-dialysis	Loading dose predialysis 2-4 mg/L dialysate*
Isoniazid	5 mg/kg post-dialysis	Daily dose post-dialysis or ½ usual dose
Imipenem	Supplemental dose post-dialysis and q12h thereafter	500 mg/day
Itraconazole	Usual regimen	Usual regimen
Kanamycin	4-5 mg/kg post-dialysis	3.75 mg/kg/day
Ketoconazole	Usual regimen	Usual regimen
Metronidazole	Usual regimen	Usual regimen
Mezlocillin	2-3 gm post-dialysis then 3-4 gm q12h	3 gm q12h
Minocycline	Usual dose	Usual dose
Moxalactam	1-2 gm post-dialysis	1-2 gm/day
Nafcillin	Usual regimen	Usual regimen
Netilmicin	2 mg/kg post-dialysis	Loading dose predialysis 3-5 mg/L dialysate*

(continued)

	Hemodialysis	Peritoneal dialysis
Ofloxacin	Usual regimen	200-400 mg/day
Oxacillin	Usual regimen	Usual regimen
Penicillin G	500,000 units post-dialysis	
Penicillin V	0.25 gm post-dialysis	
Pentamidine	Usual regimen	Usual regimen
Piperacillin	1 gm post-dialysis, then 2 gm q8h	3-6 gm/day
Pyrazinamide	Usual dose post-dialysis	(Avoid)
Rifampin	Usual regimen	Usual regimen
Streptomycin	0.5 gm post-dialysis	
Tetracycline	500 mg post-dialysis	(Use Doxycycline)
Ticarcillin	3 gm post-dialysis, then 2 gm q12h	2-3 gm q12h
Ticarcillin + clavulanic acid	3 gm (ticarcillin) post-dialysis, then 2 gm q12h	2-3 gm (ticarcillin) q12h
Tobramycin	1 mg/kg post-dialysis	Loading dose predialysis 2-4 mg/L dialysate*
Trimethoprim-sulfa	4-5 mg/kg (as trimethoprim) post-dialysis	0.16/0.8 q48h
Vancomycin	1 gm/wk	0.5-1 gm/wk
Vidarabine	Scheduled dose post-dialysis	
Zidovudine (AZT)	300 mg/day	300 mg/day

* Aminoglycosides given for prolonged periods to patients receiving continuous peritoneal dialysis have been associated with high rates of ototoxicity. Monitor level after loading dose and follow for symptoms of ototoxicity.

USE OF ANTIMICROBIAL AGENTS IN HEPATIC DISEASE

Many antimicrobial agents are metabolized by the liver and/or excreted via the biliary tract. Nevertheless, relatively few require dose modifications in hepatic disease; with few exceptions, doses are usually modified only if there is concurrent renal failure and/or the liver disease is either acute or is associated with severe hepatic failure as indicated by ascites or jaundice. The following recommendations are adopted from Drug Information 92, American Hospital Formulary Service, Amer Soc Hosp Pharmacists, Bethesda, MD, pp 33-481, 1992.

Agent: Recommended dose modification

Aztreonam: Some recommend a dose reduction of 20-25%.

Carbenicillin: Maximum of 2 gm/day for patients with severe renal and hepatic insufficiency.

Cefoperazone: Maximum dose is 4 gm/day; if higher monitor levels; with coexisting renal impairment maximum dose is 1-2 gm/day.

Ceftriaxone: Maximum daily dose of 2 gm with severe hepatic _and_ renal impairment.

Chloramphenicol: Use with caution with renal and/or hepatic failure; monitor serum levels to achieve levels of 5-20 ug/mL.

Clindamycin: Dose reduction recommended only for severe hepatic failure.

Isoniazid: Use with caution and monitor hepatic function for mild-moderate hepatic disease; acute liver disease or history of INH-associated hepatic injury is contraindication to INH.

Metronidazole: Modify dose for severe hepatic failure although specific guidelines are not provided; peak serum levels with 500 mg doses are 10-20 ug/ml.

Mezlocillin: Reduce dose by 50% or double the dosing interval.

Nafcillin: Metabolized by liver and largely eliminated in bile; nevertheless, dose modifications are suggested only for combined hepatic and renal failure.

Penicillin G: Dose reduction for hepatic failure only when accompanied by renal failure.

Rifampin: Induces hepatic enzymes responsible for inactivating methadone, corticosteroids, oral antidiabetic agents, digitalis, quinidine, cyclosporine, oral anticoagulants, estrogens, oral contraceptives and chloramphenicol. Concurrent use of these drugs with rifampin and use of rifampin in patients with prior liver disease requires careful review.

Ticarcillin: For patients with hepatic dysfunction and creatinine clearance < 10 mL/min, give 2 gm IV/day in one or two doses.

Ticarcillin/Clavulanate K: For patients with hepatic dysfunction and creatinine clearance < 10 mL/min give usual loading dose (3.1 gm) followed by 2 gm once daily.

ADVERSE REACTIONS TO ANTIMICROBIAL AGENTS

A. ADVERSE REACTIONS BY CLASS

	Frequent	Occasional	Rare
Acyclovir	Irritation at infusion site	Rash; nausea and vomiting; diarrhea; renal toxicity (esp with rapid IV infusion, prior renal disease and nephrotoxic drugs); dizziness; abnormal liver function tests; itching; headache	CNS-agitation, encephalopathy; lethargy, disorientation, seizures; hallucinations; anemia; hypotension; neutropenia; thrombocytopenia
Amantadine	Insomnia, lethargy, dizziness, inability to concentrate (5-10% of healthy young adults receiving 200 mg/day)	GI intolerance especially nausea (5-10%); rash	CNS-lethargy, tremor, confusion, obtundation, delirium, psychosis, seizures (primarily IV admin.); heart failure; eczematoid dermatitis; photosensitivity; oculogyric episodes; orthostatic hypotension; peripheral edema; bone marrow suppression
Aminoglycosides Tobramycin Gentamicin Amikacin Netilmicin Kanamycin	Renal failure: related to dose duration and hydration status (monitor creatinine 3-7x/wk and output; monitor peak levels when dose is high, treatment long or toxicity noted)	Vestibular and auditory damage; related to dose and duration (most common with prior high frequency loss, tinnitis, vertigo, renal failure and other ototoxic drugs -- note dizziness, vertigo, roaring, tinnitis, hearing loss)	Fever; rash; blurred vision; neuromuscular blockage esp with myesthenia; or Parkinson's; eosinophilia Allergic reactions -- usually due to sulfites in some preparations
Aminosalicylic acid (PAS)	GI intolerance	Liver damage; allergic reactions; thyroid enlargement	Acidosis; vasculitis; hypoglycemia (diabetes); hypokalemia; encephalopathy; decreased prothrombin activity; myalgias; renal damage; gastric hemorrhage
Amoxicillin + clavulanic acid	(Similar to amoxicillin - See penicillins)		

(continued)

	Frequent	Occasional	Rare
Amphotericin B	Fever (maximal at 1 hr) and chills (at 2 hrs) (Prevent/reduce with hydrocortisone, ibuprophen, ASA, acetominophen, meperidine); renal damage -- dose dependent and reversible in absence of prior renal damage and dose <3 gm; reduce with hydration and sodium supplementation; hypokalemia; anemia, phlebitis and pain at injection site	Hypomagnesemia; nausea, vomiting, metallic taste; headache	Hypotension; rash; pruritus; blurred vision; peripheral neuropathy; convulsions; hemorrhagic gastroenteritis; arrhythmias; diabetes insipidus; hearing loss; pulmonary edema; anaphylaxis; acute hepatic failure; eosinophilia; leukopenia; thrombocytopenia
Ampicillin + sulbactam	(Similar to those for ampicillin alone - See penicillins)		
Atovaquone		Rash (usually macro-papular and rarely treatment-limiting; nausea, vomiting, mild diarrhea; headache	Fever, elevated aminotransferases (generally mild), abdominal pain
Aztreonam	Eosinophilia	Phlebitis at infusion site; rash; diarrhea; nausea; eosinophilia; abnormal liver function tests	Thrombocytopenia; colitis; hypotension; unusual taste; seizures; chills
Bacitracin	Nephrotoxicity (proteinuria, oliguria, azotemia); pain with IM use		Rash; blood dyscrasias
Capreomycin	Renal damage (tubular necrosis esp in patients with prior renal damage): Increased creatinine, proteinuria, cylindruria, monitor UA and creatinine weekly	Ototoxicity (vestibular > auditory should: assess vestibular function before and during treatment); electrolyte abnormalities; pain, induration and sterile abscesses at injection sites	Allergic reactions; leukopenia; leukocytosis; neuromuscular blockage (large IV doses - reversed with neostigmine); hypersensitivity reactions; hepatitis?

(continued)

	Frequent	Occasional	Rare
Cephalosporins	Phlebitis at infusion sites; diarrhea (esp cefoperazone); pain at IM injection sites (less with cefazolin)	Allergic reactions (anaphylaxis rare); diarrhea and colitis; hypo-prothrombinemia (cefamandole, cefoperazone, moxalactam, cefmetazole and cefotetan); platelet dysfunction (moxalactam); eosinophilia; positive Coombs' test	Hemolytic anemia; interstitial nephritis (cephalothin); hepatic dysfunction; convulsions (high dose with renal failure); neutropenia; thrombocytopenia; serum sickness (esp cefaclor)
Chloramphenicol		GI intolerance (oral); marrow suppression (dose related)	Fatal aplastic anemia; fever; allergic reactions; peripheral neuropathy; optic neuritis
Chloroquine		Visual disturbances (related to dose and duration of treatment with dose used for rheumatoid arthritis); GI intolerance; pruritus	CNS-headache, confusion, dizziness, psychosis; peripheral neuropathy; cardiac toxicity; hemolysis (G-6-PD deficiency); marrow suppression; exacerbate psoriasis
Ciprofloxacin	(See quinolones)		
Clindamycin	Diarrhea (frequency of C. difficile toxin is 5% for all clindamycin recipients and 15-25% for those with antibiotic associated diarrhea)	Rash; colitis and PMC, usually due to C. difficile; GI intolerance (oral)	Blood dyscrasias; hepatic damage; neutropenia; neuromuscular blockage; eosinophilia; fever; metallic taste; phlebitis at IV infusion sites
Clofazimine	Ichthyosis; and dry skin; pink to brownish-black discoloration of skin, cornea, retina and urine (up to 75-100% with prolonged use, first noted in 1-4 wks, resolves 6-12 months after drug is stopped but traces may persist); GI intolerance	Persistent abdominal pain, diarrhea and weight loss (high dose over 3 months); dry, burning, irritated eyes; pruritis, rash	Bowel obstruction with does >300 mg/day (may be fatal, cause is unknown); GI bleeding; splenic infarction; eosinophilic enteritis; vision loss

(continued)

55

	Frequent	Occasional	Rare
Colistimethate	(See Polymyxins)		
Cycloserine	CNS-anxiety, confusion, depression, somnolence, disorientation, headache, hallucinations, tremor, hyper-reflexia, increased CSF protein and pressure (dose related and reversible) (Contraindicated in active alcoholics; twitching and seizures prevented with large doses pyroxidine -- 100 mg tid)	Liver damage; malabsorption; peripheral neuropathy; folate deficiency; anemia	Coma; seizures (contraindicated in epileptics); hypersensitivity reactions; heart failure, arrhythmias
Dapsone	Hemolytic anemia (dose dependent)	Blood dyscrasias (methemo-globulinemia and sulfahemo-globinemia $\pm$ G6PD deficiency); nephrotic syndrome; allergic reactions; insomnia; irritability; headache (transient); GI intolerance	Hypoalbuminemia; epidermal necrolysis; optic atrophy; agranulocytosis; peripheral neuropathy; aplastic anemia; "Sulfone syndrome" -- fever, exfoliative dermatitis, jaundice, adenopathy, methemoglobinemia and anemia -- treat with steroids
Dideoxyinosine (ddI; didanosine)	Diarrhea (15-30%) Pancreatitis (5-9%, fatal in 6% of cases) Peripheral neuropathy (pain-ful feet, 5-12%) All are dose related	Nausea; vomiting; rash; marrow suppression; hyperuricemia; hepatitis with transaminase levels >5x normal in up to 10%	Cardiomyopathy; hepatic failure
Dideoxycytidine (ddC; zalcitabine)	Peripheral neuropathy (17-31%; frequency is related to cumulative dose)	Aphthous oral and esophageal ulcers; pancreatitis (1%); flu-like complaints; hepatitis with transaminase levels > 5x normal in up to 10%	Thrombocytopenia; leukopenia
Diloxanide	Flatulence, diarrhea, nausea		Dizziness, diplopia, headache

(continued)

	Frequent	Occasional	Rare
Emetine	Arrhythmias; precordial pain; muscle weakness; phlebitis	Diarrhea; vomiting; neuropathy; heart failure	
Erythromycins	GI intolerance (oral-dose related); phlebitis (IV)	Diarrhea; stomatitis; cholestatic hepatitis (esp estolate-reversible); phlebitis (IV administration); generalized rash	Allergic reactions; colitis; hemolytic anemia; reversible ototoxicity (esp high dose and renal failure)
Ethambutol		Optic neuritis (decreased acuity, reduced color discrimination, constricted fields, scotomata -- dose related and infrequent with with 15 mg/kg); GI intolerance; confusion; precipitation of acute gout	Hypersensitivity Peripheral neuropathy; thrombocytopenia; toxic epidermal necrolysis; lichenoid skin rash
Ethionamide	GI intolerance (CNS effect)	Allergic reactions; peripheral neuropathy (prevented with pyroxidine); reversible liver damage (9%) with jaundice (1-3%) -- monitor transaminase q2-4 wks; gynecomastia; menstrual irregularity	Optic neuritis; gouty arthritis; hypothyroidism; impotence; hypothyroidism; purpura; poor diabetic control, rash
Fluconazole		Nausea; vomiting; bloating, abdominal pain; transaminase elevating to ≥ 8x normal (1%); headache; rash; diarrhea; prolonged protime with coumadin	Hepatitis; Stevens-Johnson syndrome; thrombocytopenia; anaphylaxis
Flucytosine	GI intolerance (including nausea, vomiting, diarrhea and ulcerative colitis)	Marrow suppression with leukopenia or thrombocytopenia (dose related, esp with renal failure, >100 mg/ml, or concurrent amphotericin); confusion; rash; hepatitis (dose related)	Hallucinations; eosinophilia; granulocytosis; fatal hepatitis

(continued)

	Frequent	Occasional	Rare
Foscarnet	Renal failure (usually reversible; 30% get creatinine > 2 mg/dl; discontinue if creatinine > 2.9 mg/dl)	Mineral and electrolyte changes -- (calcium, magnesium, phosphorus, ionized calcium, potassium); seizures (10%), fever, GI intolerance, anemia	Marrow suppression, arrhythmias
Furazolidone	GI intolerance	Allergic reactions; pulmonary infiltrates; headache	Hemolytic anemia (G-6-PD deficiency); hypotension; polyneuropathy; hypoglycemia; agranulocytosis
Ganciclovir (DHPG) (Cytovene)	Neutropenia (ANC < 500/mm³ in 15-20%, usually early in treatment and responds within 3-7 days to drug holiday or to G-CSF/ GM-CSF); thrombocytopenia (platelet count < 20,000/mm³ in 10%, reversible)	Anemia; fever; rash; CNS-headache, seizures, confusion; changes in mental status; abnormal liver function tests (2-3%)	Psychosis; neuropathy; impaired reproductive function (?); hematuria; renal failure; nausea; vomiting; GI bleeding or perforation myocardiopathy; hypotension; ataxia; coma; somnolence
Griseofulvin	Headache (often resolves with continued treatment)	Photosensitivity	GI disturbances; allergic reactions; paresthesias; exacerbation of lupus; liver damage; lymphadenopathy; blood dyscrasias; thrush; transient hearing loss; fatigue; dizziness; insomnia; psychosis
Imipenem		Phlebitis at infusion sites; allergic reactions; nausea; vomiting and diarrhea; eosinophilia; hepatotoxicity (transient)	Seizures; myoclonus; colitis; bone marrow suppression; renal toxicity
Interferon alpha	Flu-like illness (80% with > 5 mil units/d; fever; fatigue, anorexia, headache, myalgias, depression, abdominal pain, diarrhea	Marrow suppression -- Leukopenia, anemia ± thrombocytopenia (3-70%, dose related, usually transient and well tolerated); Neuro-psychiatric effects -- psychosis,	Edema; arrhythmias; cardiomyopathy; renal failure; hearing loss

(continued)

58

	Frequent	Occasional	Rare
Interferon alpha (continued)	Starts within 6 hrs and lasts 2-12 hrs; pretreat with NSAIA	Confusion, somnolence, anxiety); hepatitis -- dose related and up to 40% receiving high doses; alopecia (8%); rash	CNS-optic neuritis; psychosis; convulsions; toxic encephalopathy; twitching; coma; blood dyscrasias; hyperglycemia; lupus-like syndrome; keratitis; pellagra-like rash
Isoniazid	Hepatitis - age related < 20 yrs-nil; 35-6%; 45-11%; 55-18%. Patient should be warned of symptoms and drug should be discontinued if transaminase levels are 3x normal limit	Allergic reactions; fever; peripheral neuropathy (reduce with pyridoxine), esp with alcoholism, diabetes, pregnancy, malnutrition	Hepatitis (1/1000)
Itraconazole		Headache; nausea (10%); vomiting, rash (8%)	
Ketoconazole	GI intolerance (dose related) Temporary increase in transaminase levels (2-5%)	Endocrine-decreased steroid and testosterone synthesis with impotence, gynecomastia, oligospermia, reduced libido; menstrual abnormalities (prolonged use and dose related, usually ≥ 600 mg/day); headache; dizziness; asthenia; pruritus; rash	Abrupt hepatitis (1:15,000), rare cases of fatal hepatic necrosis; anaphylaxis; lethargy; arthralgias; fever; marrow suppression; hypothyroidism (genetically determined)
Mefloquine	Vertigo; light-headedness; nausea; nightmares; headache; visual disturbances (dose related)	Psychosis and seizures (dose related -- rare at doses used for prophylaxis); GI intolerance; dizziness	Prolonged cardiac conduction
Methenamine	GI intolerance; metallic taste; headache	GI intolerance; dysuria (reduced dose or acidification)	Allergic reactions; edema; tinnitus; muscle cramps
Metronidazole	GI intolerance; metallic taste; headache	Peripheral neuropathy (prolonged use-reversible); phlebitis at injection sites; Antabuse-like reaction	Seizures; ataxic encephalitis; colitis; leukopenia; dysuria; pancreatitis; allergic reactions; mutagenic in Ames test

(continued)

59

	Frequent	Occasional	Rare
Miconazole		Phlebitis at injection sites; chills; pruritus; rash; dizziness; blurred vision; hyperlipidemia; nausea; vomiting; hyponatremia	Marrow suppression - anemia and thrombocytopenia; renal damage; anaphylaxis; psychosis; cardiac arrest
Nalidixic acid	(See Quinolones)		
Nitrofurantoin	GI intolerance	Hypersensitivity reactions; pulmonary infiltrates (acute, subacute or chronic; ± fever, eosinophilia, rash or lupus-like reaction)	Peripheral neuropathy; hepatitis; hemolytic anemia (G-6-PD deficiency); lactic acidosis; parotitis; pancreatitis
Nystatin		GI intolerance	Allergic reactions
Ofloxacin	(See Quinolones)		
Penicillins	Hypersensitivity reactions; rash (esp ampicillin and amoxicillin); diarrhea (esp ampicillin)	GI intolerance (oral agents); fever; Coombs' test positive; phlebitis at infusion sites and sterile abscesses at IM sites; Jarisch-Herxheimer reaction (syphilis or other spirochetal infections)	Anaphylaxis; leukopenia; thrombocytopenia; colitis (esp ampicillin); hepatic damage; renal damage; CNS-seizures, twitching (high doses in patients with renal failure); hyperkalemia (penicillin G infusion); abnormal platelet aggregation with bleeding diathesis (carbenicillin and ticarcillin)
Pentamidine	Nephrotoxicity - in 25%, usually reversible with discontinuation Aerosol administration - cough (30%)	Hypotension (administer IV over 60 min); hypoglycemia (5-10%, usually occurs after day 5 of treatment including past treatment, may last days or weeks, treat with IV glucose), rash (including Stevens-Johnson syndrome; marrow suppression (common in AIDS patients); GI intolerance Aerosol administration - asthma reaction (5%)	Hepatotoxicity; leukopenia; thrombocytopenia; pancreatitis; hyperglycemia, insulin-dependent diabetes

(continued)

60

	Frequent	Occasional	Rare
Polymyxins	Pain and phlebitis at injection sites; neurotoxicity (ataxia, paresthesias); nephrotoxicity		Allergic reactions; neuromuscular blockade
Primaquine		Hemolytic anemia (G-6-PD deficiency); GI intolerance	Headache; pruritus
Pyrazinamide	Non-gouty polyarthralgia; asymptomatic; hyperuricemia	Hepatitis (dose related, frequency not increased when given with INH or rifampin, rarely serious); GI intolerance; gout (treat with allopurinol and probenecid)	Rash; fever; porphyria; photosensitivity
Pyrimethamine		Folic acid deficiency with megaloblastic anemia and pancytopenia (dose related and reversed with leucovorin); allergic reactions	CNS-ataxia, tremors, seizures (dose related), fatigue
Quinine		GI intolerance; cinchonism (tinnitus, headache, visual disturbances); hemolytic anemia (G-6-PD deficiency)	Arrhythmias; hypotension with rapid IV infusion; hypoglycemia; hepatitis; thrombocytopenia
Quinolones	(Animal studies show arthropathies in weight bearing joints of immature animals; significance in humans is not known, but this class is considered contraindicated in children and pregnancy)	GI intolerance; CNS-headache; malaise; insomnia; dizziness; allergic reactions	Papilledema; nystagmus; visual disturbances; diarrhea; pseudomembranous colitis; abnormal liver function tests including hepatic necrosis; marrow suppression; photosensitivity anaphylaxis; seizures; toxic psychosis; CNS stimulation -- tremors, restlessness; confusion

(continued)

	Frequent	Occasional	Rare
Rifampin	Orange discoloration of urine, tears (contact lens), sweat (See drug interactions)	Hepatitis (frequency not increased when given with INH); jaundice (usually reversible with dose reduction and/or continued use); GI intolerance; hypersensitivity reactions; increases hepatic metabolism of steroids to increase steroid requirement in adrenal insufficiency and require alternative to birth control meds (See drug interactions); flu-like syndrome with intermittent use characterized by dyspnea, wheezing	Thrombocytopenia; leukopenia; hemolytic anemia; eosinophilia; renal damage; proximal myopathy; hyperuricemia; anaphylaxis
Spectinomycin		Pain at injection site; urticaria; fever; insomnia; dizziness; nausea; headache	Anaphylaxis; fever; anemia; renal failure and abnormal liver function tests (multiple doses)
Sulfonamides	Allergic reactions - rash, pruritis (appears to be dose related), fever (usually 7-10 days of initial dose). Cross reactions noted between sulfonamides including thiazide diuretics and antidiabetic agents	Periarteritis nodosum, lupus, Stevens-Johnson syndrome, serum sickness; crystalluria with renal damage, urolithiasis and oliguria (prevent with increasing urine pH hydration and use of sulfonamide -- sulfonamide combinations); GI intolerance; photosensitivity	Myocarditis; psychosis; neuropathy; dizziness, depression; hemolytic anemia (G-6-PD deficiency); marrow suppression; agranulocytosis
Tetracyclines	GI intolerance (dose related); stains and deforms teeth in children up to 8 yrs; vertigo (minocycline); negative nitrogen balance and increased azoemia with renal failure (except doxycycline); vaginitis	Hepatotoxicity (dose related, esp pregnant women); esophageal ulcerations; diarrhea; candidiasis (thrush and vaginitis); photosensitivity (esp demeclocycline); phlebitis with IV treatment and pain with IM injection	Malabsorptions; allergic reactions; visual disturbances; aggravation of myasthenia; hemolytic anemia; colitis

(continued)

	Frequent	Occasional	Rare
Ticarcillin + clavulanic acid	Similar to those for ticarcillin alone (See Penicillins)		
Trimethoprim	GI intolerance (dose related); rash (up to 24% receiving ≥ 400 mg/d x 14 days)	Marrow suppression -- megaloblastic anemia, neutropenia, thrombocytopenia (hematologic toxicity increased with folate depletion and high doses -- treat with leucovorin, 3-15 mg/day x 3 days)	Pancytopenia; erythema multiforme, Stevens-Johnson syndrome, TEN
Trimethoprim-sulfamethoxazole	Fever, leukopenia, rash (AIDS patients); reactions noted above for sulfonamides and trimethoprim		
Vancomycin	Phlebitis at injection sites	"Red-man syndrome" (flushing over chest and face) or hypotension (infusion too rapid); rash; fever; neutropenia; eosinophilia; allergic reactions with rash	Anaphylaxis; ototoxicity and nephrotoxicity dose related); peripheral neuropathy; marrow suppression
Vidarabine		GI intolerance; phlebitis at infusion site; fluid overload	Blood dyscrasias; CNS-confusion and neurologic deterioration (esp with renal failure)
Zidovudine (AZT, Retrovir)	Marrow suppression: anemia and/or leukopenia (dose and stage related: marrow toxicity with Hgb < 7.5 g/dL or ANC < 750/ml is 3%/yr for asymptomatic patients and 40% for AIDS patients)	Subjective complaints: headaches (50%); malaise; insomnia; myalgias; nausea (often resolves with dose reduction and/or continued use); myopathy with myalgias or weakness plus elevated CPK -- responds to drug withdrawal within 2 wks	Seizures (reversible); allergy (rash, anaphylaxis); twitching: mania; hepatitis; esophageal ulceration

63

B. **Penicillin Allergy**

1. Classification of penicillin hypersensitivity reactions

Type	Mechanism	Clinical expression
I	IgE	Urticaria, angioedema, anaphylaxis, laryngeal edema, asthma frequency - 0.02%, mortality - 10%
II	Cytotoxic Ab of IgG class	Hemolytic anemia
III	Immune complexes IgG & IgM Ab	Serum sickness
IV	Cell-mediated	Contact dermititis
Idiopathic	Unknown	Maculopapular rash (common), interstitial nephritis, drug fever, eosinophilia, exfoliative dermititis, Stevens- Johnson syndrome

2. **Cross reactions** among betalactam agents
   Allergy to one penicillin indicates allergy to all.
   Allergy to penicillins may indicate allergy to cephalosporins and imipenem;
   it is generally considered safe to give cephalosporins to patients with
   non-IgE- medicated reactions to penicillins such as maculopapular rashes.
   There is no apparent cross reaction with aztreonam.

3. **Skin testing:** This is considered a safe, rapid and effective method to
   exclude an IgE mediated response with ≥ 98% assurance (MMWR 38:S13,1989)

   a. Patients with a history of severe reactions during the past year
      should be tested in the hospital setting with antigens diluted 100-
      fold; others may be tested in a physician staffed clinic.

   b. Patients with a history of penicillin allergy and a negative skin
      test should receive penicillin, 250 mg po and be observed for one
      hour prior to treatment with therapeutic doses. Those with a positive
      skin test should be desensitized.

   c. Penicillin allergy skin testing (adapted from Beall*)
      Note: If there has been a severe, generalized reaction to penicillin
      in the previous year, the antigens should be diluted 100-fold, and
      patients should be tested in a controlled environment. Both major and
      minor determinants should be available for the tests to be interpre-
      table. The patient should not have taken antihistamines in the previous
      48 hours.

Reagents

Major determinants:
  Benzylpenicilloyl-polylysine (major, Pre-Pen [Taylor Pharmacal Co., Decatur, Illinois], 6 x 10^{-5}M)
  Benzylpenicillin (10^{-2} or 6000 U/mL)
Minor determinants:
  Benzylpenicilloic acid (10^{-2}M)
  Benzylpenilloic acid (10^{-2}M)
Positive control (histamine, 1 mg/mL)
Negative control (buffered saline solution)

Dilute the antigens 100-fold for preliminary testing if there has been an immediate generalized reaction within the past year.

Procedure

Epicutaneous (scratch or prick) test: apply one drop of material to volar forearm and pierce epidermis without drawing blood; observe for 20 minutes. If there is no wheal $\geq$ 4mm, proceed to intradermal test.

Intradermal test: Inject 0.02 ml intradermally with a 27- gauge short-bevelled needle; observe for 20 minutes.

Interpretation: For the test to be interpretable, the negative (saline) control must elicit no reaction and the positive (histamine) control must elicit a positive reaction.

Positive test: A wheal > 4mm in mean diameter to any penicillin reagent; erythema must be present.

Negative test: The wheals at the site of the penicillin reagents are equivalent to the negative control.

Indeterminate: All other results

---

*Reprinted with permission from Beall GN, Penicillins, pp 205-9. In: Saxon A, moderator. Immediate hypersensitivity reactions to beta-lactam antibiotics. Ann Intern Med 1987;107:204-15.

4. Penicillin desensitization (Adapted from the Medical Letter on Drugs and Therapeutics 30:77,1988 and MMWR 38:S13,1989).

    a. Penicillin densensitization should be done in a hospital because IgE mediated reactions can occur, although they are rare. Desensitization may be done orally or intravenously, although oral administration is often considered safer, simpler and easier.

    b. Parenteral desensitization: Give 1 unit penicillin IV and then double the dose at 15 minute intervals or increase the dose 10-fold at 20-30 minute intervals.

c.   Oral-desensitization protocol (from Wendel)

Dose*	Penicillin V Suspension (units/ml)	Amount[T] ml	units	Cumulative dose (units)
1	1,000	0.1	100	100
2	1,000	0.2	200	300
3	1,000	0.4	400	700
4	1,000	0.8	800	1,500
5	1,000	1.6	1,600	3,100
6	1,000	3.2	3,200	6,300
7	1,000	6.4	6,400	12,700
8	10,000	1.2	12,000	24,700
9	10,000	2.4	24,000	48,700
10	10,000	4.8	48,000	96,700
11	80,000	1.0	80,000	176,700
12	80,000	2.0	160,000	336,700
13	80,000	4.0	320,000	656,700
14	80,000	8.0	640,000	1,296,700

Observation period: 30 minutes before parenteral administration of penicillin.
*Interval between doses, 15 minutes; elapsed time, 3 hours and 45 minutes; cumulative dose, 1.3 million units
[T]The specific amount of drug was diluted in approximately 30 ml of water and then given orally.

Adapted with permission from the New England Journal of Medicine 312:1229-32, 1985.

5.   Management of allergic reactions
      Epinephrine: IgE mediated reactions
      Antihistamines: Accelerated and late urticaria, maculopapular rashes
      Glucocorticoids: Severe urticaria, prolonged systemic anaphylaxis, serum
            sickness, contact dermatitis, exfoliative and bullous skin reactions,
            interstitial nephritis, pulmonary and hepatic reactions

6.   Anaphylactic shock

	Epinephrine dose
Initial treatment	
Subcutaneous (preferred) or intramuscular	0.3-0.5 ml (1:1000)
Repeat every 20-30 min prn up to 3x	
Severe shock or inadequate response to IM or SC; administration intravenous	3-5 ml at 5-10 min intervals (1:1000)

C. Adverse Reactions during Pregnancy (Adapted from Drug Evaluations, 6th Edition, AMA, Chicago, 1986, pp 44-46)

Agent	1st trimester (Embryonic development)	2nd & 3rd trimesters (Fetal development)	Labor-delivery
Antibacterial agents			
Aminoglycosides	8th nerve damage**	8th nerve damage**	-
Chloramphenicol	-	Gray-baby syndrome*	Gray-baby syndrome*
Dapsone	-	-	Carcinogenic*** Hemolytic reactions*
Metronidazole	Tumors***	-	-
Nitrofurantoin	-	Hyperbilirubinemia* Hemolytic anemia*	Hyperbilirubinemia* Hemolytic anemia*
Streptomycin	8th nerve damage multiple defects, micromelia*	8th nerve damage*	-
Sulfamethoxazole-trimethoprim	Malformations****	-	-
Sulfonamides	-	Hyperbilirubinemia*	Hyperbilirubinemia*
Tetracycline	Inhibit bone growth* Micromelia** Syndactyly**	Stain deciduous teeth* Inhibit bone growth* Enamel hypoplasia**	-
Antimalarial agents			
Chloroquine	8th nerve damage**	8th nerve damage**	
Quinine	Malformations, abortions, 8th nerve damage*	Deafness Thrombocytopenia	-
Antituberculous agents			
Isoniazid	CNS effects***	-	-
Rifampin	CNS effects***	-	-
Streptomycin (see above)			

* Generally well documented in humans
**Suspected in humans
*** Documented in animals only
**** Questionable effects in humans

67

D. Relative Safety of Antimicrobial Agents During Pregnancy (classification according to the Medical Letter 29:61,1987 and data from Drug Information - 1992, American Hospital Formulary Service, Amer Soc Hosp Pharmac, Bethesda, pp 33-481, 1992)

Note: Drugs are listed by category of microbes. Medical Letter classifies drugs in 3 categories: Probably safe, Use with caution, or Contraindicated. PDR and FDA recommendations usually state that any drug used in pregnant women is justified only when the medical need justifies the risk to the fetus or that safety in pregnancy is not established.

ANTIBACTERIAL AGENTS	Experimental animal studies (often 5-20x human dose)	Experience in Pregnant Women	Recommendation (including Medical Letter recommendations)
Aminoglycosides	---	Several reports of congenital deafness with streptomycin	Use only with life-threatening infections where no alternatives are available. Warn patient of risk. Med Letter: Caution
Aztreonam	Harmless except slightly reduced survival in offspring with very high doses	No studies	Use with caution. Med Letter: Probably safe
Cephalosporins	Harmless	No adverse effects reported	Use with caution. Med Letter: Probably safe
Chloramphenicol	---	Gray baby syndrome with administration in late pregnancy or labor	Use with great caution at term or labor. Med Letter: Caution
Clindamycin	---	No studies	Med Letter: Caution
Dapsone	---	No adverse effects reported	Use with caution. Med Letter: Caution
Erythromycin	Harmless	No studies	Use only when clearly needed, although CDC recommends erythromycin for treatment of chlamydia and syphilis in pregnancy. Avoid estolate. Med Letter: Probably safe
Imipenem	Harmless	No studies	Use with caution. Med Letter: Caution
Methenamine	Harmless	No adverse effects reported	Safety not definitely established. Med Letter: Probably safe
Metronidazole	Fetotoxicity (with parenteral administration only)		Contraindicated during first trimester. Med Letter: Caution

(continued)

68

ANTIBACTERIAL AGENTS	Experimental animal studies (often 5-20x human dose)	Experience in Pregnant Women	Recommendation (including Medical Letter recommendations)
Nitrofurantoin	---	Hemolytic anemia in neonate due to immature enzyme systems. Drug appears safe in early pregnancy	Contraindicated at term. Med Letter: Caution
Penicillins	Harmless	No adverse effects reported	Use only when necessary, although CDC recommends penicillin G for syphilis and gonorrhea during pregnancy. Med Letter: Probably safe
Quinolones	Arthropathy in immature animals with erosions in joint cartilage	No studies	Contraindicated. Med Letter: Contraindicated
Spectinomycin		No studies	CDC recommends for pregnant women with gonorrhea. Med Letter: Probably safe
Sulfonamides	Cleft palate and bone abnormalities with high doses	Extensive use -- no complication except one case of agranulocytosis (possibly associated) Risk of sulfa-induced kernicterus when used in last term -- risk is low	Use with caution and avoid in last trimester when feasible. Contraindicated at term. Med Letter: Caution
Tetracyclines		Retardation of skeletal development and bone growth. Enamel hypoplasia and discoloration of teeth of fetus	Contraindicated. Med Letter: Contraindicated
Trimethoprim	Teratogenic	No studies	Use with caution due to effect on folic acid metabolism. Med Letter: Caution
Trimethoprim-sulfamethoxazole	Teratogenic	No congenital abnormalities in 35 children born to women who received TMP-SMX in first trimester	Use with caution due to effect on folic acid metabolism. Contraindicated at term due to kernicterus from sulfonamides. Med Letter: Caution
Vancomycin		No studies	Use with caution. Med Letter: Caution

(continued)

ANTIFUNGAL AGENTS	Experimental animal studies (often 5-20x human dose)	Experience in Pregnant Women	Recommendation (including Medical Letter recommendations)
Amphotericin B	--	No studies	Use with caution. Med Letter: Caution
Fluconazole	--	No studies	Use with caution. Med Letter: Caution
Flucytosine	Teratogenic	No studies	Use with caution. Med Letter: Caution
Griseofulvin	Embryotoxic and teratogenic	Congenital malformations and conjoined twins reported; relationship to drug debated	Contraindicated. Med Letter: Contraindicated
Itraconazole	Embryotoxic and teratogenic	No studies	Use with caution.
Ketoconazole	Embryotoxic and teratogenic	No studies	Use with caution. Med Letter: Caution
Miconazole	Harmless	No studies	Med Letter: Caution
Nystatin	--	No complications reported	Safe. Med Letter: Probably safe

ANTIMYCO-BACTERIAL AGENTS	Experimental animal studies (often 5-20x human dose)	Experience in Pregnant Women	Recommendation (including Medical Letter recommendations)
Aminosalicylic acid (PAS)	--	No studies	Use with caution. Med Letter: Caution
Capreomycin	Teratogenic -- "wavy rib"	No studies	Use with caution. Med Letter: Caution
Ethambutol	Teratogenic	No adverse effects reported	Use with caution. Med Letter: Caution
Ethionamide	Teratogenic	No studies	Use with caution. Med Letter: Caution
Isoniazide	Embryocidal. No teratogenic effects	No adverse effects reported	AAP recommendation: Pregnant women with positive PPD should receive INH if HIV pos., recent contact or x-ray showing old TB; begin after 1st trimester if possible; otherwise delay prophylaxis until postdelivery. Give with pyridoxine. Med Letter: Caution

(continued)

ANTIMYCO-BACTERIAL AGENTS	Experimental animal studies (often 5-20x human dose)	Experience in Pregnant Women	Recommendation (including Medical Letter recommendations)
Pyrazinamide	----	No studies	Use with caution. Med Letter: Caution
Rifampin	Congenital malformations -- cleft palate, spina bifida Embryotoxicity	Isolated cases of fetal abnormalities. Administration in last weeks of pregnancy may cause postnatal hemorrhage	Use with caution. Med Letter: Caution

ANTIPARASITIC AGENTS	Experimental animal studies (often 5-20x human dose)	Experience in Pregnant Women	Recommendation (including Medical Letter recommendations)
Chloroquine	Accumulates in melanin of fetal eyes	Use with lupus: 8th nerve deficits, postcolumn defects, mental retardation. Use for malaria: No adverse effects	CDC and WHO conclude benefits outweigh risk with malaria exposure outweigh risk. Med Letter: Probably safe
Iodoquinol	----	No studies	Med Letter: Caution
Mebendazole	Embryotoxic, teratogenic	170 patients -- no adverse effects	Use with caution esp in 1st trimester and warn patient of risk. Med Letter: Caution
Mefloquine			Contraindicated: CDC advises contraception during prophylaxis and for 2 months after.
Niclosamide	Harmless	No studies	Usually can delay therapy. Med Letter: Probably safe
Oxamniquine	Embryocidal	No studies	Use with caution.
Paromomycin	----	No studies	Med Letter: Probably safe
Pentamidine	----	Spontaneous abortion reported during aerosol administration (causal relationship not established)	Avoid use of aerosolized pentamidine including those planning to become pregnant

(continued)

71

ANTIPARASITIC AGENTS	Experimental animal studies (often 5-20x human dose)	Experience in Pregnant Women	Recommendation (including Medical Letter recommendations)
Piperazine	---	Limited experience	Safety not clearly established Med Letter: Caution
Praziquantel	Harmless except increased rates of abortion	No studies	Use with caution Med Letter: Probably safe
Primaquine	---	No studies; theoretical concern is hemolytic anemia in G-6-PD deficient fetus	CDC: Chloroquine for relapsing malaria until postdelivery, then use primaquine for radical care
Pyrantel pamoate	Harmless	No studies	Self-medicate under direction of physician
Pyrimethamine	Teratogenic; stunted fetus; malformations	No reported adverse effects	Use with caution: indicated for toxoplasmosis in pregnancy. Fansidar indicated when risk of chloroquine resistant malaria cannot be avoided Med Letter: Caution
Quinacrine	Teratogenic	No studies	Usually can delay treatment of cestodiasis Med Letter: Caution
Quinine	Teratogenic	Stillbirths reported. Congenital malformations with large doses used for attempted abortions. Preferred.	Contraindicated. CDC previously recommended use for life-threatening malaria, but quinidine gluconate is now recommended Med Letter: Caution
Thiabendazole	Harmless except when suspended in olive oil	No experience	Use with caution. Med Letter: Caution

ANTIVIRAL AGENTS	Experimental animal studies (often 5-20x human dose)	Experience in Pregnant Women	Recommendation (including Medical Letter recommendations)
Acyclovir	Not teratogenic but potential to cause chromosomal damage at high doses	Limited data from BW registry -- no adverse effects; report to 1-800-722-9292	CDC: Use for life-threatening disease; do not use for treatment or prophylaxis of genital herpes. Med Letter: Caution

(continued)

72

ANTIVIRAL AGENTS	Experimental animal studies (often 5-20x human dose)	Experience in Pregnant Women	Recommendation (including Medical Letter recommendations)
Amantadine	Embryotoxic and teratogenic	Single case of 1st trimester exposure with single ventricle	Use with great caution. Med Letter: Contraindicated
Foscarnet	Skeletal abnormalities (<5%)	No studies	Use only if clearly needed.
Ganciclovir	Teratogenic and embryogenic, growth retardation, aplastic organs	No studies	Use only when necessary and warn patient of teratogenic and embryogenic effects Med Letter: Caution
Vidarabine	Teratogenic, maternal toxicity, fetal abnormalities	No studies	Use only when necessary. Med Letter: Caution
Zidovudine	Fetal resorptions; teratogenic and fetal hematologic toxicity with extremely high doses	No adverse effects with 160 patients reported to BW registry	Use only when necessary and report to registry 800-722-9292 Med Letter: Caution

DRUG INTERACTIONS
(Adapted from The Medical Letter Handbook of Adverse Drug Interactions, Medical Letter, pp 6-282, 1991; AMA Drug Evaluations and Drug Information 92; American Hospital Formulary Service; Amer Soc Hosp Pharmacists, Bethesda, MD, pp 33-481, 1992)

Drug	Effect of Interaction
Acyclovir	
Narcotics	Increased meperidine effect
Probenecid	Possible increased acyclovir toxicity
Amantadine	
Anticholinergics	Hallucination, confusion, nightmares
Thiazide diuretics	Increased amantadine toxicity with hydroclorothiazide-triamterene combination
Aminoglycosides	
Amphotericin	Increased nephrotoxicity
Bumetanide	Ototoxicity
Cephalosporins	Increased nephrotoxicity
Cisplatin*	Increased nephrotoxicity
Cyclosporine*	Increased nephrotoxicity
Enflurane*	Increased nephrotoxicity
Ethacrynic acid*	Increased ototoxicity
Furosemide*	Increased oto- and nephrotoxicity
MgSO$_4$	Increased neuromuscular blockage
Methotrexate	Possible decreased methotrexate activity with oral aminoglycosides
Vancomycin	Increased nephrotoxicity and possible increased ototoxicity
Aminosalicylic acid (PAS)	
Anticoagulants, oral	Increased hypoprothrombenia
Digitalis	Decreased digoxin effect
Probenecid	Increased PAS toxicity
Rifampin	Decreased rifampin effectiveness (give as separate doses by 8-12 hr)
Amphotericin B	
Aminoglycosides	Increased nephrotoxicity
Capreomycin	Increased nephrotoxicity
Corticosteroids	Increased hypokalemia
Cisplatin	Increased nephrotoxicity
Cyclosporine*	Increased nephrotoxicity
Digitalis	Increased cardiotoxicity (?)
Diuretics	Increased hypokalemia
Methoxyflurane	Increased nephrotoxicity
Skeletal muscle relaxants	Increased effect of relaxants
Vancomycin	Increased nephrotoxicity
AZT (Retrovir, Zidovudine)	
Amphotericin B	Increased anemia

(continued)

Drug	Effect of Interaction
Cancer chemotherapy (adriamycin, vinblastin, vincristine)	Increased marrow toxicity
Dapsone	Increased marrow toxicity
Flucytosine	Increased leukopenia
Ganciclovir*	Increased leukopenia, concurrent use contraindicated except with G-CSF
Interferon	Increased leukopenia
Phenytoin	Decreased phenytoin levels
Probenecid	Increased AZT levels (and rash)
Capreomycin	
Aminoglycosides*	Increased oto- and nephrotoxicity
Theophylline	Increased theophylline effect and toxicity
Cephalosporins	
Alcohol	Disulfiram-like reaction for those with tetrazolethiomethyl side chain: Cefamandole, cefoperazone, cefotetan, cefmetazole, moxalactam
Aminoglycosides	Possibly increased nephrotoxicity
Ethacrynic acid	Increased nephrotoxicity
Furosemide	Increased nephrotoxicity
Probenecid	Increased concentrations of most cephalosporins
Chloramphenicol	
Anticoagulants, oral	Increased hypoprothrombinemia
Chlorpropamide	Increased chlorpropamide activity
Dicumarol	Increased dicumarol activity
Phenobarbital	Decreased concentrations chloramphenicol
Phenytoin	Increased phenytoin activity
Rifampin*	Decreased concentrations chloramphenicol
Tolbutamide	Increased tolbutamide activity
Ciprofloxacin (See Fluoroquinolones)	
Clindamycin	
Antiperistaltic agents (Lomotil, loparamide)	Increased risk and severity of C. difficile colitis
Cycloserine	
Alcohol*	Increased alcohol effect or convulsions; warn patients
Ethionamide	Increased CNS toxicity
Isoniazid	CNS toxicity, dizziness, drowsiness
Phenytoin	Increased phenytoin effect (toxicity)
Dapsone	
Coumadin	Increased prothrombin time
ddI	Decreased levels of dapsone
Primaquine	Increased hemolysis with G-6-PD deficiency
Probenecid	Increased dapsone levels
Pyrimethamine	Increased marrow toxicity (Monitor CBC)
Rifampin	Decreased levels of dapsone
Trimethoprim	Increased levels of both drugs (continued)

Drug	Effect of Interaction
ddC (HIVID, zalcitabine, dideoxycytidine)	
Agents associated with peripheral neuropathy:	Cisplatin, dapsone, ddI, disulfiram, ethionamide, glutethimide, gold, hydralazine, Iodoquinol, INH, metronidazole, nitrofurantoin, phenytoin, ribivirin, vincristine
Agents associated with pancreatitis:	Pentamidine, ddI, rifampin
ddI (videx, didanosine)	
Dapsone	Decreased dapsone absorption, give ≥ 2hrs before ddI
Ketoconazole	Decreased ketoconazole absorption, give ≥ 2hrs before ddI
Tetracycline	Decreased tetracycline absorption, give ≥ 2hrs before ddI
Quinolones	Decreased quinolone absorption, give ≥ 2hrs before ddI
Note: All drugs that require gastric acidity for absorption should be given ≥ 2hrs before ddI	
Alcohol	Increased frequency of pancreatitis
Pentamidine	Increased frequency of pancreatitis
Erythromycins	
Anticoagulants (oral)	Increased hypoprothrombinemia
Carbamazepine	Increased carbamazepine toxicity
Corticosteroids	Increased effect of methylprednisolone
Cyclosporine	Increased cyclosporine toxicity (nephrotoxicity)
Digoxin	Increased digitalis toxicity
Disopyramide	Increased disopramide toxicity
Ergot alkaloids	Increased ergot toxicity
Phenytoin	Increased or decreased phenytoin effect
Seldane	Ventricular arrhythmias
Theophylline	Increased theophylline effect
Triazolam	Increased triazolam toxicity
Ethionamide	
Cycloserine	Increased CNS toxicity
Isoniazid	Increased CNS toxicity
Fluconazole	
Coumadin	Increased prothrombin time
Cyclosporine	Increased cyclosporine in renal transplant recipients
Phenytoin	Increased phenytoin effect
Sulfonylureas	Increased levels with hypoglycemia
Fluoroquinolones (ciprofloxacin, norfloxacin, ofloxacin, lomefloxacin)	
Antacids	Decreased fluoroquinolone absorption with Mg, Ca or Al containing antacids or sucralfate: Give antacid > 2hrs after fluoroquinolone
Anticoagulants (oral)	Increased hypoprothrombinemia
Caffeine	Increased caffeine effect; significance?; not noted with ofloxacin
Cyclosporine	Possible increased nephrotoxicity
Iron*	Decreased ciprofloxacin absorption

(continued)

Drug	Effect of Interaction
Nonsteroidal anti-inflammatory agents	Possible seizures and increased epileptogenic potential of theophylline, opiates, tricyclics and neuroleptics
Probenecid	Increased fluoroquinolone levels
Theophylline	Increased theophylline toxicity -- esp ciprofloxacin and enoxacin (seizures, cardiac arrest, respiratory failure)
Zinc	Decreased ciprofloxacin absorption

Foscarnet

Drug	Effect of Interaction
Aminoglycosides	Increased renal toxicity
Amphotericin B	Increased renal toxicity
Pentamidine	Increased hypocalcemia

Ganciclovir

Drug	Effect of Interaction
Azathriaprim	Increased marrow suppression
AZT (Retrovir)*	Increased leukopenia or give G-CSF
Imipenem	Increased frequency of seizures (?)

Griseofulvin

Drug	Effect of Interaction
Alcohol	Possibly potentiates effect of alcohol
Anticoagulant (oral)	Decreased anticoagulant effect
Contraceptive	Decreased contraceptive effect
Phenobarbital	Decreased griseofulvin levels

Isoniazid

Drug	Effect of Interaction
Alcohol	Increased hepatitis; Decreased INH effect in some
Antacids	Decreased INH with Al containing antacids
Anticoagulants (oral)	Possible increased hypoprothrombinemia
Benzodiazepines	Increased effects of benzodiazepines
Carbamazepine*	Increased toxicity of both drugs
Cycloserine	Increased CNS toxicity, dizziness, drowsiness
Disulfiram*	Psychotic episodes, ataxia
Ethionamide	Increased CNS toxicity
Enflurane*	Possible nephrotoxicity
Ketoconazole*	Decreased ketoconazole effect
Phenytoin	Increased phenytoin toxicity
Rifampin	Possible increased hepatic toxicity
Theophylline	Increased theophylline levels
Tyramine (rich foods & fluids)	Palpitations, sweating, urticaria, headache, vomiting, with consumption of cheese, wine, some fish

Itraconazole

Drug	Effect of Interaction
Coumadin	Increased hypoprothrombinemia
Cyclosporine	Increased cyclosporine levels
Digoxin	Increased digoxin levels
H_2 antagonists	Decreased itraconazole levels
Hypoglycemics (oral)	Severe hypoglycemia
INH	Decreased itraconazole levels
Phenytoin	Decreased itraconazole levels
Rifampin	Decreased itraconazole levels
Terfenadine	Cardiac dysrhythmias

(continued)

Drug	Effect of Interaction
Ketoconazole	
Alcohol	Possible disulfiram-like reaction
Antacids	Decreased ketoconazole effect
Anticoagulants, oral	Increased hypoprothrombinemia
Corticosteroids	Increased methylprednisolone effect
Cyclosporine	Increased cyclosporine toxicity
H2 antagonists*	Decreased ketoconazole effect; use sucralfate or antacids given 2 hrs before
Isoniazid*	Decreased ketoconazole effect
Phenytoin	Altered metabolism of both drugs
Rifampin*	Decreased activity of both drugs
Seldane*	Ventricular arrhythmias
Theophylline	Increased theophylline activity
Mebendazole	
Phenytoin and Carbamazepine	Decreased mebendazole concentrations: clinically significant only for extraintestinal helminthic infections
Metronidazole	
Alcohol	Disulfiram-like reaction
Anticoagulants, oral	Increased hypoprothrombinemia
Barbiturates	Decreased metronidazole effect with phenobarbital
Corticosteroids	Decreased metronidazole effect
Cimetidine*	Possible increased metronidazole toxicity
Disulfiram*	Organic brain syndrome
Fluorouracil	Transient neutropenia
Lithium	Lithium toxicity
Miconazole	
Aminoglycosides	Possible decreased tobramycin levels
Anticoagulant, oral	Increased hypoprothrombinemia
Hypoglycemics	Severe hypoglycemia with sulfonylurea
Phenytoin	Increased phenytoin toxicity
Nalidixic acid	
Anticoagulants, oral	Increased hypoprothrombinemia
Nitrofurantoin	
Antacids	Possible decreased nitrofurantoin effect; give 6 hrs apart
Probenecid	Decreased nitrofurantoin effect (for UTIs)
Penicillins	
Allopurinol	Increased frequency of rash with ampicillin
Anticoagulants, oral	Decreased anticoagulant effect with nafcillin and dicloxacillin
Cephalosporins	Increased cefotaxime toxicity with mezlocillin + renal failure
Contraceptives	Possible decreased contraceptive effect with ampicillin or oxacillin
Cyclosporine	Decreased cyclosporine effect with nafcillin and increased cyclosporin toxicity with ticarcillin
Lithium	Hypernatremia with ticarcillin

(continued)

Drug	Effect of Interaction
Methotrexate	Possible increased methotrexate toxicity
Probenecid	Increased concentrations of penicillins

Pentamidine

Aminoglycosides	Increased nephrotoxicity
Amphotericin B	Increased nephrotoxicity
Capreomycin	Increased nephrotoxicity
Foscarnet	Increased nephrotoxicity

Piperazine

Chlorpromazine	Possibly induces seizures

Polymyxin B and colistimethate

Aminoglycoside	Increased nephrotoxicity; increased neuromuscular blockade
Neuromuscular blocking agents	Increased neuromuscular blockade
Vancomycin	Increased nephrotoxicity

Pyrazinamide

Allopurinal*	Failure to decrease hyperuricemia

Pyrimethamine

Antacids	Possible decreased pyrimethamine absorption
Dapsone*	Agranulocytosis reported
Kaolin	Possible decreased pyrimethamine absorption
Phenothiazines	Possible chlorpromazine toxicity

Rifampin

Aminosalicylic acid (PAS)	Decreased effectiveness of rifampin; give in separate doses by 8-12 h
Anticoagulants	Increased hypoprothrombinemia
Barbiturates	Decreased barbiturate effect
Benzodiazepines	Possible decreased benzodiazepine effect
ß-adrenergic blockers	Decreased B blocker effect
Chloramphenicol*	Decreased chloramphenicol effect
Clofazimine	Reduced rifampin effect
Clofibrate	Decreased clofibrate effect
Contraceptives	Decreased contraceptive effect
Corticosteroids*	Decreased corticosteroid effect
Cyclosporine*	Decreased cyclosporine effect
Dapsone	Decreased dapsone effect (not significant with treatment of leprosy)
Digitalis	Decreased digitalis effect
Disopyramide*	Decreased disopyramide effect
Doxycycline	Decreased doxycycline effect
Estrogens	Decreased estrogen effect
Haloperidol	Decreased haloperidol effect
Hypoglycemics	Decreased hypoglycemic effect of sulfonurea
Isoniazid	Increased hepatotoxicity
Ketoconazole*	Decreased effect of ketoconazole and rifampin (concurrent use contraindicated)

(continued)

Drug	Effect of Interaction
Methadone	Methadone withdrawal symptoms
Mexiletin	Decreased antiarrhythmic effect
Phenytoin	Decreased phenytoin effect
Progestins	Decreased norethindrome effect
Quinidine	Decreased quinidine effect
Theophyllines	Decreased theophylline effect
Trimethoprim	Decreased trimethoprim levels
Verapamil	Decreased verapamil effect

Spectinomycin

Lithium	Increased lithium toxicity

Sulfonamides

Anticoagulants, oral	Increased hypoprothrombinemia
Barbiturates	Increased thiopental effect
Cyclosporine	Decreased cyclosporine effect with sulfamethazine
Digoxin	Decreased digoxin effect with sulfasalazine
Hypoglycemics	Increased hypoglycemic effect of sulfonylurea
Methotrexate	Possible increased methotrexate toxicity
Monoamine oxidase inhibitors	Possible increased phenelzine toxicity with sulfisoxazole
Phenytoin	Increased phenytoin effect except with sulfisoxazole

Tetracycline

Alcohol	Decreased doxycycline effect in alcoholics
Antacids*	Decreased tetracycline effect with antacids containing Ca^{++}, Al^{++}, Mg^{++} and $NaHCO_3$ (give 3 hrs apart)
Anticoagulants, oral	Increased hypoprothrombinemia
Antidepressants, tricyclic*	Localized hemosiderosis with amitriptyline and minocycline
Antidiarrhea agents	Agents containing kaolin and pectin or bismuth subsalicylate decrease tetracycline effect
Barbiturates*	Decreased doxycycline effect
Bismuth subsalicylate (Pepto-Bismol)	Decreased tetracycline effect
Carbamazepine (Tegretol)*	Decreased doxycycline effect
Contraceptives, oral*	Decreased contraceptive effect
Digoxin	Increased digoxin effect (10% of population)
Iron, oral	Decreased tetracycline effect (except with doxycycline) and decreased iron effect; give 3 hrs before
Laxatives	Agents containing Mg^{++} decrease tetracycline effect
Lithium	Possible increased lithium toxicity (single case)
Methotrexate	Possible increased methotrexate toxicity
Methoxyflurane anesthesia (Penthrane)	Possibly lethal nephrotoxicity
Milk	Decreased absorption of tetracycline. Does not apply to doxycycline or minocycline
Molindone	Decreased tetracycline effect
Phenformin*	Decreased doxycycline effect
Phenytoin	Decreased doxycycline effect
Rifampin	Possible decreased doxycycline effect
Theophylline	Possible increased theophylline toxicity
Zinc*	Decreased tetracycline effect	(continued)

Drug	Effect of Interaction
Thiabendazole	
Theophyllines	Increased theophylline toxicity
Trimethoprim	
Azathioprine	Leukopenia
Cyclosporine*	Increased nephrotoxicity
Dapsone	Increased levels of both drugs; increased methemoglobinemia
Digoxin	Possible increased digitalis effect
Phenytoin	Increased phenytoin effect
Thiazide diuretics	Possible increased hyponatremia with concomitant use of amiloride with thiazide diuretics
Trimethoprim-sulfamethoxazole	
Anticoagulants, oral	Increased hypothrombinemia
Mercaptopurine*	Decreased mercaptopurine activity
Methotrexate*	Megaloblastic anemia
Paromycin	Increased nephrotoxicity
Phenytoin	Increased phenytoin toxicity
Procainamide	Increased procainamide
Vancomycin	
Aminoglycosides	Increased nephrotoxicity and possible increased ototoxicity
Amphotericin B	Increased nephrotoxicity
Cisplatin	Increased nephrotoxicity
Digoxin	Possible decreased digoxin effect
Paromomycin	Increased nephrotoxicity
Polymyxin	Increased nephrotoxicity
Vidarabine	
Allopurinol	Increased neurotoxicity, nausea, pain and pruritus
Theophyllines	Increased theophylline effect

* Concurrent use to be avoided if possible

PREVENTIVE MEDICINE

A. Vaccines available in the United States, by type and recommended routes of administration (MMWR 38:207,1989)

Vaccine	Type	Route
BCG (Bacillus of Calmette and Guérin	Live bacteria	Intradermal or subcutaneous
Cholera	Inactivated bacteria	Subcutaneous or intradermal*
DTP (D=Diphtheria) (T=Tetanus) (P=Pertussis)	Toxoids and inactivated bacteria	Intramuscular
HB (Hepatitis B)	Inactive viral antigen	Intramuscular
Haemophilus influenzae b -Polysaccharide (HbPV) -or Conjugate (HbCV)	Bacterial polysaccharide or Polysaccharide conjugated to protein	Subcutaneous or intramuscular[T] Intramuscular
Influenza	Inactivated virus or viral components	Intramuscular
IPV (Inactivated Poliovirus Vaccine)	Inactivated viruses of all 3 serotypes	Subcutaneous
Measles	Live virus	Subcutaneous
Meningococcal	Bacterial polysaccharides of serotypes A/C/Y/W-135	Subcutaneous
MMR (M=Measles) (M=Mumps) (R=Rubella)	Live viruses	Subcutaneous
Mumps	Live virus	Subcutaneous
OPV (Oral Poliovirus Vaccine)	Live viruses of all 3 serotypes	Oral
Plague	Inactivated bacteria	Intramuscular
Pneumococcal	Bacterial polysaccharides of 23 pneumococcal types	Intramuscular or subcutaneous
Rabies	Inactivated virus	Subcutaneous or intradermal[§]
Rubella	Live virus	Subcutaneous
Tetanus	Inactivated toxin (toxoid)	Intramuscular‸
Td or DT** (T=Tetanus) (D or d=Diphtheria)	Inactivated toxins	Intramuscular‸
Typhoid	Inactivated bacteria	Subcutaneous[TT]
Yellow fever	Live virus	Subcutaneous

*The intradermal dose is lower.
[T]Route depends on the manufacturer; consult package insert for recommendation for specific product use.
[§]Intradermal dose is lower and used only for preexposure vaccination.
‸Preparations with adjuvants should be given intramuscularly.
** DT=tetanus and diphtheria toxoids for use in children aged <7 years. Td= tetanus and diphtheria toxoids for use in persons aged ≥7 years. Td contains the same amount of tetanus toxoid as DTP or DT but a reduced dose of diphtheria toxoid.
[TT]Boosters may be given intradermally unless acetone-killed and dried vaccine is used.

B. GUIDE FOR ADULT IMMUNIZATION
(Adapted from: Guide for Adult Immunization, American College of Physicians, 2nd Ed., Philadelphia, PA 1-178,1990; MMWR 40(RR12):1-94,1991)

Category	Vaccine	Comments
AGE		
18-24 yrs	Td* (0.5 ml IM)	Booster every 10 yrs at mid-decades (age 25, 35, 45, etc) for those who completed primary series
	Measles** (MMR, 0.5 ml SC x 1 or 2)	Post-high school institutions should require two doses of live measles vaccine (separated by 1 month), the first dose preferably given before entry
	Mumps*** (MMR, 0.5 ml SC x 1)	Especially susceptible males
	Rubella*** (MMR, 0.5 ml SC x 1)	Especially susceptible females; pregnancy now or within 3 months post-vaccination is contraindication to vaccination
	Influenza	Advocated for young adults at increased risk of exposure (military recruits, students in dorms, etc)
25-64 yrs	Td*	As above
	Mumps***	As above
	Measles** (MMR, 0.5 ml SC x 1)	Persons vaccinated between 1963 and 1967 may have received inactivated vaccine and should be revaccinated
	Rubella*** (MMR, 0.5 ml SC x 1)	Principally females $\leq$ 45 yrs with child-bearing potential; pregnancy now or within 3 months post-vaccination is contraindication to vaccination
$\geq$ 65 yrs	Td*	As above
	Influenza (0.5 ml IM)	Annually, usually in November
	Pneumococcal (23 valent, 0.5 ml IM)	Single dose; efficacy for elderly not established, but case control and epidemiology studies suggest 60-70% effectiveness in preventing pneumococcal bacteremia (NEJM 325:1453, 1991)
SPECIAL GROUPS		
Pregnancy		All pregnant women should be screened for hepatitis B surface antigen (HBsAg) and rubella antibody
		Live virus vaccines**** should be avoided unless specifically indicated
		It is preferable to delay vaccines and toxoids until 2nd or 3rd trimester
		Immune globulins are safe; most vaccines are a theoretical risk only

(continued)

83

Category	Vaccine	Comments
	Td* (0.5 ml IM)	If not previously vaccinated - dose at 0, 4 wks (preferably 2nd and 3rd trimesters) and 6-12 mo.; boost at 10 yr intervals; protection to infant is conferred by placental transfer of maternal antibody
	Measles	Risk for premature labor and spontaneous abortion; exposed pregnant women who are susceptible** should receive immune globulin within 6 days and then MMR post delivery at least 3 months after immune globulin (MMR is contraindicated during pregnancy)
	Mumps	No sequelae noted, immune globulin is of no value and MMR is contraindicated
	Rubella	Rubella during 1st 16 wks carries great risk, e.g., 15-20% rate of neonatal death and 20-50% incidence of congenital rubella syndrome; history of rubella is unreliable indicator of immunity. Women exposed during 1st 20 weeks should have rubella serology and if not immune should be offered abortion.
	Hepatitis A	Immune globulin within 2 weeks of exposure
	Hepatitis B	All pregnant women should have prenatal screening for HBsAg; newborn infants of HBsAg carriers should receive HBIG and HBV vaccine; pregnant women who are HBsAg negative and at high risk should receive HBV vaccine
	Inactivated oral polio vaccine (0.5 ml SC)	Advised if exposure is imminent in women who completed the primary series over 10 yrs ago. Unimmunized women should receive 2 doses separated by 1-2 mo.; unimmunized women at high risk who need immediate protection should receive oral live polio vaccine
	Influenza Pneumococcal vaccine	Not routinely recommended, but can be given if there are other indications
	Varicella (VZIG, 12.5 U/kg IM)	Varicella-zoster immune globulin (VZIG) may prevent or modify maternal infection
Family member exposure		**Recommendations generally apply to household contacts**
	H. influenzae type B	H. influenzae meningitis: Rifampin prophylaxis for all household contacts in households with another child <4 yrs; contraindicated in pregnant women
	Hepatitis A	Immune globulin within 2 weeks of exposure

(continued)

Category	Vaccine	Comments
	Hepatitis B	HBV vaccine (3 doses) for those with intimate contact and no serologic evidence of prior infection
	Influenza	Influenza case should be treated with amantadine to prevent spread; unimmunized high risk family members should receive amantadine (x 14 days) and vaccine
	Meningococcal infection	Rifampin or sulfonamide for family contacts of meningococcal meningitis
	Varicella-zoster	No treatment unless immunocompromised: consider VZIG

ENVIRONMENTAL SETTINGS

Residents of nursing homes

	Vaccine	Comments
	Influenza (0.5 ml IM)	Annually; vaccination rates of 80% required to prevent outbreaks
	Pneumococcal vaccine (23 valent, 0.5 ml IM)	Single dose, efficacy not clearly established
	Td* (0.5 ml IM)	Booster dose at mid-decades

Residents of institutions for mentally retarded

	Vaccine	Comments
	Hepatitis B	Screen all new admissions and long term residents: HBV vaccine for susceptibles (Seroprevalence rates are 30-80%)

Category	Vaccine	Comments
Prison inmates	Hepatitis B	As above
Homeless	Td*	
	Measles, rubella, mumps	MMR 0.5 ml SC (young adults)
	Influenza	
	Pneumococcal vaccine	

OCCUPATIONAL GROUPS

Health care workers

	Vaccine	Comments
	Hepatitis B (3 doses)	Personnel in contact with blood or blood products; serologic screening with vaccination only of seronegatives is optional; serologic studies show 5% are nonresponders (neg for anti-HBs) even with repeat vaccinations
	Influenza	Annual
	Rubella (MMR, 0.5 ml SC)	Personnel who might transmit rubella to pregnant patients or other health care workers should have documented immunity or vaccination

(continued)

Category	Vaccine	Comments
	Mumps (MMR, 0.5 ml SC)	Personnel with no documented history of mumps or mumps vaccine should be vaccinated
	Measles (MMR, 0.5 ml SC)	Personnel who do not have immunity** should be vaccinated; those vaccinated in or after 1957 should receive an additional dose and those who are unvaccinated should receive 2 doses separated by at least 1 month; during outbreak in medical setting vaccinate (or revaccinate) all health care workers with direct patient contact
	Polio	Persons with incomplete primary series should receive inactivated polio vaccine
<u>Immigrants and refugees</u>		
	Td*	Immunize if not previously done
	Rubella, Measles, Mumps	Most have been vaccinated or had these conditions, although MMR is advocated except for pregnant women
	Polio	Adults will usually be immune
	Hepatitis B	Screen for HBsAg and vaccinate family members and sexual partners of carriers; screening is especially important for pregnant women
LIFESTYLES		
<u>Homosexual men</u>		
	Hepatitis B	Prevaccination serologic screening advocated since 30-80% have serologic evidence of HBV markers
<u>IV drug abusers</u>		
	Hepatitis B	As above; seroprevalence rates of HBV marker are 50-80%
IMMUNODEFICIENCY		
<u>HIV infection</u>	Measles	Postexposure prophylaxis with immune globulin (0.25 ml/kg IM)
	Pneumococcal vaccine	Recommended
	H. influenzae b conjugate vaccine	Consider
	Influenza (0.5 ml IM)	Annual; consider amantadine during epidemics
<u>Asplenia</u>	Pneumococcal vaccine (23 valent, 0.5 ml IM)	Recommended, preferably given 2 weeks before elective splenectomy; revaccinate those who received the 14 valent vaccine and those vaccinated > 6 yrs previously
	Meningococcal vaccine	Indicated
	H. influenzae b conjugate	Consider

(continued)

Category	Vaccine	Comments
Renal failure	Hepatitis B	For patients whose renal disease is likely to result in dialysis or transplantation; double dose and periodic boosters advocated
	Pneumococcal vaccine	Pneumococcal vaccine
	Influenza	Annual
Alcoholics	Pneumococcal vaccine	
Diabetes & other high risk diseases	Influenza	
	Pneumococcal vaccine	
TRAVEL* (Recommendations of Med Lett 34:41,1992; and CDC Information for International Travel 1992, HHS Publication #92-8280)		For travelers to developed countries (Canada, Europe, Japan, Australia, New Zealand) the risk of developing vaccine-preventable disease is no greater than for traveling in the U.S.
		Each country has its own vaccine requirements
		Smallpox vaccination is no longer required and should not be given
	Yellow fever (see MMWR 39: RR6,1990)	Recommended for endemic area: Tropical S. America and most of Africa between 15° North & 15° South
		Available in U.S. only at sites designated by local or state health departments
		Contraindications: Immunocompromised host; pregnancy is a relative contraindication (live virus vaccine)
	Cholera	Not recommended since risk is low and vaccine has limited effectiveness (Lancet 1:270,1990)
	Typhoid fever	Recommended for travel to rural areas of countries where typhoid fever is endemic or any area of an outbreak. The live oral vaccine (one cap every other day x 4 starting 2 wks before travel) is preferred over the parenteral vaccine due to comparable efficacy and better tolerance (Lancet 336:891, 1990); available from Berna Products (800-533-5899)
	Hepatitis A	Immune globulin for susceptible travelers to areas with poor sanitation conditions; especially if contact with small children or work in health care areas; dose is 0.02 ml/kg (or 2 ml) IM for travel < 3 mo. and 0.06 ml/kg (or 5 ml) IM for travel > 3 mo. Repeat dose q 4-6 mo. while in endemic area. Susceptibility may be determined with tests for IgG antibody that are widely available (Lancet 1:1447,1988). (continued)

Category	Vaccine	Comments
	Hepatitis B	HBV vaccine if travel to endemic areas, and travel > 6 mo., sexual contact with local persons is likely or if contact with blood is likely. Major risk areas are Southeast Asia and sub-Saharan Asia.
	Rabies	Consider human diploid cell rabies vaccine (HDCV) or rabies vaccine absorbed (RVA) for extended travel to endemic area
	Japanese encephalitis (1 ml SC x 3 1-2 wks apart)	Vaccine recommended for > 1 mo. in rural rice-growing areas with extensive exposure to mosquitoes. Potential problem countries include Bangladesh, Cambodia, Indonesia, Laos, Malasia, Burma, Pakistan, China, Korea, Taiwan, Thailand, Vietnam, India, Nepal, Sri Lanka and the Philippines (NEJM 319: 641,1988). Available through U.S. embassies in Asia
	Measles	Susceptible persons** should receive a single dose before travel
	Meningococcal vaccine	Recommended for travel to areas of epidemics, most frequently sub-Saharan Africa (Dec-Jan), Middle East, India and Napal
	Polio	Travelers to developing countries should receive a primary series of inactivated polio vaccine if not previously immunized If protection is needed within 4 wks: single dose eIPV or trivalent (live) OPV recommended. Previously immunized travelers should receive one booster of OPV or eIPV

---

* Td - Diphtheria and tetanus toxoids absorbed (for adult use). Primary series is 0.5 ml IM at 0, 4 wks and 6-12 months; booster doses at 10-year intervals are single doses of 0.5 ml IM. Adults who have not received at least 3 doses of Td should complete the primary series. Persons with unknown histories should receive the series.

** Persons are considered immune to measles if there is documentation of receipt of two doses of live measles vaccine after the first birthday, prior physician diagnosis of measles, laboratory evidence of measles immunity or birth before 1957.

*** Persons are considered immune to mumps if they have a record of adequate vaccination, documented physician diagnosed disease, or laboratory evidence of immunity. Persons are considered immune to rubella if they have a record of vaccination after their first birthday or laboratory evidence of immunity. (A physician diagnosis of rubella is considered non-specific).

** ***The preferred vaccine for persons susceptible to measles, mumps or rubella is MMR given as 0.5 ml SC for measles (one or two doses), mumps (one dose) or rubella (one dose). Pregnant women should not be vaccinated until after delivery.

**** Live virus vaccines = measles, rubella, yellow fever, oral polio vaccine

C. SPECIFIC VACCINES

1. **Influenza Vaccine (Recommendations of the Advisory Committee on Immunization Practice: MMWR 41:315, 1992; 41 RR-9, 1992)**

<u>Preparations</u>: Inactivated egg grown viruses that may be split (chemically treated to reduce febrile reactions in children) or whole. For the 1992-93 season the FDA Vaccine Advisory Panel has recommended a trivalent vaccine with A/Texas/36/91-like (H1N1), A/Beijing/353/89-like (H3N2) and B/Panama/45/90-like viruses. Product information available from Connaught (800) 822-2463, Parke Davis (800) 223-0432 and Wyeth (800) 321-2304. A history of prior vaccination in any prior year does not preclude the need for revaccination. Remaining 1991-92 season vaccine should not be used.

<u>Administration (over 12 years)</u>: Whole or split virus vaccine, 0.5 ml x 1 IM in the deltoid muscle, preferrably in November and as early as September.

Target groups

<u>Groups at increased risk for influenza-related complications</u>
1. Persons $\geq$ 65 years
2. Residents of nursing homes and other chronic care facilities housing persons of any age with chronic medical conditions
3. Persons with chronic disorders of the pulmonary or cardiovascular system, including those with asthma
4. Adults and children who require regular medical follow-up or hospitalization during the prior year due to chronic metabolic diseases (diabetes), renal dysfunction, hemoglobulinopathies or immunosuppression
5. Children and teenagers who are receiving long-term aspirin therapy (risk of Reye's syndrome)

<u>Groups that can transmit influenza to high risk patients</u>
1. Physicians, nurses and other personnel who have contact with high risk patients
2. Employees of nursing homes and chronic care facilities who have contact with patients or residents
3. Providers of home care to high risk persons
4. Household members of high risk persons

<u>Other groups</u>
1. Persons who desire it
2. Persons who provide essential community services
3. Persons in institutional settings
4. Persons with HIV infection
5. Elderly and other high risk persons embarking on international travel: Tropics -- all year; Southern hemisphere -- April thru September

Contraindications
1. Severe allergy to eggs
2. Persons with acute febrile illness (delay until symptoms abate); persons with minor illnesses such as URIs may be vaccinated

(continued)

3. Pregnancy: There has been no excess in the influenza-associated mortality among pregnant women since the 1957-1958 pandemic. Influenza vaccine is not routinely recommended, but pregnancy is not viewed as a contraindication in women with other high risk conditions; it is preferred to vaccinate after the first trimester unless the first trimester corresponds to the influenza season.

Adverse reactions:
1. Soreness at the vaccination site for up to 2 days in about one-third.
2. Fever, malaise, etc. - infrequent and most common in those not previously exposed in influenza antigens, e.g. young children. Reactions begin 6-12 hrs post-vaccination and persist 1-2 days.
3. Allergic reactions - rare and include hives, angioedema, asthma, anaphylaxis; usually allergy to egg protein.

2. Measles Prevention: Revised recommendations of the Advisory Committee on Immunization Practices (MMWR 40 RR 12:20-21, 1991)

Category	Recommendations
Routine childhood schedule	Two doses*, 1st at 12 months (high risk area) or 15 months (most areas); 2nd dose at 4-6 yrs.
Adults	Single dose unless documentation of at least one dose of live measles vaccine ≥ 1 yr** or other evidence of immunity***
Colleges and other educational institutions	Two doses* unless documentation of receipt of two doses** live measles vaccine at ≥ 1 yr or other evidence of immunity***, ****
Medical personnel beginning employment	Two doses* for all persons who do not have proof of two** doses live measles vaccine at ≥ 1 yr or other evidence of immunity***, ****
Outbreaks in institutions or medical facilities	Two doses* for all persons born after 1956 who do not have proof of two** doses of live measles vaccine ≥ 1 yr or other evidence of immunity***, ****
Exposures	Vaccine preferred if given < 72 h after exposure. Alternative is immune globulin (0.25 ml/kg IM, maximum 15 ml), acceptable if given within 6 days. Live measle vaccine should be given 3 mo. after IG

* Usually MMR (0.5 ml SC). Two doses in adults should include 2nd dose ≥ 1 month after first.

** Single dose of live measles vaccine given at ≥ 1 yr of age should provide long-lasting immunity in 95%. In some settings a 5% rate of susceptibility provides enough non-immune persons to sustain an epidemic. Persons vaccinated with killed measles vaccine (1963-67) are considered unvaccinated.

*** Born before 1957, physician diagnosed measles or laboratory evidence of immunity (measles-specific antibody). Serologic studies in health care workers showed 9% of persons born before 1957 were not immune, and 29% of health care workers who acquired measles (1985-89) were born before 1957. Therefore, vaccine should be offered to those born before 1957 if there is reason to consider them susceptible.

3. **Rabies Vaccine (Recommendation of Advisory Committee on Immunization Practice) MMWR 40RR-3:1-16,1991)**

There are two types of immunizing products
1. Rabies vaccine to induce active immune response; this response requires 7-10 days and persists ≥ 2 years.
   a. Rabies Vaccine, Human Diploid Cell: HDCV for intramuscular or intradermal injection (Connaught Labs, 800-VACCINE).
   b. Rabies Vaccine Absorbed: RVA (distributed by Biologics Products Program, Michigan Department of Public Health (517) 335-8050.
2. Rabies immune globulins (RIG) to give rapid passive protection with half life of 21 days available from Cutter Biological and Connaught Laboratories.

Table 1. Rabies postexposure prophylaxis. United States, 1991

Animal type	Evaluation and disposition of animal	Postexposure prophylaxis recommendations
Dogs and cats	Healthy and available for 10 days observation	Should not begin prophylaxis unless animal develops symptoms of rabies*
	Rabid or suspected rabid	Immediate vaccination
	Unknown (escaped)	Consult public health officials
Skunks, raccoons, bats, foxes, and most other carnivores; woodchucks	Regarded as rabid unless geographic area is known to be free of rabies or until animal proven negative by laboratory test^r	Immediate vaccination
Livestock, rodents, and lagomorphs (rabbits and hares)	Consider individually	Consult public health officials. Bites of squirrels, hamsters, guinea pigs, gerbils, chipmunks, rats, mice, other rodents, rabbits, and hares almost never require antirabies treatment.

* During the 10-day holding period, begin treatment with HRIG and HDCV or RVA at first sign of rabies in a dog or cat that has bitten someone. The symptomatic animal should be killed immediately and tested.
^r The animal should be killed and tested as soon as possible. Holding for observation is not recommended. Discontinue vaccine if immunofluorescence test results of the animal are negative.

Table 2. Rabies postexposure prophylaxis schedule. United States, 1991

Vaccination status	Treatment	Regimen*
Not previously vaccinated	Local wound cleaning	All postexposure treatment should begin with immediate thorough cleansing of all wounds with soap and water.
	HRIG	20 IU/kg body weight. If anatomically feasible, up to one-half the dose should be infiltrated around the wound(s) and the rest should not be administered in the same syringe or into the same anatomical site as vaccine. Because HRIG may partially suppress active production of antibody, no more than the recommended dose should be given.
	Vaccine	HDCV or RVA. 1.0 ml. IM (deltoid area^T), one each on days 0, 3, 7, 14 and 28.
Previously vaccinated^TT	Local wound	All postexposure treatment should begin with immediate thorough cleansing of all wounds with soap and water.
	HRIG	HRIG should not be administered.
	Vaccine	HDCV or RVA. 1.0 ml. IM (deltoid area^T), one each on days 0 and 3.

* These regimens are applicable for all age groups, including children.
^T The deltoid area is the only acceptable site of vaccination for adults and older children. For younger children, the outer aspect of the thigh may be use. Vaccine should never be administered in the gluteal area.
^TT Any person with a history of pre-exposure vaccination with HDCV or RVA, prior postexposure prophylaxis with HDCV or RVA, or previous vaccination with any other type of rabies vaccine and a documented history of antibody response to the prior vaccination.

4. <u>Tetanus Prophylaxis</u> (MMWR 40:RR10,1991)

History of Tetanus toxoid	Clean, minor wounds		Other wounds**	
	Td*	TIG*	Td*	TIG*
Unknown or < 3 doses	Yes	No	Yes	Yes
≥ 3 doses***	No, unless > 10 yrs since last dose	No	No, unless > 5 yrs since last dose	No

*   Td = Tetanus toxoid; TIG = Tetanus immune globulin
**   Wounds contaminated with dirt, stool, soil, saliva, etc; puncture wounds; avulsions; wounds from missiles, crushing, burns and frostbite.
*** If only three doses of toxoid, a fourth should be given.

5. **Pneumococcal Vaccine** - Advisory Committee on Immunization Practices, Centers For Disease Control, American Thoracic Society, The Infectious Diseases Society of America, American College of Physicians: MMWR 40 RR-12:1-94, 1991 and Guide for Adult Immunization ACP (2nd Edition) - 91-96, 1990.

<u>Vaccine</u>: 23 valent polysaccharide vaccine for the <u>S</u>. pneumoniae contains antigens for serotypes responsible for 87% of bacteremic pneumococcal disease in the U.S. Most adults show a 2x rise in type specific antibody at 2-3 weeks after vaccination. Efficacy estimated at 45-65%; it is not established in immunosuppressed populations (NEJM 325:1453, 1991).

<u>Recommendations for adults</u>
1. Immunocompetent adults at increased risk of pneumococcal disease or its complications due to chronic illness (e.g. cardiovascular disease, pulmonary disease, diabetes, alcoholism, cirrhosis, or cerebrospinal fluid leaks) or who are ≥ 65 years old.

2. Immunocompromised adults at increased risk of pneumococcal disease or its complications (e.g. splenic dysfunction or anatomic asplenia, lymphoma, Hodgkin's disease, multiple myeloma, chronic renal failure, nephrosis organ transplant recipients, HIV infection and other conditions associated with immunosuppression).

3. Persons in special environments or social settings with identified risk of pneumococcal disease (Native Americans, homeless, etc.).

   Notations: 1) Vaccine should be given at least 2 weeks before elective splenectomy; 2) Vaccine should be given as long as possible before planned immunosuppressive treatment; 3) Hospital discharge is a convenient time for vaccination since 2/3's of patients with serious pneumococcal infections have been hospitalized within the prior 5 years; 4) May be given simultaneously with influenza vaccine (separate injection sites).

4. Patients with HIV infection should be given vaccine early in the course of disease for adequate antibody response.   (continued)

<u>Adverse reactions</u>
1. Pain and erythema at injection site: 50%
2. Fever, myalgia, severe local reaction: < 1%
3. Anaphylactoid reactions: 5/million
4. Frequency of severe reactions is increased with revaccination
    < 13 months after primary vaccination; severe reactions are
    no more frequent when revaccination occurs > 4 yrs after
    primary vaccination.

<u>Revaccination</u>: Should be strongly considered for high risk patients
    vaccinated 6 or more years previously; revaccination after 3-5 years is
    recommended for transplant recipients, patients with renal failure and
    patients with nephrotic syndrome.

6. **Hepatitis Vaccine (Recommendations of the Advisory Council on Immunization Practices)**
    (MMWR 39:RR-2, 1-26, 1990)

    a. <u>HAV</u>: Immune globulin (IG)

	Dose ml/kg IM	Frequency
(1) Pre-exposure		
Workers with non-human primates	0.06	q 4-6 mo.
Travelers to developing countries		
Visit less than 3 mo.	0.02	Once
Visit over 3 mo.	0.02	q 4-6 mo.

(2) Post-exposure (must be given within
    two weeks of exposure)

Close personal contacts and sexual
    partners
Day care centers: Staff and
    attendees when one case or at least
    two cases in families of attendees
Institutions for custodial care:
    Residents with staff with close
    contact with cases ⎫ 0.02 Once
Common source exposure: food and
    waterborne outbreaks if recognized
    within the 2 week post-exposure
    period of effectiveness
Food handlers: Other food handlers,
    but not patrons unless uncooked
    food was handled without gloves
    and patrons can be located within
    2 weeks of exposure
Hospitals: Not recommended for
    hospital personnel ⎭

b. <u>Hepatitis B</u> (MMWR 36:353-366,1987; MMWR 37:342-351,1987; MMWR
    39:1-26,1990):

<u>Vaccine preparations</u>
(1) Heptavax B: Plasma-derived vaccine available since 6/82; 20 ug
    HBsAg/ml; use is now restricted to hemodialysis patients, other
    immunocompromised hosts and persons with yeast allergy.

(2) Recombivax HB: Recombinant vaccine produced by <u>Saccharomyces cerevisiae</u> (baker's yeast) and available since 7/86; 10 or 40 μg HBsAg/ml; usual adult dose is 3 1 ml doses (10 μg) at 0,1 and 6 mo.

(3) Engerix-B: Recombinant vaccine available since 1989; 20 μg HBsAg/ml; usual adult dose regimen is 3 1 ml doses (20 μg) at 0, 1 and 6 months; alternative schedule is 4 1 ml doses (20 μg) at 0, 1, 2 and 12 mo. (for more rapid induction of immunity)

<u>Pre-exposure vaccination:</u>

(1) <u>Regimen:</u> Three IM doses (deltoid) at 0 time, 1 month and 6 months. The usual adult dose is 1 ml (20 μg Engerix B or 10 μg of Recombivax HB); hemodialysis patients and possibly other immunocompromised patients should receive 2-4x the usual adult dose (usually 40 μg doses of either recombinant vaccine preparation)

(2) <u>Response rates:</u> > 90% of healthy adults develop adequate antibody response (> 10 million Internat. Units/ml) and field trials show 80-95% efficacy.

(3) <u>Postvaccination serologic testing:</u> Recommended only when clinical management depends on knowledge of immune status, i.e., infants born to HBsAg positive mother, dialysis staff and patients, persons with HIV infection and exposed health care workers. When done, test at 1-6 mo. after last dose.

(4) <u>Revaccination:</u> Revaccination of non-responders will produce response in 15-25% with one additional dose and in 30-50% with 3 doses. 13-60% of responders lose detectable antibody within 9 years, although implications for revaccination are unclear since protective efficacy persists at least 9 years. At present, booster doses are not recommended (MMWR 40:RR-13, 1991).

(5) <u>Prevaccination serologic testing:</u> Testing groups at highest risk is usually cost effective if the prevalence of HBV markers is > 20% (see table). Routine testing usually consists of one antibody test: either anti-HBc or anti-HBs. Anti-HBc detects both carriers (HBsAg) and non-carriers (anti-HBsAg), but does not distinguish between them. Average wholesale price of 3 dose vaccine regimen is $160; usual cost of serologic testing for anti-HBs or anti-HBc is $12-$20.

<u>Prevalence of hepatitis B serologic markers</u>

Population group	Prevalence of serologic markers of HBV infection	
	HBsAg (%)	Any marker(%)
Immigrants/refugees from areas of high HBV endemicity	13	70-85
Alaskan Natives/Pacific Islanders	5-15	40-70
Clients in institutions for the developmentally disabled	10-20	35-80
Users of illicit parenteral drugs	7	60-80
Sexually active homosexual men	6	35-80
Household contacts of HBV carriers	3-6	30-60
Patients of hemodialysis units	3-10	20-80
Health-care workers - frequent blood contact	1-2	15-30
Prisoners (male)	1-8	10-80
Staff of institutions for the developmentally disabled	1	10-25

(continued)

Population group	Prevalence of serologic markers of HBV infection	
	HBsAg (%)	Any marker(%)
Heterosexuals with multiple partners	0.5	5-20
Health-care workers - no or infrequent blood contact	0.3	3-10
General population (NHANES II)		
Blacks	0.9	14
Whites	0.2	3

(6) Side-effects: Pain at injection site (3-29%) and fever > 37.7°C (1-6%). Note: These side effects are no more frequent than in placebo recipients in controlled studies. Experience in over 4 million adults shows rare cases of Guillain-Barré syndrome with plasma-derived vaccine and no serious side effects with recombinant vaccines. Adverse reactions should be reported to 1-800-822-7967.

(7) Vaccine efficacy: 80-95% for preventing HBV infection and virtually 100% if protective antibody response (≥ 10 mIU/mL is achieved

(8) Candidates for vaccination

   a. Health care workers who perform tasks involving contact with blood or bloody fluids. This should be done during training before contact with blood.

   b. Public safety personnel who perform tasks involving contact with blood or bloody fluids. If exposure is infrequent, consider timely post-exposure prophylaxis.

   c. Clients* and staff of institutions for developmentally disabled. For nonresidential day care of developmentally disabled, the staff should be vaccinated and clients "should have consideration of vaccination"

   d. Hemodialysis patients*, preferably early in the course of renal disease since patients with uremia or receiving dialysis are less likely to respond.

   e. Patients who receive clotting factor concentrates*

   f. Adoptees, foster children or unaccompanied minors* from countries where HBV is endemic. If screening serology shows HBsAg, other family members should be vaccinated.

   g. International travelers if 1) travel includes > 6 mo in HBV endemic area plus close contact with local population or 2) travel involves contact with blood or sexual contact with high risk residents. Vaccination should begin at least 6 mo. before travel; the alternative is the 4-dose schedule with 3 doses in 2 months

   h. Parenteral drug abusers* who are susceptible; documentation of antiHBsAg response recommended for those with HIV infection

   i. Sexually active gay men*; documentation of anti-HBsAg response recommended for those with HIV infection

   j. Sexually active heterosexual men and women who 1) have recently acquired STDs, 2) prostitutes and 3) more then one partner in prior 6 months

   k. Inmates of long-term correctional facilities*

   l. Household and sexual contacts of HBsAg carriers*

   * Indicates categories when prevaccination screening for susceptibility is clearly cost effective

(continued)

(9) Pregnant women (MMWR 40:RR-13, 1991). Risk of HBV transmission from HBsAg positive pregnant woman to infant is 10-85% depending on HBsAg status. Perinatal infection has a 90% risk of chronic HBV infection and 25% mortality due to liver disease -- cirrhosis or hepatocellular carcinoma. Children who do not acquire HBV perinatally are at increased risk for person-to-person spread during the first 5 years. Over 90% of these infections can be prevented using active and passive immunizations.

Recommendations: All pregnant women should be tested for HBsAg during an early prenatal visit; infants born to HBsAg positive mothers should receive HBIG (0.5 ml) 1M x 1 (preferably within 12 hrs of delivery) and HB vaccine (0.5 ml) 1M x 3 (5 μg recombinant vaccine) at 0 time (concurrent with HBIG) at 1-2 mo. and at 6 mo. Test infants for HBsAg and anti-HBs at 12-15 mo.

(10) Post-exposure vaccination (MMWR 40:RR-13,1991)
   a. Acute exposure to blood
      Definition of exposure: percutaneous (needlestick, laceration or bite) or permucosal (ocular or mucous membrane) exposure to blood. Recommendations depend on HBsAg status of source and vaccination/vaccine response of exposed person. Note: HBIG, when indicated, should be given as soon as possible and value beyond 7 days post-exposure is unclear.

Recommendations for postexposure prophylaxis for percutaneous or permucosal exposure to hepatitis B, United States

	Treatment when source is:		
Exposed person	HBsAg* positive	HBsAg negative	Source not tested or unknown
Unvaccinated	HBIG[T] x 1[$] and initiate HB‘ vaccine**	Initiate HB vaccine**	Initiate HB vaccine**
Previously vaccinated Known responder	Test exposed for anti-HBs[TT] 1. If adequate,[$$] no treatment 2. If inadequate, HB vaccine booster dose	No treatment	No treatment
Known nonresponder	HBIG x 2 or HBIG x 1 plus 1 HB vaccine	No treatment	If known high-risk source, may treat as if source were HBsAg positive
Response unknown	Test exposed for anti-HBs 1. If inadequate,[$$] HBIG x 1 plus HB vaccine booster dose 2. If adequate, no treatment	No treatment	Test exposed for anti-HBs 1. If inadequate, HB vaccine booster dose 2. If adequate, no treatment

*HBsAg = Hepatitis B surface antigen.
[T]HBIG = Hepatitis B immune globulin.
[$]HBIG dose 0.06 mL/kg IM.
‘HB = Hepatitis B.
**For HB vaccine dose, see page 93.
[TT]Antibody to hepatitis B surface antigen.
[$$]Adequate anti-HBs is 10 SRU by radioimmunoassay or positive by enzyme immunoassay.

(continued)

b. Post-exposure immunoprophylaxis with other types of exposures
(MMWR 40:RR13, pg 9, 1991)

Type of Exposure	Immunoprophylaxis	Comment
Perinatal (HBsAg positive mother)	HBIG + vaccination	HBIG plus vaccine within 12 hrs of birth
Sexual contact - Acute HBV	HBIG (0.06 ml/kg IM) ± vaccination	HBIG efficacy 75%; all susceptible partners should receive HBIG and start vaccination within 14 days of last exposure; testing susceptibility with anti-HBc recommended if it does not delay prophylaxis >14 days. Vaccination is optimal if exposed person is not in a high risk category and sex partner is HBsAg negative at 3 months
Sexual contact - Chronic carrier (HBsAg x 6 mo.)	Vaccination*	
Household contact - Acute HBV	None unless there is sexual contact or blood exposure (sharing tooth-brushes, razors, etc.)	With known exposure: HBIG ± vaccination
Household contact - Chronic carrier (HBsAg x 6 mo.)	Vaccination*	

* 1 ml IM x 3 at 0, 1, and 6 months

PROPHYLACTIC ANTIBIOTICS IN SURGERY

Antimicrobial Agents in Surgery (Adapted from the Medical Letter 31:105-108,1989 and Kaiser AB: N Engl J Med 315:1129-1138,1986; Rev Infect Dis Suppl 10, 13:S 779, 1991; Mayo Clin Proc 67:288, 1992)

Type of Surgery	Preferred regimen	Alternative	Comment
CARDIOTHORACIC			
Cardiovascular: Coronary by-pass; valve surgery	Cefazolin 2 gm IV pre-op (and 6gh x 48h)* Cefuroxime 1.5 gm IV ± q6-8h x 48h)*	Vancomycin** 15 mg/kg IV pre-op, after initiation of by-pass (10 mg/kg) (and q8h x 48h)	Single doses appear to be as effective as multiple doses providing high serum concentrations are maintained throughout the procedure (Antimicrob Ag Chemother 29:744, 1986). Some now use vancomycin routinely.
Pacemaker insertion	Cefazolin as above (see comments)	No alternative	Single doses appear to be as effective as multiple doses. Prophylaxis advocated only for centers with high infection rates.
Peripheral vascular surgery			
Abd. aorta and legs	Cefazolin 1-2 gm IV pre-op (± 1 gm q6h x 48h)*	Vancomycin** 15 mg/kg (and q8h x 48 h) Cefuroxime 1.5 gm IV q8h x 3	Recommended for procedures on abdominal aorta and procedures on leg that include groin incision. Some recommend prophylaxis for any implantation of prosthetic material or vascular access in hemodialysis (Ann Surg 188:283, 1978).
Carotid or brachial artery	None	Cefoxitin 1 gm IV	
Thoracic surgery: lobectomy, pneumonectomy	Cefazolin 1-2 gm IV pre-op (± 1 gm q8h x 48h)*		Optimal duration is unknown. Antibiotic prophylaxis is not recommended for thoracic trauma or chest tube insertion. Efficacy is not established (RID 13, Suppl 10:S869, 1991).
GASTROINTESTINAL			
Gastric surgery	Cefazolin 1-2 gm IV pre-op	Clindamycin 600 mg IV + gentamicin 1.7 mg/kg	Advocated only for high risk - bleeding ulcer, gastric cancer, gastric by-pass and percutaneous endoscopic gastrostomy. Prophylactic antibiotics are not indicated for uncomplicated duodenal ulcer surgery.

(continued)

98

Type of Surgery	Preferred regimen	Alternative	Comment
Biliary tract	Cefazolin 1-2 gm IV pre-op	Ampicillin 1 gm IV ± Gentamicin 1.7 mg/kg pre-op and q8h x 3	Advocated only for high risk - acute cholecystitis, obstructive jaundice, common duct stones, age over 70 yrs.
Colorectal and small bowel	Neomycin 1 gm po and erythromycin 1 gm po at 1 pm, 2 pm and 11 pm the day before surgery (19,18 and 11 hrs pre-op)	Cefoxitin 2 gm IV or Clindamycin 600-900 mg IV plus gentamicin 1.7 mg/kg IV or Metronidazole 1 gm IV plus gentamicin 1.7 mg/kg IV	Some advocate the combined use of an oral and parenteral prep, especially for low anterior resection. Some advocate 3 subsequent doses of parenteral agents at 8 hr intervals. Oral prep with metronidazole + neomycin or kanamycin are probably as effective as erythromycin + neomycin (RID 13, Suppl 10:S815, 1991).
Penetrating trauma abdomen	Cefoxitin 2 gm IV pre-op or Clindamycin 600 mg IV plus gentamicin 1.7 mg/kg pre-op	Antipseudomonad penicillin, ticarcillin-clavulanate or any combination of an amino-glycoside + metronidazole or clindamycin	Patients with intestinal perforation should receive these agents for 2-5 days. Most studies use suboptimal doses of aminoglycosides (RID 13, Suppl 10:S847, 1991).
Appendectomy	Cefoxitin 2 gm IV pre-op (and 1-5 days post-op - see comments)	Metronidazole 1 gm IV or clindamycin 600-900 mg IV plus gentamicin 1.7 mg/kg	For perforated or gangrenous appendix continue regimen for 3-5 days. For non-perforated appendix 1-4 doses are adequate (RID 13, Suppl 10:S813, 1991).
Laparotomy, lysis of adhesions, splenectomy, etc. without GI tract surgery	None		
GYNECOLOGY AND OBSTETRICS			
Vaginal and abdominal hysterectomy	Cefazolin 1-2 gm IV pre-op (and q6h x 2)	Doxycycline 200 mg IV or doxycycline 100 mg po hs 3-4 hr pre-op	Single dose appears to be as effective as multiple doses. Recommendation for radical hysterectomy is cefazolin 1-2 gm pre-op (RID 13, Suppl 10:S821, 1991).
Cesarean section	Cefazolin 2 gm or ampicillin 2 gm IV after clamping cord (and q6h x2)*	Cefotetan 2 gm IV after clamping cord	Advocated primarily for high risk - active labor, premature rupture of membranes, but low risk patients may also benefit (RID 13, Suppl 10:S821, 1991). (continued)

Type of Surgery	Preferred regimen	Alternative	Comment
Abortion	Doxycycline 200 mg po before and 100 mg po 12 hrs later	Doxycycline 300-400 mg po Metronidazole 400 mg x 3 doses in perioperative period period	For patients with N. gonorrhoeae or C. trachomatis, treat STD with minimum delay in abortion (Am J Ob Gyn 150:689, 1984 1984).
Hysterosalpingography	Doxycycline 200 mg po pre-procedure		(RID 13, Suppl 10:S845, 1991)
Placement of IUD	Doxycycline 200 mg po pre-procedure		(Brit J Ob Gyn 97:412, 1990)
Cervical cerclage	Cefazolin 2 gm IV pre-procedure		(Am J Ob Gyn 141:1065, 1981)
Cystocele or rectocele repair	None		
Tubal ligation	None		
HEAD AND NECK Tonsillectomy ± adenoidectomy	None		Controlled studies are limited.
Rhinoplasty	None		
Major surgery with entry via oral cavity or pharynx	Clindamycin 900 mg IV ± gentamicin 1.7 mg/kg IV pre-op and q6h x 1-2	Cefazolin 2 gm IV pre-op	Clindamycin study (J Otolaryng 19:197, 1990) Controlled study shows cefazolin dose of 2 gm superior to 0.5 gm (Ann Surg 207:108,1988).
ORTHOPEDIC SURGERY Joint replacement	Cefazolin 1-2 gm IV pre-op (± 1 gm q6h x 3 doses)*	Vancomycin** 1 gm IV Cefamandole is as effective as cefazolin	Cefazolin dose should be 2 gm for knee replacement with tourniquet (Orthop Rev 18:694, 1989). Antibiotic-impregnated cement appears to be effective (Int Orthop 11:241, 1987).

(continued)

Type of Surgery	Preferred regimen	Alternative	Comment
Open reduction of fracture/internal fixation	Cefazolin 1 gm IV (± 1 gm q6h x 3 doses)*	Vancomycin 1 gm IV q12h Clindamycin 900 mg IV q8h	Nafcillin or cephalothin x 48-72 hr appears effective for preventing post-op wound infections in closed hip fractures (J Bone Joint Surg 62:A-457, 1980).
Compound fracture	Cefazolin 1-2 gm IV q8h x 5-10 days or Nafcillin 1-2 gm q4h		Start treatment immediately and continue 5-10 days.
Amputation of leg	Cefoxitin 1-2 gm IV within 1 hr (± 2 gm q6h x 48h)*	Cefazolin 1-2 gm IV (± 1 gm q6h x 48h)*	(J Bone & Joint Surg 67:800, 1985)
NEUROSURGERY			
Cerebrospinal fluid shunt	Trimethoprim 160 mg plus sulfamethoxazole 800 mg IV pre-op and q12 h x 3 doses	Nafcillin or oxacillin ± rifampin x 1-2 days	Efficacy of antimicrobials not established (Ped Neurosci 15:111, 1989; RID 13, Suppl 10:S858, 1991)
Craniotomy	Vancomycin 1 gm IV ± gentamicin 1.5 mg/kg x 1	Clindamycin 300 mg IV and at 4 hr; cefazolin 1.5 gm plus gentamicin 1.5 mg/kg x 1; cefotaxime 2 gm x 2 repeated at 6 hr	Efficacy not clearly established, but advocated even for low risk procedures except where infection rates are <0.1% (Neurosurg 24:401, 1989)
Spinal surgery	None		
Ocular	Gentamicin or tobramycin topically for 2-24 hrs before surgery	Neomycin, gramicidin and polymyxin B topically 2-24 hrs pre-op	Some give subconjunctival injection (gentamicin, 10-20 mg ± cefazolin 100 mg) at end of surgery.
UROLOGY			
Prostatectomy Sterile urine	None (see Comment)		Cefazolin sometimes advocated for open prostatectomy (Urol Clin N Amer 17:595, 1990).
Infected urine	Continue agent active in vitro or give single pre-operative dose		Sterilization of urine before surgery is preferred.

(continued)

101

Type of Surgery	Preferred regimen	Alternative	Comment
Prostatic biopsy	None		
Dilation of urethra	None		
MISCELLANEOUS			
Inguinal hernia repair	Cefazolin 1gm IV pre-op (see Comment)		One study showed benefit of cefonicid, 1 gm IV 30 min. pre-op (R. Platt et al. NEJM 322:153,1990); sequel study showed diverse antibiotics (primarily cefazolin) in high risk patients was beneficial (R. Platt et al, JID 166:556, 1992).
Mastectomy	Cefazolin 1 gm IV pre-op (see Comment)		One study showed benefit of cefonicid for breast surgery (R. Platt et al. NEJM 322: 153,1990); sequel study (see above). Greatest risks were radical mastectomy and axillary node dissection.
Traumatic wound	Cefazolin 1 gm IV q8h		

* Single dose generally considered adequate; for dirty surgery, treatment should be continued 5-10 days.

** Vancomycin preferred for hospitals with a high rate of wound infections caused by methicillin-resistant S. aureus or S. epidermidis. and for patients with allergy to penicillins or cephalosporins.

102

PREVENTION OF BACTERIAL ENDOCARDITIS
Recommendations by the American Heart Association
(JAMA 264:2919,1990)

CARDIAC CONDITIONS

Cardiac conditions considered at risk (not all inclusive)
- Prosthetic cardiac valve, including bioprosthetic and homograph valves
- Prior endocarditis
- Most congenital malformations
- Rheumatic and other acquired valvular dysfunction
- Hypertrophic cardiomyopathy
- Mitral valve prolapse with valve regurgitation (Patients with mitral valve prolapse associated with thickening and/or redundancy of the valve may be at increased risk, esp. men $\geq$ 45 yrs.)

Prophylaxis not recommended
- Isolated secundum atrial septal defect
- Surgical repair without residual > 6 months of secundum atrial defect, ventricular septal defect or patent ductus
- Prior coronary by-pass surgery
- Mitral valve defect without regurgitation (see above)
- Physiologic or functional heart murmurs
- Prior rheumatic fever without valve disease
- Cardiac pacemakers and implanted defibrillators
- Prior Kawasaki disease without valve dysfunction

PROCEDURES

Procedures that confer risk and require prophylaxis
- Dental procedures that induce gingival or mucosal bleeding including professional cleansing
- Tonsillectomy and adenoidectomy
- Surgical procedures that involve the intestinal or respiratory mucosa
- Bronchoscopy with a rigid bronchoscope
- Sclerotherapy for esophageal varicies
- Esophageal dilatation
- Gallbladder surgery
- Cystoscopy
- Urethral dilatation
- Urethral catheterization with urinary tract infection (include treatment for likely urinary pathogen)
- Urinary tract surgery if urinary tract infection (include treatment for likely urinary pathogen)
- Prostatic surgery
- Incision and drainage of infected tissue (include treatment for likely pathogen)
- Vaginal hysterectomy
- Vaginal delivery in presence of infection (include treatment for likely pathogens)

103

<u>Endocarditis prophylaxis not recommended*</u>

    Dental procedures not likely to cause bleeding such as adjustment of
        orthodontic appliances or fillings above the gum line

    Injection of local intraoral anesthetic except intraligamentary injections

    Shedding primary teeth

    Tympanostomy tube insertion

    Bronchoscopy with flexible bronchoscopy with or without biopsy

    Endoscopy of GI tract with or without biopsy

    Cardiac catheterization

    Cesarean section

    Absence of infection for urethral catheterization, dilatation and curettage,
        uncomplicated vaginal delivery, therapeutic abortion, sterilization
        procedures or insertion or removal of intrauterine device

*   Patients at high risk may receive prophylactic antibiotics even for low risk
procedures involving the lower respiratory, genitourinary or gastrointestinal
tracts; these include patients with prosthetic valves, a history of endocarditis or surgically constucted systemic - pulmonary shunts or conduits.

RECOMMENDED REGIMENS

<u>Recommended regimens for dental, oral and upper respiratory procedures</u>

<u>Standard</u>
    Amoxicillin: 3.0 gm orally 1 hr pre-procedure; then 1.5 gm 6 hr after first
    dose

<u>Amoxicillin or penicillin allergy</u>
    Erythromycin: Erythromycin ethylsuccinate, 800 mg or erythromycin
    stearate, 1 gm po 2 hr pre-procedure; then 1/2 initial dose 6 hr later
    Clindamycin: 300 mg orally 1 hr pre-procedure; 150 mg 6 hr later

<u>Unable to take oral medications</u>
    Ampicillin: 2.0 gm IM or IV 30 min pre-procedure; 1.0 gm ampicillin IM or
    IV or 1.5 gm amoxicillin orally 6 hr later

<u>Amoxicillin or penicillin allergy and unable to take oral meds</u>
    Clindamycin: 300 mg IV 30 min pre-procedure; then 150 mg IV or po 6 hr
    later

<u>Patient considered high risk* and not a candidate for standard regimen</u>
    Ampicillin: 2 gm IV <u>plus</u> gentamicin, 1.5 mg/kg 30 min pre-procedure; 1.5 gm
    amoxicillin po 6 hr later <u>or</u> repeat parenteral regimen 8 hr later

<u>Amoxicillin or penicillin allergy in patient considered high risk*</u>
    Vancomycin: 1 gm IV over 1 hr starting 1 hr pre-procedure; no repeat dose

Regimens for genitourinary and gastrointestinal procedures

Standard
Ampicillin, 2 gm IV or IM plus gentamicin, 1.5 mg/kg (not to exceed 80 mg) 30 min pre-procedure; amoxicillin, 1.5 gm po 6 hr later or repeat parenteral regimen 8 hr later

Ampicillin or penicillin allergy
Vancomycin, 1 gm IV over 1 hr plus gentamicin, 1.5 mg/kg IV or IM 1 hr pre-procedure; may be repeated once 8 hr later

Alternate low risk patient* regimen
Amoxicillin, 3.0 gm po 1 hr pre-procedure; 1.5 gm 6 hr later

* High risk: Prosthetic valve, history of endocarditis or surgically constructed systemic - pulmonary shunts or conduits

PROPHYLAXIS FOR DENTAL PATIENTS WITH PROSTHETIC JOINTS

1. Analysis by Gillespie showed no evidence of benefit (Infect Dis Clin N Amer 4:465, 1990).

2. Position statement of the American Academy of Oral Medicine (Oral Surg, Oral Med, Oral Path 66:430, 1988):

> It is the opinion of the American Academy of Oral Medicine that there is insufficient scientific evidence to support routine antibiotic prophylaxis for patients with prosthetic joints who are receiving dental care. Therefore it appears that a blanket recommendation for antibiotic coverage would be inappropriate at this time. This decision should be determined by the dentist's clinical judgment or in consultation with the patient's surgeon.

3. Position of C.W. Norden (RID 13, S10, S845, 1991): Antibiotic prophylaxis is not recommended for routine dental work. Antibiotic prophylaxis is recommended for such individuals with periodontal or potential dental infections using an oral cephalosporin or clindamycin 1 hr before dental work and two subsequent doses.

PREVENTION OF DISEASES ASSOCIATED WITH TRAVEL

A.   INTERNATIONAL TRAVELER'S HOTLINE

CDC 24 hr/day automated telephone system with advice for international travelers concerning malaria, food and water precautions, traveler's diarrhea, immunizations for children < 2 years, pregnant travelers disease outbreaks and vaccine requirements by geographic area. Call (404) 639-1610. Health Information for International Travel 1990 edition is available at $5.00/copy from Superintendent of Documents, U.S. Government Printing Office, Washington, D.C. 20402, (202) 783-3238, stock no. 017-023-00187-6.

B.   TRAVELER'S DIARRHEA (Adapted from NIH Consensus Development Panel, 1985. See JAMA 253:2700,1985; and Medical Letter 34:41-44,1992)

Risk: High risk areas (incidence 20-50%): developing countries of Latin America, Africa, Middle East and Asia

Intermediate risk: Southern Europe and some Caribbean islands

Low risk: Canada, Northern Europe, Australia, New Zealand, United States

Agents

Bacteria	Viruses
E. coli (enterotoxigenic,* enteroinvasive, enteroadherent)	Norwalk agent Rotavirus (?)
Salmonella	
Shigella	Parasites
Campylobacter jejuni	Giardia lamblia
Aeromonas hydrophila	Entamoeba histolytica
Plesiomonas shigelloides	Cryptosporidia
Vibrio cholerae (non-01)	
Vibrio fluvialis	
Vibrio parahaemolytica	

* Most common

Prevention

Food and beverages: Risky foods - Raw vegetables, raw meat or raw seafood, tapwater, ice, unpasteurized milk and dairy products and unpeeled fruit; safe foods -- cooked foods that are still hot, fruits peeled by traveler, carbonated bottled water and other beverages.

Preventative agents with documented efficacy (efficacy of 50-85%)

Doxycycline: 100 mg po/day (photosensitivity reactions)

Sulfa-trimethoprim: 1 DS (double strength) tab po/day (serious skin reactions and hematological reactions reported).

Trimethoprim: 200 mg po/day

Ciprofloxacin: 500 mg po/day

Norfloxacin: 400 mg po/day

Bismuth subsalicylate (Pepto-Bismol): 2 300 mg tabs qid

Treatment

Oral intake to maintain fluid and electrolyte balance:
Potable fruit juice, caffeine-free soft drinks, salted crackers.
For severe symptoms: WHO Oral Rehydration Salts may be formulated
by - Ingredients/L or qt. water
NaCl: 3.5 gm (3/4 tsp)
NaHCO$_3$ (baking soda): 2.5 gm (1 tsp)
KCl: 1.5 g (1 cup orange juice or 2 bananas)
Sucrose (table sugar): 40 gm (4 level tbsp)
*May be ordered from: Jianas Bros, 2533 S.W. Blvd, Kansas City,
MO; phone (816) 412-2880, fax (816) 421-2883*
Antimotility drugs
Diphenoxylate (Lomotil) (2.5 mg tabs po 3-4 x daily)
Loperamide (Imodium) (4 mg, then 2 mg after each loose stool to
maximum of 16 mg/day)
Bismuth subsalicylate (Pepto-Bismol) (30 ml or 2 tabs q 30 min x 8)
Antimicrobial agents (empiric selection)
Sulfa-trimethoprim: 1 DS tab bid x 5 days or 2 DS x 1
Trimethoprim: 200 mg po bid x 5 days
Doxycycline: 100 mg po bid x 5 days
Ciprofloxacin: 500 mg po bid x 5 days
Norfloxacin: 400 mg po bid x 5 days
Combination: Sulfa-trimethoprim, 1 DS bid x 3 days plus Loperamide
(above dose), appears more effective than either drug alone
(JAMA 263:257,1990)

Panel Recommendations

1. Prophylactic drugs are not recommended (but prophylactic anti-
    microbial agents appear most cost-effective; see Reves RR et al:
    Arch Intern Med 148:2421,1988).

2. Travelers to risk areas should carry antimotility drugs (diphen-
    oxylate or loperamide) or bismuth subsalicylate and an antimicrobial
    agent (sulfa-trimethoprim, trimethoprim, doxycycline or fluroquinolone).
    a. Mild diarrhea (less than 3 stools/day, without blood, pus or
        fever): Loperamide, diphenoxylate or bismuth subsalicylate in
        doses noted above.
    b. Moderate or severe diarrhea: Antimicrobial agent (regimens
        noted above -- but some feel these are antiquated).
        *Note: Medical Letter Consultants (34:41, 1992) recommends combined
        treatment for symptomatic adults using Imodium plus TMP-SMX 1
        DS bid, ciprofloxacin 500 mg bid, norfloxacin 400 mg bid or
        olfloxacin 300 mg bid for up to 3 days.*
        Many underdeveloped countries now have high rates of resistance among
        Enterotoxigenic E. coli, Shigella and other enteric bacterial pathogens. This
        accounts for the preference for fluoroquinolones for travel to many
        countries; TMP-SMX should still be appropriate for Mexico. Children
        <18 yrs should not take fluoroquinolones; furazolidine is a possible
        substitute.
    c. Persistent diarrhea with serious fluid loss, fever or stools
        showing blood or mucus: Seek medical attention.

3. Instruct patients regarding:
   Dietary precautions for prevention
   Oral rehydration
   Use of drugs including side effects

<u>Cholera epidemic</u>: South and Central America (see JAMA 267:1495, 1992)

The cholera epidemic has involved primarily Peru (297,000 cases in 1991), Ecuador (42,000), Columbia (11,000), Guatemala (2,900), Mexico (2,400), Panama (1,000), El Salvador (900) and Brazil (600). Travelers should be warned to a) avoid raw or partially cooked seafood, b) drink only boiled or bottled, carbonated water, c) avoid food or drinks from street vendors and d) avoid uncooked vegetables. Cholera vaccine is marginally effective and is not recommended. There are no cholera vaccine requirements with entry or exit into Peru, Equador or the U.S. Call the traveler's hotline for updated review: (404) 332-4559.

C. **IMMUNIZATIONS:** See pages 87-88

D. **MALARIA PROPHYLAXIS AND TREATMENT (MMWR 39:1-10,1990, 40:727, 1991) and The Medical Letter on Drugs and Therapeutics 31:13,1990)**

Centers for Disease Control Malaria Hotline: (404) 332-4555

Risk areas: Most areas of Central and South America, Hispaniola, sub-Saharan Africa, the Indian Subcontinent, Southeast Asia, the Middle East and Oceania. During 1980-1990 there were 2,109 cases of P. falciparum in U.S. civilians: 1,721 (82%) acquired in sub-Saharan Africa; 162 (8%) in Asia; 111 (5%) in the Caribbean and South America, and 115 (5%) in other areas. All 43 cases of fatal infections were acquired in Africa south of the Sahara.

Drug resistance of P. falciparum to chloroquine (CRFP) is probable or confirmed in all countries with P. falciparum except Central America -- west of the Panama Canal Zone, Mexico, Haiti, the Dominican Republic, and most of the Middle East. Resistance to both chloroquine and Fansidar is widespread in Thailand, Burma, Cambodia and the Amazon basin area of South America, and has been reported in sub-Saharan Africa.

Advice to travelers
1. Personal protection:
   Transmission is most common between dusk and dawn.
   Precautions include remaining in well-screened areas and using mosquito nets, clothing that covers most of the body, insect repellent containing DEET on exposed areas, and pyrethrum-containing insect spray for environs and clothing.
2. Chemoprophylaxis (see Table 1 for doses)
   a. Travel to areas with no chloroquine-resistant P. falciparum:
      Chloroquine beginning 1-2 weeks before travel and 4 weeks after leaving risk area.
      Alternative: Hydroxychloroquine (for persons who do not tolerate chloroquine).

b.   Travel to areas with chloroquine-resistant P. falciparum:
        Mefloquine, 250 mg as a single dose taken weekly beginning one week
        before travel; prophylaxis is continued weekly during travel in malarious
        areas and for four weeks after leaving such areas.
        Alternatives: Doxycycline beginning 1-2 days before travel
            and for 4 weeks after leaving risk area. Chloroquine advocated for
            persons with contraindication to mefloquine and doxycycline,
            especially pregnant females and children. If chloroquine is
            used, the traveler should take a single dose (Table 2) of
            Fansidar to take for prompt use with a febrile illness if
            professional medical care is not available.
c.   Contraindications to mefloquine: pregnant women and travelers with a
        history of epilepsy or psychiatric disorders; rare serious side effects are
        psychosis and seizures.
3.   Primaquine: This drug may be given after the traveler has left the
        risk area to prevent relapses due to P. vivax and P. ovale.
        Primaquine prophylaxis is usually given during the last 2 weeks
        of the 4 week period of prophylaxis after exposure. Indications are
        not clear, but best advised when the traveler has prolonged
        exposure, such as missionaries and Peace Corp volunteers. (Primaquine is now
        available from Winthrop Pharmaceuticals and is no longer available from the
        CDC).

Distribution of Malaria and Chloroquine-resistant *Plasmodium falciparum*, 1991

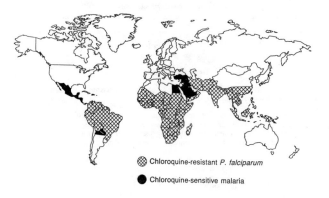

⊗ Chloroquine-resistant *P. falciparum*

● Chloroquine-sensitive malaria

Health Information for International Travel 1992; US Department of Health and Human
Services, June 1992, pg 99.

Doses of antimalarial agents for treatment and prophylaxis

TABLE 1. Drugs used in the prophylaxis of malaria

Drug	Adult dose
Chloroquine phosphate* (Aralen)	300 mg base (500 mg salt) orally, once/week *(Travelers to Africa should also take Proguanil and should carry Fansidar (3 tabs) for empiric treatment of a febrile illness if professional medical care is not available.)*
Hydroxychloroquine sulfate (Plaquenil)	310 mg base (400 mg salt) orally, once/week
Mefloquine (Lariam)	228 mg base (250 mg salt) orally, once/week
Doxycycline*	100 mg orally, once/day
Proguanil	200 mg orally, once/day in combination with weekly chloroquine (not available in U.S.; obtain in Canada, Europe and many African countries)
Primaquine	15 mg base (26.3 mg salt) orally, once/day for 14 days

*   Alternatives to Mefloquine for travel to countries where drug resistant P. falciparum is endemic

TABLE 2. Drug used in the presumptive treatment of malaria

Drug	Adult dose
Pyrimethamine-sulfadoxine (Fansidar*)	3 tablets (75 mg pyrimethamine and 1500 mg sulfadoxine), orally as a single dose

Treatment of Malaria

(See pages 137-138) revised guidelines for quinidine gluconate for severe P. falciparum infection (MMWR 40 RR-4:21, 1991).

1.   Quinidine gluconate has replaced quinine dihydrochloride as the preferred agent for parenteral treatment of severe infections caused by P. falciparum.

2.   Indications for parenteral treatment: a) prominent vomiting, b) signs or symptoms of neurologic dysfunction, or c) peripheral asexual parasitemia (parasite index) of ≥5% of red blood cells.

3.   Administration: loading dose of 10 mg (6.2 mg quinidine base)/kg given over 1-2 hrs; then constant infusion with 0.02 mg/kg/min (quinidine gluconate).

4.   Monitor in ICU with attention to hydration, blood glucose, EKGs and quinidine levels. Slow infusion if levels >6 mcg/mL, QT >0.6 sec or QRS widened to >25% of baseline.

5.   Continue IV treatment until parasitic index is <1% and/or oral meds tolerated. Treatment is continued (oral plus parenteral) for 3-7 days; additional tetracycline (250 mg po q 6h x 7 days) is recommended.

TREATMENT OF FUNGAL SYSTEMIC INFECTIONS

Adapted from NIAID Mycosis Study Group Reports (Ann Intern Med 98:13,1983; Ann Intern Med 103:861,1985; Chest 93:848,1987), recommendations of the American Thoracic Society (Amer Rev Respir Dis 138:1078,1988), consultants of the Medical Letter 32:58,1990, and Mayo Clin Proc 67:69, 1992

Fungus	Form	Preferred Treatment	Dose, alternative agent(s), comment
Aspergillus	Bronchopulmonary	Corticosteroids	
	Aspergilloma (fungus ball)	Usually none	Massive hemoptysis - surgical resection with perioperative amphotericin. Progressive invasive disease - amphotericin B IV, 30-40 mg/kg
	Invasive pulmonary or extrapulmonary	Amphotericin B IV	Total dose: 30-40 mg/kg Most patients require rapid advance in daily dose to 0.5-1.0 mg/kg; for neutropenic patients the usual dose is 1.0-1.5 mg/kg Flucytosine or rifampin sometimes added, but efficacy is not established Itraconazole appears promising: 100-400 mg/day
Blastomyces	Acute pulmonary (immunocompetent)	Usually none	
	Acute pulmonary - severe or progressive	Itraconazole po Ketoconazole po	200-400 mg/day 400 mg/day, with unfavorable clinical response - increase to 600-800 mg/day Alternative: Amphotericin B IV, 30-40 mg/kg
	Chronic pulmonary	Itraconazole po Ketoconazole po	200-400 mg/day 400 mg/day, up to 600-800 mg/day
	Disseminated (immunocompetent without renal or CNS involvement)	Itraconazole po Ketoconazole po	200-400 mg/day 400 mg/day, up to 600-800 mg/day
	Disseminated with GU involvement	Itraconazole po Ketoconazole po	200-400 mg/day 600-800 mg/day Alternative: Amphotericin B IV, 30-40 mg/kg (continued)

111

Fungus	Form	Preferred Treatment	Dose, alternative agent(s), comment
Blastomyces (continued)	Disseminated Immunosuppressed or CNS involvement	Amphotericin B IV Itraconazole po	Total dose: 30-40 mg/kg 200-400 mg/day
Candida	Localized - mucocutaneous		
	Oral (thrush)	Nystatin S&S Clotrimazole troche Ketoconazole po Fluconazole po	500,000 units 3-5x/day x 10-14 days 10 mg troches 3-5x/day x 10-14 days 200 mg po bid, 5-7 days 200 mg, then 100 mg/day (50 mg/day is also effective) AIDS: Continue any of above regimens indefinitely or use prn
	Vaginal	Miconazole topical Nystatin topical Clotrimazole topical Ketoconazole po Fluconazole po Itraconazole po	Intravaginal cream (2%) or suppository (100 mg) qd x 7 days Intravaginal cream or tablet (100,000 units) bid x 7 days Intravaginal cream (1%) or tablet (100 mg) qd x 7 days (available without prescription) 200 mg po bid x 5-7 days 150 mg po x 1 400 mg po, 200 mg/day x 2 days
	Cutaneous - intertrigo balanitis, paronychia	Nystatin, ciclopirox, clotrimazole, miconazole,	Topical treatment, keep area dry and clean with maximal exposure to air
	Chronic mucocutaneous	Ketoconazole po	200 mg po bid x 3-12 months Alternative: Intermittent amphotericin B ± topical anti-Candida agent or fluconazole
	Esophageal	Fluconazole	100 mg po qd (up to 400 mg/day) x > 3wks (and >2 wks post-resolution of symptoms) Alternative: Amphotericin B (0.2-0.4 mg/kg/day) x 7-14 days or ketoconazole, 200 mg po bid x 10-21 days AIDS: Maintenance fluconazole 100-200 mg po qd (continued)

Fungus	Form	Preferred Treatment	Dose, alternative agent(s), comment
Candida (continued)	Peritoneal (peritoneal dialysis)	Amphotericin B topical or IV ± flucytosine	Topical treatment: 2-4 ug/L in dialysate fluid Flucytosine: 50-100 mg/L dialysate fluid Catheter may require removal
	Peritoneal - (post op, perforated viscus, etc)	Amphotericin B IV	Total dose: 3-10 mg/kg (Indications to treat are often unclear)
		Fluconazole	200-400 mg/day
	Urinary	No treatment or amphotericin B topically	Remove catheter or use for bladder instillations of amphotericin B: 50 mg/L in D5W and infuse 1 L/day via closed triple lumen catheter x 5 days Alternative: Flucytosine: 25/mg/kg po qid or fluconazole: 200 mg po/day Fungus ball: Surgical removal and amphotericin B IV
	Bloodstream Septicemia	Amphotericin B IV	Total dose: 3-10 mg/kg Remove or change IV lines Line sepsis: Remove line and treat with amphotericin B (≥3 mg/kg) ± flucytosine
		Fluconazole	400 mg, then 200 mg/day
	Disseminated or metastatic (deep organ infection)	Amphotericin B IV ± flucytosine po	Total dose: 20-40 mg/kg (0.3-0.8 mg/kg/day) 150 mg/kg/day (flucytosine) Indications for flucytosine: Normal marrow and renal function or clinical deterioration with amphotericin B Alternative: Fluconazole: 200-400 mg/day (best results with peritonitis, UTI, and hepatosplenic abscesses for patients who refuse or cannot tolerate amphotericin B)

(continued)

Fungus	Form	Preferred Treatment	Dose, alternative agent(s), comment
Candida (*continued*)	Endocarditis	Amphotericin B IV ± flucytosine po	Total dose: 30-40 mg/kg 150 mg/kg/day (flucytosine) Surgery required
Chromoblastomycosis		Flucytosine po	100 mg/kg/day x 8-12 wks Alternatives: Ketoconazole po 400 mg/day x 3-6 mo, thiabendazole, intra-lesional amphotericin B or combination of flucytosine and one of these; itraconazole promising, 100-200 mg/day Small lesions usually respond to flucytosine; large lesions should be surgically excised with perioperative flucytosine
Coccidioides	Pulmonary - acute	Usually none	
	Pulmonary - severe, cavitary or progressive infiltrate	Ketoconazole po Amphotericin B IV Itraconazole po	400-600 mg/day x 6-18 mo. 7-20 mg/kg (amphotericin) 400 mg/day x 6-18 mo Fluconazole: Preliminary experience with 200 mg/day is promising
	Pulmonary cavitary disease - giant cavities (>5 cm), sub-pleural location, serious hemoptysis and secondary infection	Surgical excision	Perioperative amphotericin B often advocated (500 mg)
	Disseminated (non-meningeal, immunocompetent)	Amphotericin B IV	Total dose: 30-40 mg/kg (amphotericin) Alternative is ketoconazole in dose of 400-800 mg/day x 6-18 mo. or longer, but response rates are low, relapse rates in responders is high *Note: Itraconazole: Preliminary results with 400 mg/day x 12 mo are promising* (Lancet 340:648, 1992).
	Disseminated - immuno-suppressed non-meningeal	Amphotericin B IV	Total dose: 30-40 mg/kg Fluconazole: Preliminary results with 400 mg/day are promising. Itraconazole: 400 mg/day is promising

(continued)

Fungus	Form	Preferred Treatment	Dose, alternative agent(s), comment
Coccidioides (*continued*)	Meningitis	Amphotericin B IV and topically	Total dose: 30-40 mg/kg IV Intrathecal: 0.5-0.7 mg 2x/wk Alternative: Miconazole or ketoconazole (1200-2400 mg/day) ± intrathecal Amphotericin B
Cryptococcus	Pulmonary - stable and immunocompetent	Usually none	Exclude extrapulmonary disease: culture blood, urine and CSF; follow x-rays q 1-2 mo. x 1 yr
	Pulmonary - progressive and/or immunosuppressed host	Amphotericin B IV ± flucytosine	Total dose: 15-20 mg/kg (amphotericin) Alternative for immunocompetent host with progressive pulmonary or extrapulmonary non-meningeal is ketoconazole 200-800 mg po/day
	Extrapulmonary non-meningeal	Amphotericin B ± flucytosine	Total dose: 2-3 gm (amphotericin B) Alternative for immunocompetent patient is ketoconazole 400 mg/day or fluconazole 200 mg/day (up to 400 mg/day) or itraconazole 400 mg/day
	Disseminated including meningeal without AIDS	Amphotericin B ± flucytosine	Standard: Amphotericin (0.3 mg/kg/day) + flucytosine (150 mg/kg/day) x 6 weeks Four week regimen: Immunocompetent host without neurologic complications, pretreatment CSF WBC > 20/mm3 + Ag < 1:32; and post-therapy CSF Ag < 1:8 + neg India ink
	Meningitis AIDS patients	Amphotericin B, 0.5-0.7 mg/kg/day ± flucytosine, (100 mg/kg/day) until 15 mg/kg Amphotericin B + neg CSF culture. Amphotericin B (0.7 mg/kg/day) x 10-14 days, then fluconazole (400 mg/day po) x 8-10 wks, then fluconazole (200 mg/day)	Fluconazole 200-400 mg/day (considered safe for initial treatment only if mental status is normal) Maintenance treatment with fluconazole (200 mg/day) required for all patients. Maintenance dose of amphotericin B (for fluconazole failures) is 1 mg/kg/wk or itraconazole 200-400 mg/day

(continued)

Fungus	Form	Preferred Treatment	Dose, alternative agent(s), comment
Histoplasma	Pulmonary - acute ± erythema nosodum	Usually none	Severe/acute: Some recommend amphotericin B (500 mg over 2-3 wks) + corticosteroids or ketoconazole (400 mg/day) x 6 mo.
	Pulmonary - chronic	Itraconazole po Ketoconazole po	200-400 mg/day x 6-12 mo. 400 mg/day x 6-12 mo. (up to 800 mg/day) Amphotericin B (30-40 mg/kg) for patients who are seriously ill, or immunosuppressed (AIDS patients) or fail ketoconazole
	Pulmonary - cavitary Stable, minimal Sx, thin wall cavity	None	
	Persistent, thick walled cavity (>2 mm) or progressive sx	Itraconazole po Ketoconazole po	200-400 mg/day x 6-12 mo. 400 mg/day x 6-12 mo. (up to 800 mg/day) Alternative: Amphotericin B IV, 30-40 mg/kg Surgery for intractable hemoptysis despite medical Rx
	Disseminated - immuno-competent, without CNS involvement	Itraconazole po Ketoconazole po	200-400 mg/day x 6-12 mo. 400 mg/day x 6-12 mo. (up to 800 mg/day) Patients with severe illness, AIDS or immunosuppression should receive amphotericin B
	Disseminated - CNS involvement or immunosuppressed	Amphotericin B IV	Total dose: 30-40 mg/kg AIDS: Amphotericin in dose of 0.5-1.0 gm, then maintenance itraconazole po 400 mg/day or amphotericin B IV 1.0-1.5 mg/kg/wk
	Mediastinal granuloma or fibrosis	Surgical resection if symptomatic	Invasive disease into airways, esophagus, etc (rare): Treat with ketoconazole, itraconazole or amphotericin B
	Ocular	Laser photocoagulation Intraocular steroids Retinal irradiation	Appears to be immune-mediated disease

(continued)

116

Fungus	Form	Preferred Treatment	Dose, alternative agent(s), comment
Paracoccidioides	Pulmonary or mucocutaneous	Ketoconazole po Itraconazole po	200-400 mg/day x 6-12 mo. 100 mg/day x 6 mo. Alternative: Amphotericin B IV, 30-35 mg/kg (preferred for severe disease) or sulfonamides;
Phycomycetes Absidia Mucor (Mucormycosis) Rhizopus	Pulmonary and extrapulmonary including rhinocerebral	Amphotericin B IV	Total dose: 30-40 mg/kg Most patients require rapid increase to daily dose of 0.5-1.0 mg/kg Rhinocerebral: Surgical debridement required
Pseudoallescheria boydii	Sinusitis, endophthalmitis	Ketoconazole po or miconazole IV	200-600 mg/day x 1-12 mo. 200-1200 mg q8h
Sporothrix (Sporotrichosis)	Lymphocutaneous	SSKI po Heat	1 ml (1 gm/ml) tid increasing to 12-15 ml/day x 6-8 wks Alternative: Ketoconazole, 400-800 mg/day or fluconazole, 400 mg/day or itraconazole, 100 mg/day
	Extracutaneous	Amphotericin B IV	Total dose: 30-35 mg/kg (0.5 mg/kg/day) Alternative: Ketoconazole, 400-800 mg/day or fluconazole, 400 mg/day or itraconazole, 100 mg/day

TREATMENT OF DERMATOPHYTIC FUNGAL INFECTIONS

Condition	Agents	Location	Treatment
Tinea corporis (Ringworm)	T. rubrum T. mentagrophytes M. canis E. floccosum	Circular, erythema well demarcated with scaly, vesicular or pustular border Non-hairy skin Pruritic	Topical agents: Miconazole, clotrimazole, econazole, naftifine, ciclopirox bid or ketoconazole, oxiconazole, sulconazole qd for ≥ 4 wks. If no response: griseofulvin x 4 wks
Tinea cruris (Jock itch)	E. floccosum T. rubrum T. mentagrophytes	Erythema and scaly Groin and upper thighs Pruritic	Topical agents as above. Loose fitting clothes. Absorbant powder. Unresponsive cases: griseofulvin x 2-4 wks
Tinea pedis (Athlete's foot)	T. rubrum T. mentagrophytes E. floccosum	Foot, esp fissures between toes; scaly, vesicles, pustules ± nail involvement	Topical agents as above. Keep feet dry and cool. Unresponsive cases: griseofulvin 6-8 wks. Nail involvement: oral griseofulvin or ketoconazole 6-24 mo (until new nail) or itraconazole (100 mg/day) x 3-6 mo.
Tinea capitis (Ringworm -- scalp	T. tonsurans T. mentagrophytes T. verrucosum M. canis	Scaling and erythematous area on scalp with broken hairs and localized alopecia	Griseofulvin x 4-8 wks + 2.5% selenium sulfide shampoo 2x/wk. Alternative to griseofulvin is ketoconazole
Tinea versicolor	Malassezia furfur	Scaling oval macular and patchy lesions on upper trunk and arms; dark or light, fail to tan	Topical 2.5% selenium sulfide applied as thin layer over entire body x 1-2 hrs or overnight for 1-2 wks, then wash off. Alternatives: Topical clotrimazole, econazole, ketoconazole, naftifine or haloprogin or oral ketoconazole

TREATMENT OF VIRAL INFECTIONS

A. Herpesvirus Group (Adapted from: Medical Letter 32:73,1990)

Virus	Regimen	Comment
HERPES SIMPLEX		
Genital-primary	<u>Acyclovir</u>: Oral - 200 mg 5 x daily x 10 days; IV - 15 mg/kg/day x 5 days	Mild lesions and symptoms are usually not treated (NEJM 308:916, 1983)
Genital-recurrent	<u>Acyclovir</u>: 200 mg po 5 x daily x 5 days	Initiate during prodrome or at first sign of lesions
Genital-prophylaxis	<u>Acyclovir</u>: 200 mg po, 2-5 x/day or 400 mg po bid	Indicated only with ≥ 6 recurrences/yr Good efficacy and good safety profile with treatment up to 5 yrs (JAMA 265:747, 1991) Contraindicated in pregnancy
Perirectal	<u>Acyclovir</u>: 400 mg po 5 x daily x 10 days	
Encephalitis	<u>Acyclovir</u>: IV - 10 mg/kg q8h x 10-14 days	(NEJM 314:144, 1986)
Mucocutaneous progressive	<u>Acyclovir</u>: IV - 5-10 mg/kg q8h x 7-14 days; oral - 200-400 mg po 5 x/day x 7-14 days or 400 mg 5x/day	AIDS patients often require preventative therapy with acyclovir 200-400 mg po 3-5 x/day indefinitely
Burn wound	<u>Acyclovir</u>: IV - 5 mg/kg q8h x 7 days; oral - 200 mg 5 x/day x 7-14 days	
Prophylaxis - high risk patients	<u>Acyclovir</u>: IV - 5 mg/kg q8h; oral - 200 mg 3-5 x/daily	Organ and bone marrow transplant recipients; treat seropositive patients for 1-3 mo. post-transplant (NEJM 320:1381, 1989)
Keratitis	<u>Trifluridine</u>: Topical (1%) 1 drop q2h up to 9 drops/day (3%) ointment	Ophthalmologist should supervise treatment
Acyclovir - resistant strains	<u>Foscarnet</u>: IV 60 mg/kg q8h	Thymidine kinase deficient strains, usually from immunosuppressed patients unresponsive to acyclovir

(continued)

119

Virus	Regimen	Comment
VARICELLA-ZOSTER		
Chickenpox, Adult	<u>Acyclovir</u>: 800 mg po 5x/day x 7-10 days	Must treat within 24 hrs of exantham; efficacy established (Ann Intern Med 117:358, 1992)
Chickenpox, Children	<u>Acyclovir</u>: 20 mg/kg up to 800 mg/po q6h x 5 days	Must treat within 24 hrs of exantham; no reduction in serologic response noted; considered cost effective due to decrease in parent work-time lost (NEJM 325:1539, 1991)
Pneumonia	<u>Acyclovir</u>: IV - 10-12 mg/kg q8h x 7 days; oral - 800 mg 5 x daily x 10 days	Efficacy not clearly established, but appears best if treatment is initiated within 36 hrs of admission (RID 12:788, 1990)
Dermatomal Immuno-suppressed	<u>Acyclovir</u>: IV 10-12 mg/kg q8h x 7 days	Indications to treat are greater for severe disease, early disease or zoster in immunosuppressed host (NEJM 308:1448, 1983; Am J Med 85 Suppl 2A:84, 1988)
Normal host	<u>Acyclovir</u>: Oral 800 mg 5 x daily x 7-10 days	Acyclovir and/or corticosteroids (prednisone 40 mg/day x 7 days, then taper over 3 wks) may reduce post-herpetic neuralgia. Steroids usually reserved for persons >40 years Acyclovir should be started ≤ 4 days from onset or while lesions are still forming Post-herpetic neuralgia: Amitriptyline
Ophthalmic zoster	<u>Acyclovir</u>: Oral 600-800 mg 5 x daily x 10 days	Consult ophthalmologist (Ophthalmology 93:763, 1986)
Disseminated zoster or varicella (immuno-suppressed host)	<u>Acyclovir</u>: IV 10-12 mg/kg q8h x 7 days	Alternatives are Foscarnet (60 mg/kg q8h) or vidarabine (10 mg/kg/day IV) x 5-7 days (NEJM 308:1448, 1983; NEJM 314:208, 1986)
Acyclovir resistant strains	<u>Foscarnet</u>: 60 mg/kg q8h IV	
Exposure (zoster or chickenpox)		
Immunosuppressed	<u>Varicella-zoster</u> immune globulin	(Ann Intern Med 108:221, 1988)
Susceptible health care workers	None	Must refrain from patient contact from days 10-21
Prophylaxis in transplant recipients	<u>Acyclovir</u>: 5 mg/kg IV q8h or 200 mg po q6h day 8-35	(Lancet 2:706, 1983; NEJM 320: 1381, 1989)

(continued)

120

Virus	Regimen	Comment
CYTOMEGALOVIRUS		
Immunocompetent	None	
Immunosuppressed		
Retinitis	Ganciclovir: Induction - 5 mg/kg IV bid x 14-21 days. Maintenance - 5 mg/kg IV qd Foscarnet: Induction - 60 mg/kg IV q8h x 14-21 days Maintenance - 90 mg/kg IV qd	Efficacy of ganciclovir and foscarnet established. Comparative trial in AIDS patients showed equal effectiveness vs CMV; Foscarnet recipients lived an average of 3 mo. longer possibly due to current AZT treatment and/or anti-HIV activity of foscarnet (NEJM 326:213, 1992). Most recommend foscarnet if AZT is to be continued or there is leukopenia; most recommend ganciclovir for elderly patients and those with renal failure. Failure with progressive CMV retinitis is treated by reinduction or use of the alternative agent
Colitis, enteritis esophagitis, viremia, mucocutaneous lesions, encephalitis, neuritis	As above (Ganciclovir preferred for non-AIDS patients)	Efficacy in these settings is less well established including indications for treatment and need for life-long maintenance
Pneumonitis AIDS patients		Up to 50% of BAL specimens yield CMV; most have alternative cause of pneumonitis; indications for treatment in absence of alternative pathogen are not clear
Marrow transplant recipients	Ganciclovir: 7.5-10 mg/kg/day IV x 20 days ± maintenance: 5 mg/kg 3-5 x/wk for 8-20 doses with or without CMV hyperimmune globulin or IV gamma globulin 500 mg/kg qod x 10 doses or 400 mg/kg on days 1, 4, 8 and 200 mg/kg on day 14	Ganciclovir-IVIG efficacy best supported for marrow recipients (Ann Intern Med 109:777, 1988; 109: 783, 1988; Transplantation 46:905 1988; JID 158:488, 1988) Ganciclovir monotherapy: Response rates: marrow - 22-50%; solid organs - 50-100% (reviews of 14 reports - Pharmacotherapy 12:300, 1992). IVIG monotherapy: Mortality 79% (JID 156:641, 1987)
Solid organ transplants	Ganciclovir: 7.5-10 mg/kg/day x 10-20 days	Response rates in heart, liver and renal transplant recipients in 14 reports: 67/85 (79%) (Pharmacotherapy 12:300, 1992). Maintenance therapy used in 2 of 14 reports

(continued)

Virus	Regimen	Comment
Pneumonitis (continued)		
Prophylaxis Marrow	Acyclovir: 500 mg/M^2 q8h day 5-30 ± maintenance with 800 mg po qid to day 180 (HSV prophylaxis concurrently)(NEJM 318:70, 1988)	Indications: 1) CMV pos autograft and allograft recipients; 2) seronegative allograft recipients of seropos donor; 3) asymptomatic patients with CMV pos BAL on day 35.
	Acyclovir: 200 mg po q6h day 8-35 (HSV prophylaxis concurrently) (NEJM 2:706, 1983)	Acyclovir: Value in prophylaxis vs HSV and VZV established; for CMV data are conflicting with some negative reports (Br J Cancer 59: 434, 1989)
	Ganciclovir: 5 mg/kg IV bid 5 days/ wk starting days 35-120 in patients with CMV pos BAL. Patients also received IV gamma globulin q2wks to day 180 (NEJM 324:1005, 1991; NEJM 325:1601, 1991)	Ganciclovir: Major complication is neutropenia
	Ganciclovir: 2.5 mg/kg IV q8h 7 days pretx, 6 mg/kg 3x/wk when ANC >500 to day 70 (Blood 76, Suppl 574a, 1990)	CMV poor blood products: Benefit may be restricted to seroneg donor and recipient
	Foscarnet: 40 mg/kg IV q8h days 7-30, then 60 mg/kg IV qd to day 75 (JID 166:473, 1992)	
Organ transplant recipients	Acyclovir: 800 mg po 5x/day (Ann Intern Med 114:598, 1991) Ganciclovir: 5 mg/kg IV q12h day to 14, then 6 mg/kg 5 days/wk to day 28 (NEJM 326:1182, 1992).	Indications: Best results are with ganciclovir in CMV seropositive heart recipients. Results with CMV-IVIG and oral acyclovir are disappointing (Transplant Proc 23:1170, 1991, and 23:1498, 1991).
EPSTEIN-BARR VIRUS		
Oral hairy leukoplakia	Acyclovir: 800 mg po 5x/day	Efficacy established. Relapse rates high
EBV associated lymphomas	No antiviral agent	Acyclovir confers no benefit (NEJM 311:1163, 1984)
Infectious mononucleosis	No antiviral agent	Prednisone (80 mg/d x 2-3 days, then taper over 2 wks) advocated for impending airway closure and prolonged course with high fever or persistent morbidity (JAMA 256: 1051, 1986)

B. **Influenza A: Amantadine**
   1. <u>Recommendations</u> (Advisory Council on Immunization Practices: MMWR 37:361,1988; 39:RR-7, 1-15 and 41:RR9, 12, 1992)
      a. <u>Prophylaxis</u>: 70-90% effective in preventing influenza A infection.
         Highest priority - Control presumed influenza A outbreaks in institutions with high risk persons; administer to all residents regardless of vaccination status as soon as possible after outbreak recognized and as long as there is influenza activity in community. This form of prophylaxis should also be offered to unvaccinated staff who provide care for high risk patients.

Other recommendations - 1) As adjunct to late vaccination of high risk persons (2 weeks required for vaccine response); **2)** Unvaccinated persons providing care to high risk persons in the home or in care facilities; continue until vaccine induces immunity (2 wks) or continue throughout epidemic if employee cannot be vaccinated or; **3)** Consider for vaccinated health care personnel if outbreak involves strain not covered in the vaccine; **4)** Immunodeficient persons who are expected to have a poor antibody response to the vaccine, especially high risk persons with contraindications to influenza vaccine.

   b. <u>Treatment</u>: Amantadine can reduce the severity and duration of influenza, but is not known to prevent complications in high risk patients. Consequently, no specific recommendation is made. If given, it should be started within 48 hrs of the onset of symptoms and should be discontinued when clinically warranted, usually within 3-5 days. In closed populations, persons who have influenza and are treated should be separated from those receiving amantadine for prophylaxis.

   c. Amantidine resistant strains of influenza A may emerge with amantidine treatment and may be transmitted to others.

2. <u>Dose</u> (MMWR 37:373,1988)
   a. <u>Prophylaxis</u>: 100 mg/day (all adults)

   b. <u>Treatment</u>: Age 10-64 - 200 mg/day in one or two doses; Age > 65 yrs - 100 mg/day as single daily dose; Seizure disorder - 100 mg/day

   c. Creatinine clearance in ml/min/1.73 M^2 (<u>use 1/2 dose when 100 mg/day indicated</u>).
      > 80: 200 mg/day
      60-80: 200 mg alternating with 100 mg/day
      40-60: 100 mg/day
      30-40: 200 mg twice weekly
      20-30: 100 mg three times weekly
      10-20: 200 mg alternating with 100 mg weekly

3. <u>Side effects</u> (dose related): Anxiety, insomnia, dizziness, drunk feeling, slurred speech, ataxia, depression, lightheadedness, inability to concentrate. Incidence is 5-10% for healthy young adults taking 200 mg/day; lower prophylactic dose presumably decreases side effects and retains efficacy. Less frequent side effects include seizures and confusion; seizures and behavioral change are most common in the elderly, those with poor renal function and patients with a pre-existing seizure disorder or psychiatric condition. Dose reduction reduces frequency.

4. <u>Information source (CDC)</u>: Technical Information Services, Center for Prevention Services, Mailstop E06, CDC, Atlanta, GA 30333, (404) 639-1819.

C. HIV: Antiretroviral therapy

Agent	Indication (FDA)	Dose	Side Effects
AZT (Retrovir, Zidovudine)	CD 4 count <500/cu mm	Usual dose: 500 mg po q4h while awake (500 mg/d) or 200 mg po tid (600 mg/d). Lowest effective dose: 300 mg/d. HIV associated dementia: 1000-1200 mg/d HIV associated ITP: 1000-1200 mg/d	Major: Marrow toxicity with severe anemia or leukopenia that is related to dose, duration of treatment and stage of disease. Monitor therapy with CBC and suspend treatment for Hgb <7.5 gm% or ANC <750/mm³. Frequency is 3%/yr in asymptomatic patients and 40%/yr with AIDS. Other: Headache, insomnia, myalgias and nausea (usually resolve with continued use) Cardiomyopathy: Late stage disease Myopathy: Long-term use Contraindications: Toxicity with Hg<7.5gm% or absolute neutrophil count (ANC) <750/mm³; concurrent use with ganciclovir
ddI (dideoxyinosine, Videx)	Adults with advanced HIV infection and prolonged prior treatment with AZT	Must take 2 tabs for buffering action >60 kg: 200 mg bid <60 kg: 125 mg bid	Major: 1) Pancreatitis in 5-9%, which is fatal in 6% (0.35% of all recipients); rates are higher in patients with advanced HIV infection (AIDS or CD4 <100) and with conditions associated with pancreatitis. 2) Peripheral neuropathy 5-12% related to cumulative dose. Other: Diarrhea in 30-35%. Rare: leuokpenia, anemia, hepatic failure, cardiomyopathy
ddC (dideoxytidine HIVID Zalcitabine)	Two criteria: 1)CD4 cell count <300/cu mm. 2) Prior treatment with AZT alone showing "clinical or immunologic deterioration." FDA approved only for use in combination with AZT	0.750 mg tid	Major: Peripheral neuropathy in 17-31% related to cumulative dose. Other: Pancreatitis (1%), oral or esophageal ulcers, cardiomyopathy, nausea, vomiting, diarrhea, rash, fever, headache, fatigue, arthralgias, mialgias

D. Hepatitis Viruses

Interferon alpha-2b (Medical Letter 32:1-2,1990 and 32:76-77,1990)

Chronic hepatitis C: Four studies showed interferon alfa-2b (2-3 million units SC 3x/wk x 6 mo) produced a statistically significant improvement in ALT; the three using 3 million units 3x/wk showed normal or near-normal ALT levels in about 50% of treated patients compared to 10% of controls. About 50% of responders relapsed within 6 months after treatment was discontinued (NEJM 321:1501,1506,1989). Enrollment criteria in these trials required compensated liver disease (no encephalopathy, ascites, variceal bleed; pro time <3 sec prolonged; bilirubin <2 mg/dl). Indications for treatment and therapeutic regimen to use are controversial. Some authorities suggest criteria include 1) Positive HCV serology, 2) exclusion of autoimmune hepatitis, 3) symptomatic hepatitis, 4) liver biopsy (best results with chronic persistent hepatitis; chronic active hepatitis or cirrhosis are relative contraindications). Initial treatment is 3 million units 3x/wk, treatment is continued for at least 3 months to determine response according to serum aminotransferase levels and treatment is continued for 6-12 months in responders. Some responders may require life-long treatment with 1-2 doses/week. Responders often show transient increases in ALT so that decision to retreat should be delayed 1-3 months.

<u>Hepatitis B</u>: Initial studies show interferon alfa-2b (5 million units SC daily x 4 mo) led to sustained loss of HBV DNA and HBeAg in one-third and return of liver function tests to normal in 40% (Perrillo RP et al, New Engl J Med 323:295, 1990). Enrollment criteria in these trials were compensated liver disease, chronic HBV (HBsAg >6 mo.) elevated ALT and evidence of HBV replication (HBeAg). Follow-up at 3-7 yrs shows prolonged remission in 20 of 23 who responded, 3 had reappearance of HBsAg within 1 yr, and 13 became negative for HBsAg (Korenman J et al Ann Intern Med 114:629,1991). Indications for treatment are arbitrary: most use the criteria in the trials including compensated liver disease, liver biopsy showing chronic hepatitis, ALT levels $\geq$ 2x normal and presence of HBeAg.

a.   Recommended regimen is 5 million units/day or 10 million units 3x/wk x 4 mo. Lower doses are less effective and higher doses are usually too toxic.

b.   Response rates: 30-40%. Predictors of response are e antigen (HBeAg), high AST (>100 U/L), persistence of HBV DNA at low initial levels (<100 pg/ml) and biopsy showing increased necroinflammation.

c.   Monitoring: Clinical and laboratry review at 2-4 wk intervals. Lab monitoring should include CBC, platelet count, liver function tests, TSH, and albumin prior to treatment and at treatment weeks 1,2,4,8,12 and 16. HBsAg and HBeAg should be measured at baseline, end of treatment and at 3 and 6 months.

<u>Preparations of Interferons:</u>

alpha-2a	"Roferon A"	Hoffmann-LaRoche
alfa-2b	"Intron A"	Schering Corp.
alfa-nl	"Wellferon"	Burroughs-Wellcome

<u>Adverse reactions</u>: About 50% experience flu-like symptoms of fever, malaise, myalgias and headache; Sx often respond to acetaminophen and decrease with continued treatment. Later side effects include fatigue, muscle aches, irritability, autoimmune reactions, granulocytopenia and thrombocytopenia, psychiatric symptoms, thyroid disorders and alopecia. Most side effects are dose related. Adverse reactions sufficiently severe to interfere with daily activities in 20-50% receiving 30 million units/week. Severe psychological reactions are more common in those with prior CNS disease or psychiatric problems. Long term effects are unknown and treatment requires subcutaneous injections. Wholesale cost to pharmacist is $25/3 million units.

TREATMENT OF MYCOBACTERIAL INFECTIONS

I. **TREATMENT OF TUBERCULOSIS:** Official statement of the American Thoracic Society and the Centers for Disease Control (Amer Rev Resp Dis 134:355-363,1986;136:492-496,1987, AMA Drug Evaluation, Section 15 pp 1:1-1:7,1990, MMWR 41RR-10, 1992)

New guidelines to be issued by CDC, ATS and IDSA in late 1992 include 2 major changes to the guideline summarized below:
1) All patients should receive initial treatment with four drugs unless they are from a geographic area in which resistance is nil.
2) All patients should have observed treatment until the patient can demonstrate compliance.

Classification of drugs:
Major: INH and rifampin
Adjunctive: Pyrazinamide, ethambutol, streptomycin
Second line: Ethionamide, capreomycin, kanamycin, amikacin, cycloserine, PAS
Experimental: Fluoroquinolones, clofazimine, amoxicillin-clavulante, clarithromycin azithromycin

A. Treatment of tuberculosis in adults
   1. TB without HIV infection
      Option 1: INH, rifampin, pyrazinamide and ethambutol or streptomycin is continued until susceptibility to INH and rifampin is demonstrated. These four drugs are continued 8 weeks followed by INH and rifampin for 16 weeks given daily, 2x/week or 3x/week (See B for doses). Continue treatment at least 6 months total and at least 3 months beyond culture conversion.
      Option 2: INH, rifampin, pyrazinamide and ethambutol or streptomycin daily for 2 weeks, then 2x/wk for 6 wks, then INH and rifampin for 16 weeks.
      Option 3: INH, rifampin, pyrazinamide, ethambutol or streptomycin with directly observed treatment 3x/wk for 6 months.

   2. Tuberculosis with HIV infection: Options 1, 2, and 3 are appropriate, but treatment must continue a total of at least 9 months and at least 6 months beyond culture conversion. (In general, TB is treated 50% longer in patients with HIV infection.)

   3. Tuberculosis with resistant strains (or contraindication to first line agent)
      a. Resistant to INH or rifampin: Treatment with INH or rifampin, ethambutol pyrazinamide plus streptomycin x 6 mo (non-AIDS) or 9 mo (AIDS). (Some advocate INH or rifampin, ethambutol and pyrazinamide x 18 mo.)
      b. Resistant to INH and rifampin: Treat with multiple drug regimen including at least two agents active in vitro x 18-24 mo.
      Note: 1) Intermittent therapy: Treatment 2x/wk appears to be as effective as 3x/wk; need for daily drugs for ≥2 wks at inception of treatment is not established.
      2) Aminoglycoside: Streptomycin preferred and may be given intravenously; capreomycin, kanamycin or amikacin may be preferred on basis of in vitro sensitivity tests; cost of amikacin is about 100 x that of streptomycin
      3) Utility of inclusion of INH (or rifampin) in regimen despite in vitro resistance is debated
      4) When resistance suspected, give 3 drugs not previously used pending in vitro sensitivity tests; never add a single drug when resistance suspected.
      5) Hospitalized patients with multiply resistant strains should not be discharged home until sputum smear is negative.

126

B. Recommended first line agents (Table 1)
(Amer Rev Resp Dis 134:355-363,1986 and Medical Letter 34:10,1992, MMWR 41:RR-10, pg 14, 1992)

Agent	Forms	Daily dose (maximum)	Twice/Thrice* weekly dose (maximum)	Cost/mo. (daily regimen)	Adverse reactions	Comment
Isoniazid	Tabs: 100 mg, 300 mg Syrup: 50 mg/5 ml Vials: 1 gm (1M)	5 mg/kg po or IM (300 mg)**	15 mg/kg (900 mg)*	$ 0.60	Elevated hepatic enzymes, peripheral neuropathy, hepatitis, *** hypersensitivity	Peripheral neuropathy is uncommon with dose of 5 mg/kg. Puridoxine (50 mg/day) suggested for those with diabetes, HIV, uremia, alcoholism, malnutrition, pregnancy or seizure disorder
Rifampin	Caps: 150 mg, 300 mg Vials: 600 mg (IV)	10-20 mg/kg po (600 mg)** IV (600 mg)	10 mg/kg (600 mg)*	$118.00	Orange discoloration of secretions & urine, nausea, vomiting, fever, hepatitis,*** purpura (rare)	May be given as 10 mg/ml suspension or intravenously. Accelerates clearance of methadone, coumadin, corticosteroids, estrogens, digitalis, ketoconazole, cyclosporine, dilantin, oral hypoglycemics (see Drug Interactions, pp. 79 and 80)
Pyrazinamide	Tabs: 500 mg	15-30 mg/kg po (2 gm)**	50-70 mg/kg	$121.00	Hepatitis,*** hyperuricemia, arthralgias, rash, GI intolerance	Hyperuracemia is common, gout is rare
Streptomycin	Vials: 1 gm, 4 gm	15 mg/kg IM (1 gm)** pts > 40 yrs: 10 mg/kg IM (500-750 mg)**	25-30 mg/kg pts > 40 yrs: 20 mg/kg	$118.00	Ototoxicity and possible nephrotoxicity	Decrease dose for renal failure
Ethambutol	Tabs: 100 mg, 400 mg	15-25 mg/kg po (2.5 gm)**	50 mg/kg (2x/wk) 25-30 mg/kg (3x/wk)	$106.00	Optic neuritis, skin rash	25 mg/kg/day 1st 1-2 months or if strain is INH resistant. Decrease dose for renal failure

* Dosage for treatment 2x/week and 3x/week are the same except for ethambutol.

** Usual dose for adults.

***All patients receiving INH, rifampin and/or pyrazinamide should be instructed to report immediately any symptoms of hepatitis: anorexia, nausea, vomiting, jaundice, malaise, fever >3 days or abdominal tenderness.

127

C.   Second line antituberculous drugs (Table 2)

Agent	Forms	Daily dose (maximum)	Adverse reactions	Monitoring
Capreomycin	Vials: 1 gm	15-30 mg/kg IM (1 gm)*	Auditory, vestibular, and renal toxicity	Audiometry, vestibular function, renal function
Kanamycin	Vials: 75 mg, 500 mg and and 1 gm	13-30 mg/kg IM (1 gm)*	Auditory, vestibular (rare), and renal toxicity	Audiometry, vestibular function, renal failure
Ethionamide	Tabs: 250 mg	15-20 mg/kg PO (1 gm)*	Gastrointestinal intolerance, hepatotoxicity, hypersensitivity	Hepatic enzymes
PAS	Tabs: 500 mg, 1 gm	12 gm	Gastrointestinal intolerance, hepatotoxicity, sodium load, hypersensitivity	
Cycloserine	Caps: 250 mg	1 gm	Psychosis, rash, convulsions	Assess mental status

* Usual daily dose of adult

D.   Monitoring Treatment (Table 3)

1.   Drug toxicity
   a.   Baseline tests: Hepatic enzymes, bilirubin, serum creatinine or BUN, CBC, platelet count or estimate.
        Pyrazinamide: uric acid; ethambutol: visual acuity.
        Frequency of INH hepatitis by age: 25 yrs - 1%; 35 yrs - 6%; 45 yrs - 11%; 55 yrs - 18%; 65 yrs - 11% (Goldberg MJ. Med Clin N Amer 72:661,1988).

   b.   During treatment: Clinical monitoring with assessment at least once monthly; laboratory monitoring is not recommended except for symptoms suggesting toxicity. The purpose of monthly monitoring is to determine compliance, determine symptoms of neuropathy (paresthesias) and determine symptoms of hepatotoxicity (anorexia, nausea, vomiting, dark urine, jaundice malaise, fever >3 days or abdominal tenderness).

2.   Evaluation of response: Sputum examination (smear and culture): Twice monthly until conversion is documented. Positive sputum at 3 months: Review compliance and drug susceptibility.

Table 3: Monitoring treatment (MMWR 41:RR-10, pg 15, 1992)

	Month 1	Month 2	Month 3 to completion
Medical evaluation	At least twice	Twice monthly	Once monthly if asymptomatic and smear/culture negative
Bacteriology*	Initially 3-6 sputum samples for diagnosis. Susceptibility testing of all strains	Sputum smear and culture 2x/month until sputum smear negative and patient asymptomatic	Sputum smear and culture 2x/month until sputum smear negative* and patient asymptomatic, then monthly
Drug monitoring**	Baseline lab studies in patients >35 years of age. Question and observe for evidence of toxicity; test if they occur	Question and observe for evidence of toxicity; test if they occur	Question and observe for evidence of toxicity; test if they occur

* Cultures should be obtained at least monthly until negative. This is the most reliable method for detecting treatment failure. Sputum conversion should occur within 3 months. Patients with treatment failure need to be evaluated for compliance and drug resistance

** Toxicity monitoring should be individualized based on drugs used, age and other factors such as alcohol consumption and concurrent drugs

E.   Special considerations

   1.   Extrapulmonary tuberculosis

      a.   Nine-month two-drug regimen recommended for sensitive strains; consider longer treatment for lymphadenitis, bone and joint tuberculosis.

      b.   Six-month regimen is "probably effective."

      c.   Some authorities recommend corticosteroids for tuberculosis pericarditis and meningitis. (See Recommendations of IDSA, pg 169)

   2.   Pregnancy and lactation

      a.   INH plus rifampin; ethambutol should be added for suspected resistant strains.

      b.   Streptomycin is only antituberculous drug with established fetal toxicity (interferes with ear development and causes congenital deafness); kanamycin and capreomycin presumably share this toxic potential.

      c.   Breast feeding should not be discouraged.

3. Treatment failures (persistent positive cultures after 5-6 months)

   a. Susceptibility tests on current isolate while continuing same regimen or augmenting this with two additional drugs.

   b. Sensitive strain: Consider treatment under direct observation.
      Resistant strain: At least 2 active drugs x 18-24 mo.

4. Relapse after treatment

   a. INH + rifampin regimen previously: Organism at time of relapse is usually sensitive if the original strain was. Therefore, give same regimen initially, measure susceptibility, modify the regimen accordingly and consider observed treatment.

   b. Regimen not containing INH and rifampin: Presume new isolate is resistant to agents used. See 3b above.

5. Multiply resistant strains of M. tuberculosis

   a. Definition: Resistance to INH and rifampin

   b. Epidemiology: Sporadic cases are usually acquired in third world countries, reflect non-compliance with standard treatment regimens for active tuberculosis or represent acquisition from one of these sources. Epidemics have been reported primarily through airborne spread from undiagnosed cases in AIDS patients in correctional facilities, shelters, nursing homes, crack houses and health care facilities in New York, New Jersey and Miami (NEJM 324:1644, 1991; NEJM 326:1514, 1992)

   c. Incidence (MMWR 41:RR-11, 1992): Susceptibility data for first quarter 1991

	U.S.	NYC
Resistance to INH or rifampin	14%	33%
Resistance to INH and rifampin	3%	19%

   d. Treatment (Medical Letter 34:10, 1992; NEJM 324:289, 1991): Regimens that include at least two drugs active in vitro for 18-24 mo. This combination often includes pyrazinamide, ethambutol, streptomycin and ciprofloxacin (750 mg po bid) or ofloxacin (400 mg po bid); other drugs besides standard first and second line agents include imipenem and amikacin. Strains resistant to INH and rifampin are often also resistant to ethambutol and streptomycin; about half are resistant to pyrazinamide.

   e. Outcome: Cure rates in all persons are <60%; mortality rates ascribed to tuberculosis in AIDS patients with multiply resistant strains are 72-89% and the median survival rate is 4-16 weeks. In 172 patients without AIDS the sputum conversion rate with multidrug regimens given under observation was about 65% and many convertors subsequently relapsed; the overall success rate was 56% (M. Goble et al, data presented at ICAAC, Anaheim, CA, Oct, 1992).

II.   **PREVENTATIVE TREATMENT FOR TUBERCULOSIS INFECTION IN THE U.S.**
(Recommendations of the Advisory Committee for Elimination of Tuberculosis,
MMWR 39:#RR-8, pp 9-15, 1990)

A.   **Indications**

1.   High risk groups (persons in any category should be treated regardless
of age unless previously treated).

a.   Persons with HIV infection with PPD ≥ 5 mm and persons at risk for
HIV whose serologic status is unknown but HIV is suspected.

b.   Close contacts of newly diagnosed cases with PPD ≥ 5 mm. Children and
adolescents with neg PPD who have been close contacts with infectious
persons within past 3 months are candidates until there is a negative
repeat PPD at 12 weeks post contact.

c.   Recent seroconverters with PPD ≥ 10 mm increase within 2 yr period for
persons < 35 yrs and ≥ 15 mm increase for persons over 35 years.

d.   Persons with x-ray showing fibrotic lesions likely to represent healed TB
and PPD ≥ 5 mm.

e.   Intravenous drug abusers known to be HIV seronegative and PPD
≥ 10 mm.

f.   Persons with medical conditions that have been associated with increased
risk of TB and PPD ≥ 10 mm: silicosis; diabetes mellitus (esp if poorly
controlled); corticosteroid treatment (≥ 15 mg/day prednisone for over 2-
3 wks); other immunosuppressive treatment; hematologic and
lymphoproliferative diseases such as leukemia and Hodgkin's disease; end
stage renal disease, and conditions associated with rapid weight loss or
chronic malnutrition including gastrectomy, jejunoileal by-pass and weight
loss of 10% or more below ideal body weight.

2.   Persons under 35 years with PPD ≥ 10 mm.

a.   Foreign born persons from high prevalence countries.

b.   Medically underserved low-income populations including blacks,
Hispanics and Native Americans.

c.   Residents of long term care facilities.

B.   **Preventative treatment**

1.   Usual regimen: Isoniazid, 300 mg/day for 6-12 months.

a.   Persons with HIV infection and those with stable chest x-rays compatible
with past TB should be treated for 12 months.

b.   Others: 6-12 months

2.   Directly observed therapy: Isoniazid in dose of 15 mg/kg (up to 900 mg) twice
weekly.

3.   Multiply resistant strains: Decision to treat should be based on extent of exposure,
host factors and in vitro sensitivities of the contact strain. Health care workers
with HIV infection are 40 x more likely to develop active disease. Recommended
regimens depending on sensitivity test results are pyrazinamide + fluoroquinolone
or pyrazinamide + ethambutol. Duration is 12 mo. for HIV infected persons and
6 mo. for all others.

C.   <u>Monitoring</u>: Patients should be monitored in person by trained personnel at monthly intervals. Black and Hispanic women, especially postpartum, may be at greatest risk for serious or fatal reaction and should be monitored more frequently. Purpose of monitoring is to evaluate compliance and evaluate toxicity: peripheral neuropathy and hepatotoxicity.

III.   **SCREENING FOR TUBERCULOSIS**
(Recommendations of Advisory Committee for Elimination of Tuberculosis, MMWR 39:#RR-8, pp 1-8, 1990)

A.   **Background**
1.   It is estimated that > 90% of patients with active tuberculosis have harbored <u>M</u>. tuberculosis for over 1 year.
2.   The estimated number of persons in the U.S. with latent infection is 10-15 million.
3.   Preventative treatment with isoniazid is 90-95% effective when compliance is good.

B.   **Populations to be screened**
1.   Persons with HIV infection.
2.   Close contacts with persons known or suspected to have tuberculosis.
3.   Persons with medical risks known to increase the risk of disease if infection has occurred.
4.   Foreign born persons from countries with high prevalence of TB.
5.   Medically underserved low income populations, e.g., blacks, Hispanics and Native Americans.
6.   Alcoholics and IV drug abusers.
7.   Residents of long term care facilities including correctional facilities, nursing homes, mental institutions, etc.

C.   **Screening**
1.   PPD: 5 units given intracutaneously is the preferred test.
2.   Persons with signs or symptoms of pulmonary tuberculosis should have chest x-ray regardless of skin test results.

D.   **PPD-Tuberculin anergy and HIV infection** (MMWR 40RR-5, 27, 1991)
1.   Anergy with delayed-type hypersensitivity (DTH) skin test antigens in persons with HIV infection is inversely related to CD4 cell counts. Anergy to each of 2 or 3 skin test antigens (Candida albicans, mumps and tetanus) is <10% with healthy persons and HIV infected persons with CD4 counts >500 mm^3; it is >80% for HIV infected persons with CD4 counts <50/mm^3.
2.   Recommendations for DTH testing
    a.   Persons with HIV infection should have concurrent anergy testing in conjunction with PPD testing.
    b.   Degree of immunosuppression should not influence decisions regarding anergy testing.
    c.   Recommended testing is with two DTH skin test antigens, i.e., Candida, mumps or tetanus toxoid (Multitest CMI not recommended).
    d.   Interpretation: Any induration to DTH antigens is considered positive at 48-72 hrs.
3.   Treatment recommendations for persons with HIV infection.
    a.   PPD >5 mm induration: INH prophylasis*. Some believe 2 mm of induration should be the cutoff (JAMA 267:369, 1992), but this has not been generally accepted (JAMA 267:409, 1992)

b. PPD negative plus anergy: INH prophylaxis* for those who are contacts of persons with TB and those with a risk of ≥10% of TB: IVDU's, prisoners, homeless persons, migrant workers and the persons born in Asia, Africa and Latin America.

---

* INH x ≥ 1 year; must have x-ray and clinical evaluation to exclude active TB.

IV. ATYPICAL MYCOBACTERIA (See Wolinsky E, CID 15:1, 1992)

Agent	Condition	Treatment
M. kansasii	Pulmonary Osteomyelitis Disseminated	3 drugs x 18 mo: INH, rifampin and ethambutol or these three agents for 12 mo. plus streptomycin (1 gm IM 2x/wk) x 3 mo.* Also consider ciprofloxacin, clarithromycin
M. avium complex (MAC)	Immunocompetent host: Pulmonary Lymphadenitis Osteomyelitis	3-5 drugs: INH, rifampin, ethambutol x 18-24 mo. plus streptomycin x 2-4 mo.* Also consider clarithromycin, ciprofloxacin, clofazimine, cycloserine, ethionamide lymphadenitis and amikacin. Use of INH is controversial
	Immunosuppressed host: Disseminated disease (AIDS etc)	3-5 drugs: Rifampin, ethambutol, clofazimine, clarithromycin, ciprofloxacin, amikacin or kanamycin. Alternative is clarithromycin + ethambutol or clofazimine. Clofazimine usually reserved for extra-pulmonary disease
M. marinum	Skin soft tissue	Ethambutol + rifampin ± streptomycin*, minocycline or doxycycline* or sulfa-trimethoprim*. Also consider ciprofloxacin. Surgery often required for deep infections
M. xenopi	Pulmonary	3 drugs: Rifampin, INH + ethambutol* ± streptomycin. Also consider ethionamide, cycloserine, clarithromycin, ciprofloxacin
M. malmoense	Pulmonary	Same as MAC (Rifampin, INH + ethambutol)
M. simiae	Pulmonary	Same as MAC (often refractory)
M. scrofulaceum	Lymphadenitis Disseminated	Same as MAC (usually very resistant, with lymphadenitis-resection)
M. fortuitum	Pulmonary Disseminated Skin/soft tissue iatrogenic infections	Amikacin, ciprofloxacin + sulfonamide*. Also consider clofaximine, clarithromycin (or erythromycin), doxycycline, imipenem, cefoxitin, ciprofloxacin
M. bovis	Pulmonary	Same as M. tuberculosis, but resistant to pyrazinamide
M. szulgai	Pulmonary and extrapulmonary	Same as M. kansasii

(continued)

Agent	Condition	Treatment
M. haemophilum	Skin/soft tissue	Rifampin, clofazimine, doxycycline, sulfa-trimethoprim
M. chelonae ss abscessus	Skin/soft tissue esp post-op augmentation mammoplasty, median sternotomy and other iatrogenic infections	Amikacin* + cefoxitin. Also consider clofazimine, clarithromycin
M. chelonea ss chelonea	Same	Tobramycin or amikacin + cefoxitin*. Also consider clofazimine, clarithromycin, doxycycline, erythromycin
M. smegmatis	Soft tissue, bone, etc.	Ethambutol, amikacin, ciprofloxacin sulfonamides, clofazimine, imipenem

* Regimens with established efficacy

DRUGS FOR TREATMENT OF PARASITIC INFECTIONS
(Reprinted from The Medical Letter on Drugs and
Therapeutics 34:18-25,1992 with permission)

Infection		Drug	Adult Dosage*	Pediatric Dosage*
AMEBIASIS (Entamoeba histolytica)				
asymptomatic				
Drug of choice:		Iodoquinol[1]	650 mg tid x 20d	30-40 mg/kg/d in 3 doses x 20d
	OR	Paromomycin	25-30 mg/kg/d in 3 doses x 7d	25-30 mg/kg/d in 3 doses x 7d
Alternative:		Diloxanide furoate[2]	500 mg tid x 10d	20 mg/kg/d in 3 doses x 10d
mild to moderate intestinal disease				
Drugs of choice:		Metronidazole[3]	750 mg tid x 10d	35-50 mg/kg/d in 3 doses x 10d
	OR	Tinidazole[4]	2 grams/d x 3d	50 mg/kg (max. 2 grams) qd x 3d
		followed by iodoquinol[1]	650 mg tid x 20d	30-40 mg/kg/d in 3 doses x 20d
	OR	paromomycin	25-30 mg/kg/d in 3 doses x 7d	25-30 mg/kg/d in 3 doses x 7d
severe intestinal disease				
Drugs of choice:		Metronidazole[3]	750 mg tid x 10d	35-50 mg/kg/d in 3 doses x 10d
	OR	Tinidazole[4]	600 mg bid x 5d	50 mg/kg (max. 2 grams) qd x 3d
		followed by iodoquinol[1]	650 mg tid x 20d	30-40 mg/kg/d in 3 doses x 20d
	OR	paromomycin	25-30 mg/kg/d in 3 doses x 7d	25-30 mg/kg/d in 3 doses x 7d
Alternatives:		Dehydroemetine[2,5]	1 to 1.5 mg/kg/d (max. 90 mg/d) IM for up to 5d	1 to 1.5 mg/kg/d (max. 90 mg/d) IM in 2 doses for up to 5d
		followed by iodoquinol[1]	650 mg tid x 20d	30-40 mg/kg/d in 3 doses x 20d
hepatic abscess				
Drugs of choice:		Metronidazole[3]	750 mg tid x 10d	35-50 mg/kg/d in 3 doses x 10d
	OR	Tinidazole[4]	800 mg tid x 5d	60 mg/kg (max. 2 grams) qd x 3d
		followed by iodoquinol[1]	650 mg tid x 20d	30-40 mg/kg/d in 3 doses x 20d
Alternatives:		Dehydroemetine[2,5]	1 to 1.5 mg/kg/d (max. 90 mg/d) IM for up to 5d	1 to 1.5 mg/kg/d (max. 90 mg/d) IM in 2 doses for up to 5d
		followed by chloroquine phosphate	600 mg base (1 gram)/d x 2d, then 300 mg base (500 mg)/d x 2-3 wks	10 mg base/kg (max. 300 mg base)/d x 2-3 wks
		plus iodoquinol[1]	650 mg tid x 20d	30-40 mg/kg/d in 3 doses x 20d
AMEBIC MENINGOENCEPHALITIS, PRIMARY				
Naegleria				
Drug of choice:		Amphotericin B[6,7]	1 mg/kg/d IV, uncertain duration	1 mg/kg/d IV, uncertain duration
Acanthamoeba				
Drug of choice:		see footnote 8		
Ancylostoma duodenale, see HOOKWORM				
ANGIOSTRONGYLIASIS				
Angiostrongylus cantonensis				
Drug of choice:		Mebendazole[7,9,10]	100 mg bid x 5d	100 mg bid x 5d
Angiostrongylus costaricensis				
Drug of choice:		Thiabendazole[7,9]	75 mg/kg/d in 3 doses x 3d[11] (max. 3 grams/d)	75 mg/kg/d in 3 doses x 3d[11] (max. 3 grams/d)
ANISAKIASIS (Anisakis)				
Treatment of choice:		Surgical or endoscopic removal		
ASCARIASIS (Ascaris lumbricoides, roundworm)				
Drug of choice:		Mebendazole	100 mg bid x 3d	100 mg bid x 3d
	OR	Pyrantel pamoate	11 mg/kg once (max. 1 gram)	11 mg/kg once (max. 1 gram)
	OR	Albendazole	400 mg once	400 mg once
BABESIOSIS (Babesia)				
Drugs of choice:[12]		Clindamycin[7]	1.2 grams bid parenteral or 600 mg bid oral x 7d	20-40 mg/kg/d in 3 doses x 7d
		plus quinine	650 mg tid oral x 7d	25 mg/kg/d in 3 doses x 7d

Infection	Drug	Adult Dosage*	Pediatric Dosage*
BALANTIDIASIS (Balantidium coli)			
Drug of choice:	Tetracycline[7]	500 mg qid x 10d	40 mg/kg/d in 4 doses x 10d (max. 2 grams/d)[13]
Alternatives:	Iodoquinol[1,7]	650 mg tid x 20d	40 mg/kg/d in 3 doses x 20d
	Metronidazole[3,7]	750 mg tid x 5d	35-50 mg/kg/d in 3 doses x 5d
BAYLISASCARIASIS (Baylisascaris procyonis)			
Drug of choice:	See footnote 14		
BLASTOCYSTIS hominis infection			
Drug of choice:	See footnote 15		
CAPILLARIASIS (Capillaria philippinensis)			
Drug of choice:	Mebendazole[7]	200 mg bid x 20d	200 mg bid x 20d
Alternatives:	Albendazole	200 mg bid x 10d	200 mg bid x 10d
	Thiabendazole[7]	25 mg/kg/d in 2 doses x 30d	25 mg/kg/d in 2 doses x 30d
Chagas' disease, see TRYPANOSOMIASIS			
Clonorchis sinensis, see FLUKE infection			
CRYPTOSPORIDIOSIS (Cryptosporidium)			
Drug of choice:	See footnote 16		
CUTANEOUS LARVA MIGRANS (creeping eruption)			
Drug of choice:[17]	Thiabendazole	Topically and/or 50 mg/kg/d in 2 doses (max. 3 grams/d) x 2-5d[11]	Topically and/or 50 mg/kg/d in 2 doses (max. 3 grams/d) x 2-5d[11]
Cysticercosis, see TAPEWORM infection			
DIENTAMOEBA fragilis infection			
Drug of choice:	Iodoquinol[1]	650 mg tid x 20d	40 mg/kg/d in 3 doses x 20d
OR	Paromomycin	25-30 mg/kg/d in 3 doses x 7d	25-30 mg/kg/d in 3 doses x 7d
OR	Tetracycline[7]	500 mg qid x 10d	40 mg/kg/d in 4 doses x 10d (max. 2 grams/d)[13]
Diphyllobothrium latum, see TAPEWORM infection			
DRACUNCULUS medinensis (guinea worm) infection			
Drug of choice:	Metronidazole[3,7,18]	250 mg tid x 10d	25 mg/kg/d (max. 750 mg/d) in 3 doses x 10d
Alternative:	Thiabendazole[7,18]	50-75 mg/kg/d in 2 doses x 3d[11]	50-75 mg/kg/d in 2 doses x 3d[11]
Echinococcus, see TAPEWORM infection			
Entamoeba histolytica, see AMEBIASIS			
ENTAMOEBA polecki infection			
Drug of choice:	Metronidazole[3,7]	750 mg tid x 10d	35-50 mg/kg/d in 3 doses x 10d
ENTEROBIUS vermicularis (pinworm) infection			
Drug of choice:	Pyrantel pamoate	11 mg/kg once (max. 1 gram); repeat after 2 weeks	11 mg/kg once (max. 1 gram); repeat after 2 weeks
OR	Mebendazole	A single dose of 100 mg; repeat after 2 weeks	A single dose of 100 mg; repeat after 2 weeks
OR	Albendazole	400 mg once, repeat in 2 weeks	400 mg once, repeat in 2 weeks
Fasciola hepatica, see FLUKE infection			
FILARIASIS			
Wuchereria bancrofti, Brugia malayi			
Drug of choice:[19]	Diethylcarbamazine[20]	Day 1: 50 mg, oral, p.c.	Day 1: 1 mg/kg, oral, p.c.
		Day 2: 50 mg tid	Day 2: 1 mg/kg tid
		Day 3: 100 mg tid	Day 3: 1-2 mg/kg tid
		Days 4 through 21: 6 mg/kg/d in 3 doses[21]	Days 4 through 21: 6 mg/kg/d in 3 doses[21]
Loa loa			
Drug of choice:	Diethylcarbamazine[20]	Day 1: 50 mg, oral, p.c.	Day 1: 1 mg/kg, oral, p.c.
		Day 2: 50 mg tid	Day 2: 1 mg/kg tid
		Day 3: 100 mg tid	Day 3: 1-2 mg/kg tid
		Days 4 through 21: 9 mg/kg/d in 3 doses[21]	Days 4 through 21: 9 mg/kg/d in 3 doses[21]
Mansonella ozzardi			
Drug of choice:	See footnote 19		
Mansonella perstans			
Drug of choice:[22]	Mebendazole[7]	100 mg bid x 30d	
Tropical Pulmonary Eosinophilia (TPE)			
Drug of choice:	Diethylcarbamazine	6 mg/kg/d in 3 doses x 21d	6 mg/kg/d in 3 doses x 21d
Onchocerca volvulus			
Drug of choice:	Ivermectin[2]	150 µg/kg oral once, repeated every 6 to 12 months	150 µg/kg oral once, repeated every 6 to 12 months

Infection	Drug	Adult Dosage*	Pediatric Dosage*
FLUKE, hermaphroditic, infection			
Clonorchis sinensis (Chinese liver fluke)			
Drug of choice:	Praziquantel	75 mg/kg/d in 3 doses	75 mg/kg/d in 3 doses
Fasciola hepatica (sheep liver fluke)			
Drug of choice:[23]	Bithionol[2]	30-50 mg/kg on alternate days x 10-15 doses	30-50 mg/kg on alternate days x 10-15 doses
Fasciolopsis buski (intestinal fluke)			
Drug of choice:	Praziquantel[7]	75 mg/kg/d in 3 doses x 1d	75 mg/kg/d in 3 doses x 1d
	OR Niclosamide[7]	a single dose of 4 tablets (2 g), chewed thoroughly	11-34 kg: 2 tablets (1 g) >34 kg: 3 tablets (1.5 g)
Heterophyes heterophyes (intestinal fluke)			
Drug of choice:	Praziquantel[7]	75 mg/kg/d in 3 doses x 1d	75 mg/kg/d in 3 doses x 1d
Metagonimus yokogawai (intestinal fluke)			
Drug of choice:	Praziquantel[7]	75 mg/kg/d in 3 doses x 1d	75 mg/kg/d in 3 doses x 1d
Nanophyetus salmincola			
Drug of choice:	Praziquantel[7]	60 mg/kg/d in 3 doses x 1d	60 mg/kg/d in 3 doses x 1d
Opisthorchis viverrini (liver fluke)			
Drug of choice:	Praziquantel	75 mg/kg/d in 3 doses x 1d	75 mg/kg/d in 3 doses x 1d
Paragonimus westermani (lung fluke)			
Drug of choice:	Praziquantel[7]	75 mg/kg/d in 3 doses x 2d	75 mg/kg/d in 3 doses x 2d
Alternative:	Bithionol[2]	30-50 mg/kg on alternate days x 10-15 doses	30-50 mg/kg on alternate days x 10-15 doses
GIARDIASIS (*Giardia intestinalis*, formerly *G. lamblia*)			
Drug of choice:	Quinacrine HCl	100 mg tid p.c. x 5d	6 mg/kg/d in 3 doses p.c. x 5d (max. 300 mg/d)
Alternatives:	Metronidazole[3,7]	250 mg tid x 5d	15 mg/kg/d in 3 doses x 5d
	Tinidazole[4]	2 grams once	50 mg/kg once (max. 2 grams)
	Furazolidone	100 mg qid x 7-10d	
	Paromomycin[24]	25-30 mg/kg/d in 3 doses x 7d	6 mg/kg/d in 4 doses x 7-10d
GNATHOSTOMIASIS (*Gnathostoma spinigerum*)			
Treatment of choice:	Surgical removal		
	OR Mebendazole[7]	200 mg q3h x 6d	
HOOKWORM infection (*Ancylostoma duodenale, Necator americanus*)			
Drug of choice:	Mebendazole	100 mg bid x 3d	100 mg bid x 3d
	OR Pyrantel pamoate[7]	11 mg/kg (max. 1 gram) x 3d	11 mg/kg (max. 1 gram) x 3d
	OR Albendazole	400 mg once	400 mg once
Hydatid cyst, see TAPEWORM infection			
Hymenolepis nana, see TAPEWORM infection			
ISOSPORIASIS (*Isospora belli*)			
Drug of choice:	Trimethoprim-sulfa-methoxazole[7,25]	160 mg TMP, 800 mg SMX qid x 10d, then bid x 3 wks	
LEISHMANIASIS (*L. mexicana, L. tropica, L. major, L. braziliensis, L. donovani* [Kala-azar])			
Drug of choice:[26]	Stibogluconate sodium[2]	20 mg Sb/kg/d IV or IM x 20-28d[27]	20 mg Sb/kg/d IV or IM x 20-28d[27]
	OR Meglumine antimoniate	20 mg Sb/kg/d x 20-28d[27]	20 mg Sb/kg/d x 20-28d[27]
Alternatives:[28]	Amphotericin B[7]	0.25 to 1 mg/kg by slow infusion daily or every 2d for up to 8 wks	0.25 to 1 mg/kg by slow infusion daily or every 2d for up to 8 wks
	Pentamidine isethionate[7]	2-4 mg/kg/d IM for up to 15 doses[27]	2-4 mg/kg/d IM for up to 15 doses[27]
	Topical treatment[29]		
LICE infestation (*Pediculus humanus, capitis, Phthirus pubis*)[30]			
Drug of choice:	1% Permethrin[31]	Topically	Topically
	OR 0.5% Malathion	Topically	Topically
Alternatives:	Pyrethrins with pipero-nyl butoxide	Topically[32]	Topically[32]
	Lindane	Topically[32]	Topically[32]
MALARIA, Treatment of (*Plasmodium falciparum, P. ovale, P. vivax,* and *P. malariae*)			
All *Plasmodium* except Chloroquine-Resistant *P. falciparum*			
ORAL			
Drug of choice:	Chloroquine phosphate[33,34]	600 mg base (1 gram), then 300 mg base (500 mg) 6 hrs later, then 300 mg base (500 mg) at 24 and 48 hrs	10 mg base/kg (max. 600 mg base), then 5 mg base/kg 6 hrs later, then 5 mg base/kg at 24 and 48 hrs
PARENTERAL			
Drug of choice:[35]	Quinidine gluconate[7,36]	10 mg/kg loading dose (max. 600 mg) in normal saline slowly over 1 hr, followed by continuous infusion of 0.02 mg/kg/min for 3 days maximum	Same as adult dose
	OR Quinine dihydro-chloride[37]	20 mg salt/kg loading dose in 10 ml/kg 5% dextrose over 4 hrs, followed by 10 mg salt/kg over 2-4 hrs q8h (max. 1800 mg/d) until oral therapy can be started	Same as adult dose

Infection	Drug	Adult Dosage*	Pediatric Dosage*
Chloroquine-resistant _P. falciparum_[38]			
ORAL			
Drugs of choice:[39]	Quinine sulfate[40,41] plus	650 mg tid x 3d	[†]25 mg/kg/d in 3 doses x 3d
	pyrimethamine-sulfadoxine[42]	3 tablets at once on last day of quinine	<1 yr: ¼ tablet 1-3 yrs: ½ tablet 4-8 yrs: 1 tablet 9-14 yrs: 2 tablets
OR	plus tetracycline[7,13]	250 mg qid x 7d	20 mg/kg/d in 4 doses x 7d[13]
OR	plus clindamycin[7]	900 mg tid x 3d	20-40 mg/kg/d in 3 doses x 3d

MALARIA, Treatment of Chloroquine-resistant _P. falciparum (continued)_			
ORAL _(continued)_			
Alternatives:	Mefloquine[43,44]	1250 mg once[45]	25 mg/kg once[46] (<45 kg)
	Halofantrine[47]	500 mg q6h x 3 doses	8 mg/kg q6h x 3 doses (<40 kg)
PARENTERAL			
Drug of choice:	Quinidine gluconate[7,36]	same as above	same as above
OR	Quinine dihydrochloride[37]	same as above	same as above

Prevention of relapses: _P. vivax_ and _P. ovale_ only			
Drug of choice:	Primaquine phosphate[48]	15 mg base (26.3 mg)/d x 14d or 45 mg base (79 mg)/wk x 8 wks	0.3 mg base/kg/d x 14d

MALARIA, Prevention of[49]			
Chloroquine-sensitive areas			
Drug of choice:	Chloroquine phosphate[50]	300 mg base (500 mg salt) orally, once/week beginning 1 week before and continuing for 4 weeks after last exposure	5 mg/kg base (8.3 mg/kg salt) once/week, up to adult dose of 300 mg base
Chloroquine-resistant areas[38]			
Drug of choice:[51]	Mefloquine[44,50,52]	250 mg oral once/week[53]	15-19 kg: ¼ tablet 20-30 kg: ½ tablet 31-45 kg: ¾ tablet >45 kg: 1 tablet
OR	Doxycycline[7,50,54]	100 mg daily	>8 years of age: 2 mg/kg/d orally, up to 100 mg/day
OR	Chloroquine phosphate[50]	as above	as above
	plus pyrimethamine-sulfadoxine[42] for presumptive treatment[55]	Carry a single dose (3 tablets) for self-treatment of febrile illness when medical care is not immediately available	<1 yr: ¼ tablet 1-3 yrs: ½ tablet 4-8 yrs: 1 tablet 9-14 yrs: 2 tablets
	or plus proguanil[56] (in Africa south of the Sahara)	200 mg daily during exposure and for 4 weeks afterwards	<2 yrs: 50 mg daily 2-6 yrs: 100 mg daily 7-10 yrs: 150 mg daily 10 yrs: 200 mg daily

* The letter d stands for day.

MICROSPORIDIOSIS			
Enterocytozoon bieneusi			
Drug of choice:	none[57]		
Encephalitozoon hellem			
Drug of choice:	none[58]		

Mites, see SCABIES

MONILIFORMIS _moniliformis_ infection			
Drug of choice:	Pyrantel pamoate[7]	11 mg/kg once, repeat twice, 2 wks apart	11 mg/kg once, repeat twice, 2 wks apart

Naegleria species, see AMEBIC MENINGOENCEPHALITIS, PRIMARY

Necator americanus, see HOOKWORM infection

Onchocerca volvulus, see FILARIASIS

Opisthorchis viverrini, see FLUKE infection

Paragonimus westermani, see FLUKE infection

Pediculus capitis, humanus, Phthirus pubis, see LICE

Pinworm, see ENTEROBIUS

Infection	Drug	Adult Dosage*	Pediatric Dosage*
PNEUMOCYSTIS carinii pneumonia[59]			
Drug of choice:	Trimethoprim-sulfámethoxazole	TMP 15-20 mg/kg/d, SMX 75-100 mg/kg/d, oral or IV in 3 or 4 doses x 14-21d	Same as adult dose
OR	Pentamidine	3-4 mg/kg IV qd x 14-21 days	Same as adult dose
Alternatives:	Trimethoprim[7] plus dapsone[7,60]	5 mg/kg PO qid x 21 days 100 mg PO qd x 21 days	
	Primaquine[7,48] plus clindamycin[7]	15 mg base PO qd x 21 days 600 mg IV q6h x 21 days, or 300-450 mg PO q6h x 21 days	
	Trimetrexate plus folinic acid	45 mg/m² IV qd x 21 days 20 mg/m² PO or IV q6h x 21 days	
Primary and secondary prophylaxis			
Drug of Choice:	Trimethoprim-sulfamethoxazole	1 DS[61] tab qd, bid, or 3x/week	
Alternatives:	Dapsone[7,60]	25-50 mg PO qd, or 100 mg PO 2 x week	
	Aerosol pentamidine	300 mg inhaled monthly via Respirgard II nebulizer	
Roundworm, see ASCARIASIS			
SCABIES (Sarcoptes scabiei)			
Drug of choice:	5% Permethrin	**Topically**	**Topically**
Alternatives:	Lindane[32]	**Topically**	**Topically**
	10% Crotamiton	**Topically**	**Topically**
SCHISTOSOMIASIS (Bilharziasis)			
S. haematobium			
Drug of choice:	Praziquantel	40 mg/kg/d in 2 doses x 1d	40 mg/kg/d in 2 doses x 1d
S. japonicum			
Drug of choice:	Praziquantel	60 mg/kg/d in 3 doses x 1d	60 mg/kg/d in 3 doses x 1d
S. mansoni			
Drug of choice:	Praziquantel	40 mg/kg/d in 2 doses x 1d	40 mg/kg/d in 2 doses x 1d
Alternative:	Oxamniquine[62]	15 mg/kg once[63]	20 mg/kg/d in 2 doses x 1d[63]
S. mekongi			
Drug of choice:	Praziquantel	60 mg/kg/d in 3 doses x 1d	60 mg/kg/d in 3 doses x 1d
Sleeping sickness, see TRYPANOSOMIASIS			
STRONGYLOIDIASIS (Strongyloides stercoralis)			
Drug of choice:[64]	Thiabendazole	50 mg/kg/d in 2 doses (max. 3 grams /d) x 2d[11,65]	50 mg/kg/d in 2 doses (max. 3 grams/d) x 2d[11,65]
OR	Ivermectin[2]	200 µg/kg/d x 1-2d	
OR	Albendazole	400 mg qd x 3d	400 mg qd x 3d
TAPEWORM infection — Adult (intestinal stage)			
Diphyllobothrium latum (fish), *Taenia saginata* (beef), *Taenia solium* (pork), *Dipylidium caninum* (dog)			
Drug of choice:	Praziquantel[7]	10-20 mg/kg once	10-20 mg/kg once
OR	Niclosamide	A single dose of 4 tablets (2 grams), chewed thoroughly	11-34 kg: a single dose of 2 tablets (1 gram); >34 kg: a single dose of 3 tablets (1.5 grams)
Hymenolepis nana (dwarf tapeworm)			
Drug of choice:	Praziquantel[7]	25 mg/kg once	25 mg/kg once
Alternative:	Niclosamide	A single daily dose of 4 tablets (2 g), chewed thoroughly, then 2 tablets daily x 6d	11-34 kg: a single dose of 2 tablets (1 g) x 1d, then 1 tablet (0.5 grams) /d x 6d; >34 kg: a single dose of 3 tablets (1.5 g) x 1d, then 2 tablets (1 gram)/d x 6d
— Larval (tissue stage)			
Echinococcus granulosus (hydatid cyst)			
Drug of choice:	Albendazole[66]	400 mg bid x 28 days, repeated as necessary	15 mg/kg/d x 28 days, repeated as necessary
Echinococcus multilocularis			
Treatment of choice:	See footnote 67		
Cysticercus cellulosae (cysticercosis)			
Drug of choice:[68]	Praziquantel[7]	50 mg/kg/d in 3 doses x 15d	50 mg/kg/d in 3 doses x 15d
OR	Albendazole	15 mg/kg/d in 3 doses x 8d, repeated as necessary	15 mg/kg/d in 3 doses x 8d, repeated as necessary
Alternative:	Surgery		
Toxocariasis, see VISCERAL LARVA MIGRANS			
TOXOPLASMOSIS (Toxoplasma gondii[69])			
Drugs of choice:	Pyrimethamine[70]	25-100 mg/d x 3-4 wks	2 mg/kg/d x 3d, then 1 mg/kg/d (max. 25 mg/d) x 4 wks[71]
	plus sulfadiazine	1-2 grams qid x 3-4 wks	100-200 mg/kg/d x 3-4 wks
Alternative:	Spiramycin	3-4 grams/d[72]	50-100 mg/kg/d x 3-4 wks

Infection	Drug	Adult Dosage*	Pediatric Dosage*
Drugs of choice:	Steroids for severe symptoms		
	plus mebendazole[7,73]	200-400 mg tid x 3d, then 400-500 mg tid x 10d	

TRICHOMONIASIS (*Trichomonas vaginalis*)

Infection	Drug	Adult Dosage*	Pediatric Dosage*
Drug of choice:[74]	Metronidazole[3]	2 grams once or 250 mg tid orally x 7d	15 mg/kg/d orally in 3 doses x 7d
OR	Tinidazole[4]	2 grams once	50 mg/kg once (max. 2 grams)

TRICHOSTRONGYLUS infection

Infection	Drug	Adult Dosage*	Pediatric Dosage*
Drug of choice:	Pyrantel pamoate[7]	11 mg/kg once (max. 1 gram)	11 mg/kg once (max. 1 gram)
Alternative:	Mebendazole[7]	100 mg bid x 3d	100 mg bid x 3d
OR	Albendazole	400 mg once	400 mg once

TRICHURIASIS (*Trichuris trichiura*, whipworm)

Infection	Drug	Adult Dosage*	Pediatric Dosage*
Drug of choice:	Mebendazole	100 mg bid x 3d	100 mg bid x 3d
OR	Albendazole	400 mg once[75]	400 mg once[75]

TRYPANOSOMIASIS

T. cruzi (South American trypanosomiasis, Chagas' disease)

Infection	Drug	Adult Dosage*	Pediatric Dosage*
Drug of choice:	Nifurtimox[2,76]	8-10 mg/kg/d orally in 4 doses x 120d	1-10 yrs: 15-20 mg/kg/d in 4 doses x 90d; 11-16 yrs: 12.5-15 mg/kg/d in 4 doses x 90d
Alternative:	Benznidazole[77]	5-7 mg/kg/d x 30-120d	

TRYPANOSOMIASIS (*continued*)

T. brucei gambiense; T. b. rhodesiense (African trypanosomiasis, sleeping sickness)

hemolymphatic stage

Infection	Drug	Adult Dosage*	Pediatric Dosage*
Drug of choice:	Suramin[2]	100-200 mg (test dose) IV, then 1 gram IV on days 1,3,7,14, and 21	20 mg/kg on days 1,3,7,14, and 21
OR	Eflornithine	see footnote 78	
Alternative:	Pentamidine isethionate[7]	4 mg/kg/d IM x 10d	4 mg/kg/d IM x 10d

late disease with CNS involvement

Infection	Drug	Adult Dosage*	Pediatric Dosage*
Drug of choice:	Melarsoprol[2,79]	2-3.6 mg/kg/d IV x 3 doses; after 1 wk 3.6 mg/kg per day IV x 3 doses; repeat again after 10-21 days	18-25 mg/kg total over 1 month; initial dose of 0.36 mg/kg IV, increasing gradually to max. 3.6 mg/kg at intervals of 1-5d for total of 9-10 doses
OR	Eflornithine	see footnote 78	
Alternatives:	Tryparsamide	One injection of 30 mg/kg (max. 2g) IV every 5d to total of 12 injections; may be repeated after 1 month	
	plus suramin[2]	One injection of 10 mg/kg IV every 5d to total of 12 injections; may be repeated after 1 month	

VISCERAL LARVA MIGRANS[80]

Infection	Drug	Adult Dosage*	Pediatric Dosage*
Drug of choice:[81]	Diethylcarbamazine[7]	6 mg/kg/d in 3 doses x 7-10d	6 mg/kg/d in 3 doses x 7-10d
Alternatives:	Thiabendazole[7]	50 mg/kg/d in 2 doses x 5d (max. 3 grams/d)[11]	50 mg/kg/d in 2 doses x 5d (max. 3 grams /d)[11]
	Mebendazole[7]	100-200 mg bid x 5d[82]	

Whipworm, see TRICHURIASIS

Wuchereria bancrofti, see FILARIASIS

* The letter d stands for day.

1. Dosage and duration of administration should not be exceeded because of possibility of causing optic neuritis; maximum dosage is 2 grams/day.

2. In the USA, this drug is available from the CDC Drug Service, Centers for Disease Control, Atlanta, Georgia 30333; telephone: 404-639-3670 (evenings, weekends, and holidays: 404-639-2888).

3. Metronidazole is carcinogenic in rodents and mutagenic in bacteria; it should generally not be given to pregnant women, particularly in the first trimester.

4. A nitroimidazole similar to metronidazole, but not marketed in the USA; tinidazole appears to be at least as effective as metronidazole and better tolerated. Ornidazole, a similar drug, is also used outside the USA.

5. Contraindicated in pregnancy

6. One patient with a *Naegleria* infection was successfully treated with amphotericin B, miconazole, and rifampin (JS Seidel et al, N Engl J Med, 306:346, 1982).

7. An approved drug, but considered investigational for this condition by the U.S. Food and Drug Administration.

8. Strains of *Acanthamoeba* isolated from fatal granulomatous amebic encephalitis are usually sensitive *in vitro* to pentamidine, ketoconazole (*Nizoral*), 5-fluorocytosine, and (less so) to amphotericin B (RJ Duma et al, Antimicrob Agents Chemother, 10:370, 1976). For treatment of keratitis caused by *Acanthamoeba*, concurrent topical use of 0.1% propamidine isethionate (*Brolene* – Rhône-Poulenc Rorer, Canada) plus neosporin, or oral itraconazole (*Sporanox* – Janssen) plus topical miconazole, has been successful (MB Moore and JP McCulley, Br J Ophthalmol, 73:271, 1989; Y Ishibashi et al, Am J Ophthalmol, 109:121, 1990).

9. Effectiveness documented only in animals

10. Most patients recover spontaneously without antiparasitic drug therapy. Analgesics, corticosteroids, and careful removal of CSF at frequent intervals can relieve symptoms (J Koo et al, Rev Infect Dis, 10:1155, 1988). Albendazole, levamisole (*Ergamisol*), or ivermectin has also been used successfully in animals.

11. This dose is likely to be toxic and may have to be decreased.

12. Azithromycin (*Zithromax*) 150 mg/kg plus quinine has been reported to cure an infection with *B. divergens* (D Raoult et al, Ann Intern Med, 107:944, 1987).

13. Not recommended for children less than eight years old.

14. Drugs that could be tried include diethylcarbamazine, levamisole, and fenbendazole (KR Kazacos, J Am Vet Med Assoc, 195:894, 1989) and ivermectin. Steroid therapy may be helpful, especially in eye or CNS infection. Ocular baylisascariasis has been treated successfully using laser therapy to destroy intraretinal larvae.

15. Clinical significance of these organisms is controversial, but metronidazole 750 mg tid x 10d or iodoquinol 650 mg tid x 20d anecdotally have been reported to be effective (RA Miller and BH Minshew, Rev Infect Dis, 10:930, 1988; PW Doyle et al, J Clin Microbiol, 28:116, 1990).

16. Infection is self-limited in immunocompetent patients. In AIDS patients with large-volume intractable diarrhea, octreotide (*Sandostatin*) 300–500 µg tid subcutaneously may control the diarrhea, but not the infection (DJ Cook et al, Ann Intern Med, 108:708, 1988). Paromomycin may be helpful in some patients (K Clezy et al, AIDS, 5:1146, 1991; J Gathe, Jr et al, Int Conf AIDS, 6:384, 1990).

17. Albendazole 200 mg bid x 3 days has also been reported to be effective (SK Jones et al, Br J Dermatol, 122:99, 1990).

18. Not curative, but decreases inflammation and facilitates removing the worm. Mebendazole 400-800 mg/d for 6d has been reported to kill the worm directly.

19. A single dose of ivermectin, 25–200 µg/kg, has been reported to be effective for treatment of microfilaremia due to *W. bancrofti* and *M. ozzardi* (EA Ottesen et al, N Engl J Med, 322:1113, 1990; M Sabry et al, Trans R Soc Trop Med Hyg, 85:640, 1991; TB Nutman et al, J Infect Dis, 156:662, 1987).

20. Antihistamines or corticosteroids may be required to decrease allergic reactions due to disintegration of microfilariae in treatment of filarial infections, especially those caused by *Loa loa*. Diethylcarbamazine should be administered with special caution in heavy infections with *Loa loa* because it may provoke an encephalopathy (B Carme et al, Am J Trop Med Hyg, 44:684, 1991). Apheresis has been reported to be effective in lowering microfilarial counts in patients heavily infected with loiasis. Diethylcarbamazine, 300 mg once weekly, has been recommended for prevention of loiasis (TB Nutman et al, N Engl J Med, 319:752, 1988).

21. For patients with no microfilaremia in the blood or skin, full doses can be given from day one.

22. Ivermectin may also be effective.

23. Unlike infections with other flukes, *hepatica* infections may not respond to praziquantel. Limited data, however, indicate that triclabendazole (*Fasinex*), a veterinary fasciolide, is safe and effective in a single oral dose of 10 mg/kg (L Loutan et al, Lancet, 2:383, 1989).

141

24. Not absorbed; may be useful for treatment of giardiasis in pregnant women.

25. In sulfonamide-sensitive patients, such as some patients with AIDS, pyrimethamine 50-75 mg daily has been effective (LM Weiss et al, Ann Intern Med, 109:474, 1988). In immunocompromised patients, it may be necessary to continue therapy indefinitely.

26. Limited data indicate that ketoconazole, 400 to 600 mg daily for four to eight weeks, may be effective for treatment of cutaneous and mucosal leishmaniasis (RE Saenz et al, Am J Med, 89:147, 1990).

27. May be repeated or continued. A longer duration may be needed for some forms of visceral leishmaniasis.

28. Recent studies indicate that stibogluconate (pentavalent antimony)-resistant L. donovani may respond to recombinant human gamma interferon in addition to antimony (R Badaro et al, N Engl J Med, 322:16, 1990), pentamidine followed by a course of antimony (CP Thakur et al, Am J Trop Med Hyg, 45:435, 1991), or ketoconazole (JP Wali et al, Lancet, 336:810, 1990). Recently, liposomal encapsulated amphotericin B (AmBisome, Vestar, San Dimas, CA) was used successfully to treat multiple-drug-resistant visceral leishmaniasis (RN Davidson et al, Lancet, 337:1061, 1991).

29. Application of heat 39°C to 42°C directly to the lesion for 20 to 32 hours over a period of 10 to 12 days has been reported to be effective in cutaneous L. tropica (JA Neva et al, Am J Trop Med Hyg, 33:800, 1984).

30. For infestation of eyelashes with crab lice, use petrolatum.

31. FDA-approved only for head lice

32. Some consultants recommend a second application one week later to kill hatching progeny. Seizures have been reported in association with the use of lindane. Do not use higher than recommended doses and avoid warm baths before application (IM Tenenbein, J Am Geriatr Soc, 39:394, 1991). Prolonged use of lindane has been associated with aplastic anemia (AE Rauch et al, Arch Intern Med, 150:2393, 1990).

33. If chloroquine phosphate is not available, hydroxychloroquine sulfate is as effective; 400 mg of hydroxychloroquine sulfate is equivalent to 500 mg of chloroquine phosphate.

34. In P. falciparum malaria, if the patient has not shown a response to conventional doses of chloroquine in 48-72 hours, parasitic resistance to his drug should be considered. P. vivax with decreased susceptibility to chloroquine has been reported from Papua New Guinea (KH Rieckmann et al, Lancet, 2:1183, 1989) and from Indonesia (IK Schwartz et al, N Engl J Med, 324:927, 1991). Intramuscular injection of chloroquine can be painful and has been reported to cause abscesses.

35. A recent study found artemether, a Chinese drug, effective for parenteral treatment of severe malaria in children (NJ White et al, Lancet, 339:317, 1992).

36. Some experts consider quinidine more effective than quinine. EKG monitoring is necessary to detect arrhythmias. Oral drugs should be substituted as soon as possible.

37. Not available in the USA. P. falciparum infections with a high parasitemia may require a loading dose of 20 mg/kg (NJ White et al, Am J Trop Med Hyg, 32:1, 1983). IV administration of quinine dihydrochloride can be hazardous; constant monitoring of the pulse and blood pressure is necessary to detect arrhythmia or hypotension. Use of parenteral quinine may also lead to severe hypoglycemia; blood glucose should be monitored. Oral drugs should be substituted as soon as possible.

38. Chloroquine-resistant P. falciparum infections have been reported in all areas that have malaria except Central America north of Panama, Mexico, Haiti, the Dominican Republic, and the Middle East (including Egypt). In pregnancy, chloroquine prophylaxis has been used extensively and safely, but the safety of other prophylactic antimalarial agents in pregnancy is unclear. Therefore, travel during pregnancy to chloroquine-resistant areas should be discouraged. For chloroquine-resistant parasitemia > 10%, exchange transfusion has been used (KD Miller et al, N Engl J Med, 321:65, 1989; M Saddler et al; K Vachon et al; KD Miller et al, N Engl J Med, 322:58, 1990).

39. Chloroquine-resistant falciparum malaria acquired outside of Southeast Asia, East Africa, Bangladesh, Oceania and the Amazon basin is likely to respond to quinine (or quinidine) plus pyrimethamine-sulfadoxine. In pregnancy, quinine (or quinidine) plus clindamycin is a reasonable alternative.

40. Although quinine will usually control an attack of resistant falciparum malaria, in a substantial number of infections from Southeast Asia, Bangladesh, Oceania, East Africa, and the Amazon region it fails to prevent recurrence. In these regions, there may be pyrimethamine-sulfadoxine resistance, and addition of tetracycline or clindamycin may decrease the rate of recurrence.

41. In Southeast Asia, there is a relative increase in resistance to quinine and the usual treatment dose should be extended to seven days.

42. Fansidar tablets contain 25 mg of pyrimethamine and 500 mg of sulfadoxine.

43. At this dosage, adverse effects including nausea, vomiting, diarrhea, dizziness, disturbed sense of balance, toxic psychosis, and seizures can occur. Mefloquine is teratogenic in animals. It should not be given together with quinine or quinidine, and caution is required in using quinine or quinidine to treat patients with malaria who have taken mefloquine for prophylaxis. The pediatric dosage has not been approved by the FDA.

44. In the USA, a 250-mg tablet of mefloquine contains 228 mg of mefloquine base. Outside the USA, each 274-mg tablet contains 250 mg base.

45. Outside the USA, the manufacturer recommends dividing the 1250-mg dose into 750 mg dose followed 6-8 hours later by 500 mg (ID Kingston, Med J Aust, 153:235, 1990).

46. NJ White, Eur J Clin Pharm, 34:1, 1988

47. May be effective in multiple-drug-resistant *falciparum* malaria (ed., Lancet, 2:537, 1989). Failures in treatment of multiple-drug-resistant malaria have, however, been reported (GD Shanks et al, Am J Trop Med Hyg, 45:488, 1991). For patients with minimal previous exposure to malaria, a second course of therapy is recommended one week after the first courses.

48. Primaquine phosphate can cause hemolytic anemia, especially in patients whose red cells are deficient in glucose-6-phosphate dehydrogenase. This deficiency is most common in Blacks, Orientals, and Mediterranean peoples. Patients should be screened for G-6-PD deficiency before treatment. Primaquine should not be used during pregnancy.

49. At present, no drug regimen guarantees protection against malaria. If fever develops within a year (particularly within the first two months) after travel to malarious areas, travelers should be advised to seek medical attention. Insect repellents, insecticide-impregnated bed nets, and proper clothing are important adjuncts for malaria prophylaxis.

50. For prevention of attack after departure from areas where *P. vivax* and *P. ovale* are endemic, which includes almost all areas where malaria is found (except Haiti), some experts in addition prescribe primaquine phosphate 15 mg base (26.3 mg)/d or, for children, 0.3 mg base/kg/d during the last two weeks of prophylaxis. Others prefer to avoid the toxicity of primaquine and rely on surveillance to detect cases when they occur, particularly when exposure was limited or doubtful. See also footnote 48.

51. For prophylaxis where both chloroquine and pyrimethamine/sulfadoxine resistance coexist, mefloquine is the usual drug of choice. In mefloquine-resistant areas, such as Thailand, doxycycline is recommended.

52. The pediatric dosage has not been approved by the FDA, and the drug has not been approved for use during pregnancy. Women should take contraceptive precautions while taking mefloquine and for two months after the last dose. Mefloquine is not recommended for children weighing less than 15 kg, or for patients taking beta-blockers, calcium-channel blockers, or other drugs that may prolong or otherwise alter cardiac conduction. Patients with a history of seizures or psychiatric disorders and those whose occupation requires fine coordination or spatial discrimination should probably avoid mefloquine (Medical Letter, 32:13, 1990).

53. Beginning one week before travel and continuing weekly for the duration of stay and for four weeks after leaving.

54. Beginning one day before travel and continuing for the duration of stay and for four weeks after leaving. The FDA considers use of tetracyclines as antimalarials to be investigational. Use of tetracyclines is contraindicated in pregnancy and in children less than eight years old. Physicians who prescribe doxycycline as malaria chemoprophylaxis should advise patients to use an appropriate sunscreen (Medical Letter, 31:59, 1989) to minimize the possibility of a photosensitivity reaction and should warn women that *Candida* vaginitis is a frequent adverse effect.

55. Resistance to *Fansidar* should be anticipated in Southeast Asia, Bangladesh, Oceania, the Amazon basin, and in east Africa. Use of *Fansidar* is contraindicated in patients with a history of sulfonamide or pyrimethamine intolerance. In pregnancy at term and in infants less than two months old, pyrimethamine-sulfadoxine may cause hyperbilirubinemia.

56. Proguanil (*Paludrine* – Ayerst, Canada; ICI, England), which is not available in the USA but is widely available overseas, is recommended mainly for use in Africa south of the Sahara. Failures in prophylaxis with chloroquine and proguanil have, however, been reported in travelers to Kenya (AJ Barnes, Lancet, 338:1338, 1991)

57. In a limited number of patients with severe diarrhea, albendazole 400 mg bid for 4-6 weeks was reported to produce remission (C Blanchard et al, Int J Cancer, 48:296, 1991). Octreotide (*Sandostatin*, Sandoz) has provided symptomatic relief (JP Cello et al, Ann Intern Med, 115:705, 1991).

58. A keratopath. In an AIDS patient was treated successfully with surgical debridement, topical antibiotics, and itraconazole (*Sporanox* – Janssen) (RW Yee et al, Ophthalmology, 98:196, 1991).

59. AIDS patients should be treated for 21 days. In moderate or severe PCP with room air PO₂ ≤70 mmHg or Aa gradient ≥35 mmHg prednisone should also be used (Medical Letter, 33:101, 1991).

60. Assay for G-6-PD deficiency recommended at start of therapy.

61. Each double-strength tablet contains 160 mg TMP and 800 mg SMX

62. Contraindicated in pregnancy. Neuropsychiatric disturbances and seizures have been reported in some patients (H Stokvis et al, Am J Trop Med Hyg, 35:330, 1986).

63. In east Africa, the dose should be increased to 30 mg/kg, and in Egypt and South Africa, 30 mg/kg/d x 2d. Some experts recommend 40-60 mg/kg over 2-3 days in all of Africa (KC Shekhar, Drugs, 42:379, 1991).

64. In immunocompromised patients it may be necessary to continue therapy or use other agents.

65. In disseminated strongyloidiasis, thiabendazole therapy should be continued for at least five days.

143

66. With a fatty meal to enhance absorption. Some patients may benefit from or require surgical resection of cysts (RK Tompkins, Mayo Clin Proc, 66:1281, 1991). Praziquantel may also be useful preoperatively or in case of spill during surgery.

67. Surgical excision is the only reliable means of treatment, although some reports have suggested use of albendazole or mebendazole (JF Wilson et al, Am J Trop Med Hyg, 37:162, 1987; A Davis et al, Bull WHO, 64:383, 1986).

68. Corticosteroids should be given for two to three days before and during drug therapy. Any cysticercoidal drug may cause irreparable damage when used to treat ocular or spinal cysts, even when corticosteroids are used.

69. In ocular toxoplasmosis, corticosteroids should also be used for anti-inflammatory effect on the eyes.

70. Pyrimethamine is teratogenic in animals. To prevent hematological toxicity from pyrimethamine, it is advisable to give leucovorin (folinic acid), about 10 mg/day, either by injection or orally. Some clinicians use pyrimethamine 50 to 100 mg daily after a loading dose of 200 mg with a sulfonamide also to treat CNS toxoplasmosis in patients with AIDS and, when sulfonamide sensitivity developed, have given clindamycin 1.8 to 2.4 g/d in divided doses instead of the sulfonamide. In AIDS patients, chronic suppressive treatment with lower dosage should continue indefinitely (Medical Letter, 34:95, 1991; B Danneman et al, Ann Intern Med, 116:33, Jan 1, 1992).

71. Congenitally infected newborns should be treated with pyrimethamine every two or three days and a sulfonamide daily for about one year (JS Remington and G Desmonts in JS Remington and JO Klein, eds, *Infectious Disease of the Fetus and Newborn Infant*, 3rd ed, Philadelphia:Saunders, 1990, page 89).

72. For treatment during pregnancy, continue the drug until delivery.

73. Albendazole or flubendazole (not available in the USA) may also be effective for this indication.

74. Sexual partners should be treated simultaneously. Outside the USA, ornidazole has also been used for this condition. Metronidazole-resistant strains have been reported; higher doses of metronidazole for longer periods are sometimes effective against these strains (J Lossick, Rev Infect Dis, 12:S665, 1990).

75. In heavy infection it may be necessary to extend therapy for 3 days.

76. The addition of gamma interferon to nifurtimox for 20 days in a limited number of patients and in experimental animals appears to have shortened the acute phase of Chagas' disease (RE McCabe et al, J Infect Dis, 163:912, 1991).

77. Limited data

78. In T. b. *gambiense* infections, eflornithine is highly effective in both the hemolymphatic and CNS stages. Its effectiveness in T. b. *rhodesiense* infections has been variable. Some clinicians have given 400 mg/kg/d IV in 4 divided doses for 14 days, followed by oral treatment with 300 mg/kg/d for 3-4 wks (F Doua et al, Am J Trop Med Hyg, 37:525, 1987).

79. In frail patients, begin with as little as 18 mg and increase the dose progressively. Pretreatment with suramin has been advocated for debilitated patients. Corticosteroids have been used to prevent arsenical encephalopathy (J Pepin et al, Lancet, 1:1246, 1989)

80. For severe symptoms or eye involvement, corticosteroids can be used in addition.

81. Ivermectin or albendazole may also be effective (D Stürchler et al, Ann Trop Med Parasitol, 83:473, 1989).

82. One report of a cure using 1 gram tid for 21 days has been published (A Bakhti, Ann Intern Med, 100:463, 1984).

144

ADVERSE EFFECTS OF SOME ANTIPARASITIC DRUGS*

ALBENDAZOLE *(Zentel)*
Occasional: diarrhea; abdominal pain; migration of *ascaris* through mouth and nose
Rare: leukopenia; alopecia; increased serum transaminase activity

BENZNIDAZOLE *(Rochagan)*
Frequent: allergic rash; dose-dependent polyneuropathy; gastrointestinal disturbances; psychic disturbances

BITHIONOL *(Bitin)*
Frequent: photosensitivity reactions; vomiting; diarrhea; abdominal pain; urticaria
Rare: leukopenia; toxic hepatitis

CHLOROQUINE HCl and CHLOROQUINE PHOSPHATE *(Aralen, and others)*
Occasional: pruritus; vomiting; headache; confusion; depigmentation of hair; skin eruptions; corneal opacity; weight loss; partial alopecia; extraocular muscle palsies; exacerbation of psoriasis, eczema, and other exfoliative dermatoses; myalgias; photophobia
Rare: irreversible retinal injury (especially when total dosage exceeds 100 grams); discoloration of nails and mucus membranes; nerve-type deafness; peripheral neuropathy and myopathy; heart block; blood dyscrasias; hematemesis

CROTAMITON *(Eurax)*
Occasional: rash; conjunctivitis

DEHYDROEMETINE
Frequent: cardiac arrhythmias; precordial pain; muscle weakness; cellulitis at site of injection
Occasional: diarrhea; vomiting; peripheral neuropathy; heart failure; headache; dyspnea

DIETHYLCARBAMAZINE CITRATE USP *(Hetrazan)*
Frequent: severe allergic or febrile reactions in patients with microfilaria in the blood or the skin; GI disturbances
Rare: encephalopathy

DILOXANIDE FUROATE *(Furamide)*
Frequent: flatulence
Occasional: nausea; vomiting; diarrhea
Rare: diplopia; dizziness; urticaria; pruritus

EFLORNITHINE *(Difluoromethylornithine, DFMO, Ornidyl)*
Frequent: anemia; leukopenia
Occasional: diarrhea; thrombocytopenia; seizures
Rare: hearing loss

FLUBENDAZOLE – similar to mebendazole

FURAZOLIDONE *(Furoxone)*
Frequent: nausea; vomiting
Occasional: allergic reactions, including pulmonary infiltration, hypotension, urticaria, fever, vesicular rash; hypoglycemia; headache
Rare: hemolytic anemia in G-6-PD deficiency and neonates; disulfiram-like reaction with alcohol; MAO-inhibitor interactions; polyneuritis

HALOFANTRINE *(Halfan)*
Occasional: diarrhea; abdominal pain; pruritus

IODOQUINOL *(Yodoxin)*
Occasional: rash; acne; slight enlargement of the thyroid gland; nausea; diarrhea; cramps; anal pruritus
Rare: optic atrophy, loss of vision, peripheral neuropathy after prolonged use in high dosage (for months); iodine sensitivity

IVERMECTIN *(Mectizan)*
Occasional: Mazzotti-type reaction seen in onchocerciasis, including fever, pruritus, tender lymph nodes, headache, and joint and bone pain
Rare: hypotension

LINDANE *(Kwell; and others)*
Occasional: eczematous rash; conjunctivitis
Rare: convulsions; aplastic anemia

MALATHION *(Ovide)*
Occasional: local irritation

MEBENDAZOLE *(Vermox)*
Occasional: diarrhea; abdominal pain; migration of *ascaris* through mouth and nose
Rare: leukopenia; agranulocytosis; hypospermia

MEFLOQUINE *(Lariam)*
Frequent: vertigo; lightheadedness; nausea; other gastrointestinal disturbances; nightmares; visual disturbances; headache
Occasional: confusion
Rare: psychosis; hypotension; convulsions; coma

MEGLUMINE ANTIMONIATE *(Glucantime)* Similar to stibogluconate sodium

MELARSOPROL *(Arsobal)*
Frequent: myocardial damage; albuminuria; hypertension; colic; Herxheimer-type reaction; encephalopathy; vomiting; peripheral neuropathy
Rare: shock

METRONIDAZOLE *(Flagyl, and others)*
Frequent: nausea; headache; dry mouth; metallic taste
Occasional: vomiting; diarrhea; insomnia; weakness; stomatitis; vertigo; paresthesias; rash; dark urine; urethral burning; disulfiram-like reaction with alcohol
Rare: seizures; encephalopathy; pseudomembranous colitis; ataxia; leukopenia; peripheral neuropathy; pancreatitis

NICLOSAMIDE *(Niclocide)*
Occasional: nausea; abdominal pain

NIFURTIMOX *(Lampit)*
Frequent: anorexia; vomiting; weight loss; loss of memory; sleep disorders; tremor; paresthesias; weakness; polyneuritis
Rare: convulsions; fever; pulmonary infiltrates and pleural effusion

ORNIDAZOLE *(Tiberal)*
Occasional: dizziness; headache; gastrointestinal disturbances
Rare: reversible peripheral neuropathy

OXAMNIQUINE *(Vansil)*
Occasional: headache; fever; dizziness; somnolence; nausea; diarrhea; rash; insomnia; hepatic enzyme changes; ECG changes; EEG changes; orange-red discoloration of urine
Rare: seizures; neuropsychiatric disturbances

PAROMOMYCIN *(Humatin)*
Frequent: GI disturbances
Rare: eighth-nerve damage (mainly auditory); renal damage

PENTAMIDINE ISETHIONATE *(Pentam 300, NebuPent)*
Frequent: hypotension; hypoglycemia often followed by diabetes mellitus; vomiting; blood dyscrasias; renal damage; pain at injection site; GI disturbances
Occasional: may aggravate diabetes; shock; hypocalcemia; liver damage; cardiotoxicity; delirium; rash
Rare: Herxheimer-type reaction; anaphylaxis; acute pancreatitis; hyperkalemia

145

PERMETHRIN *(Nix, Elimite)*
Occasional: burning; stinging; numbness; increased pruritus; pain; edema; erythema; rash

PRAZIQUANTEL *(Biltricide)*
Frequent: malaise; headache; dizziness
Occasional: sedation; abdominal discomfort; fever; sweating; nausea; eosinophilia; fatigue
Rare: pruritus; rash

PRIMAQUINE PHOSPHATE USP
Frequent: hemolytic anemia in G-6-PD deficiency
Occasional: neutropenia; GI disturbances; methemoglobinemia in G-6-PD deficiency
Rare: CNS symptoms; hypertension; arrhythmias

PROGUANIL *(Paludrine)*
Occasional: oral ulceration; hair loss; scaling of palms and soles
Rare: hematuria (with large doses); vomiting; abdominal pain; diarrhea (with large doses)

PYRANTEL PAMOATE *(Antiminth)*
Occasional: GI disturbances; headache; dizziness; rash; fever

PYRETHRINS and PIPERONYL BUTOXIDE *(RID, others)*
Occasional: allergic reactions

PYRIMETHAMINE USP *(Daraprim)*
Occasional: blood dyscrasias; folic acid deficiency
Rare: rash; vomiting; convulsions; shock; possibly pulmonary eosinophilia

QUINACRINE HCl USP *(Atabrine)*
Frequent: dizziness; headache; vomiting; diarrhea
Occasional: yellow staining of skin; toxic psychosis; insomnia; bizarre dreams; blood dyscrasias; urticaria; blue and black nail pigmentation; psoriasis-like rash
Rare: acute hepatic necrosis; convulsions; severe exfoliative dermatitis; ocular effects similar to those caused by chloroquine

QUININE DIHYDROCHLORIDE and SULFATE
Frequent: cinchonism (tinnitus, headache, nausea, abdominal pain, visual disturbance)
Occasional: deafness; hemolytic anemia; other blood dyscrasias; photosensitivity reactions; hypoglycemia; arrhythmias; hypotension; drug fever
Rare: blindness; sudden death if injected too rapidly

SPIRAMYCIN *(Rovamycine)*
Occasional: GI disturbances
Rare: allergic reactions

STIBOGLUCONATE SODIUM *(Pentostam)*
Frequent: muscle pain and joint stiffness; nausea; transaminase elevations; T-wave flattening or inversion
Occasional: weakness; colic; liver damage; bradycardia; leukopenia
Rare: diarrhea; rash; pruritus; myocardial damage; hemolytic anemia; renal damage; shock; sudden death

SURAMIN SODIUM *(Germanin)*
Frequent: vomiting; pruritus; urticaria; paresthesias; hyperesthesia of hands and feet; photophobia; peripheral neuropathy
Occasional: kidney damage; blood dyscrasias; shock; optic atrophy

THIABENDAZOLE *(Mintezol)*
Frequent: nausea; vomiting; vertigo
Occasional: leukopenia; crystalluria; rash; hallucinations; olfactory disturbance; erythema multiforme; Stevens-Johnson syndrome
Rare: shock; tinnitus; intrahepatic cholestasis; convulsions; angioneurotic edema

TINIDAZOLE *(Fasigyn)*
Occasional: metallic taste; nausea; vomiting; rash

TRIMETREXATE (with "leucovorin rescue")
Occasional: rash; peripheral neuropathy; bone marrow depression; increased serum aminotransferase concentrations

TRYPARSAMIDE
Frequent: nausea; vomiting
Occasional: impaired vision; optic atrophy; fever; exfoliative dermatitis; allergic reactions; tinnitus

Table 1: HIV INFECTION AND AIDS

INDICATOR CONDITIONS IN CASE DEFINITION OF AIDS (1987-92, ADULTS)

Candidiasis, of esophagus, trachea, bronchi or lungs
Coccidioidomycosis, extrapulmonary *
Cryptococcosis, extrapulmonary
Cryptosporidiosis with diarrhea > 1 month
Cytomegalovirus of any organ other than liver, spleen or lymph nodes
Herpes simplex with mucocutaneous ulcer > 1 month or bronchitis,
    pneumonitis, esophagitis
Histoplasmosis, extrapulmonary*
HIV-associated dementia*: Disabling cognitive and/or motor dysfunction
    interfering with occupation or activities of daily living
HIV-associated wasting*: Involuntary weight loss > 10% of baseline plus
    chronic diarrhea ($\geq$ 2 loose stools/day $\geq$ 30 days) or chronic weakness and
    documented enigmatic fever $\geq$ 30 days
Isosporosis with diarrhea > 1 mo*
Kaposi sarcoma in patient under 60 yrs (or over 60 yrs*)
Lymphoma of brain in patient under 60 yrs (or over 60 yrs*)
Lymphoma, non-Hodgkins of B cell or unknown immunologic phenotype and
    histology showing small, noncleaved lymphoma or immunoblastic sarcoma
<u>Mycobacterium avium</u> or <u>M</u>. <u>kansasii</u>, disseminated
<u>Mycobacterium tuberculosis</u>, disseminated*
Nocardiosis*
<u>Pneumocystis carinii</u> pneumonia
Progressive multifocal leukoencephalopathy
Salmonella septicemia (non-typhoid), recurrent*
Strongyloidosis, extraintestinal
Toxoplasmosis of internal organ

---

*   Requires positive HIV serology

Table 2: PROPOSED EXPANDED AIDS SURVEILLANCE CASE DEFINITION FOR ADOLESCENTS AND ADULTS

CD4 cell Categories	Clinical Categories		
	A Asymptomatic, or PGL or Acute HIV Infection	**B** Symptomatic** (not A or C)	**C*** AIDS Indicator Condition (1987)
1) >500/cu mm	A 1	B 1	C 1
2) 200-499/cu mm	A 2	B 2	C 2
3) <200/cu mm	A 3	B 3	C 3

* All patients in the shaded categories would be reported as having AIDS based on the prior AIDS-indicator conditions (Table 1) and/or a CD4 cell count <200/cu mm.

** Includes but is not limited to bacterial infections (pneumonia, meningitis, endocarditis or sepsis); vulvovaginal candidiasis persistent >1 month and poorly responsive to treatment; thrush, oral hairy leukoplakia; severe cervical dysplasia or carcinoma; shingles with two episodes or >1 dermatome; ITP; listeriosis; nocardiosis; PID; peripheral neuropathy; constitutional symptoms such as fever (38.5°C or diarrhea for >1 month).

TABLE 3: SEROPREVALENCE RATES OF HIV IN THE U. S.

Category	Reference	Rate	Comment
Gay men	Am J Epid 126:568,1987 J AIDS 2:77,1989	14-50%	Average in MACS (5000 participants) was 36% at entry with 1% annual seroconversion rate
IV drug abusers	JAMA 261:2677,1989	1-60%	Review of 92 studies showed great variation by location: NYC: 34-61%; New Jersey: 17-29%; Boston: 28%; Puerto Rico: 45-59%; Detroit: 8-12%; San Francisco: 5-16%; Miami: 5%; New Orleans: 1%; Atlanta: 10%; Denver: 1-5%; Los Angeles: 2-5%; Minn: 1%; Annual seroconversion rate in Baltimore: 5%
Methadone clinic clients	NEJM 326:375,1992	9.2%	Eight city surveys with rates ranging from 0.7% (Seattle) to 28.6% (Newark)
Hemophilia	JAMA 253:3409,1985	Type A-70% Type B-35%	Applies to hemophiliacs who received clotting factors before 1985
Regular sex partners of HIV-infected persons	Arch Intern Med 149:645,1989 Amer J Med 85:472,1988 JAMA 266:1664,1991	0-58%	Average is 20-25% for wives of hemophiliac men with HIV infection; discordant couple study shows efficiency of transmission 20x greater for male-female transmission
Prostitutes	MMWR 36:157,1987 JAMA 263:60,1990	0-57%	Great variation by location and confounding variable of IVDU: Newark: 57%; Wash. DC: 50%; Miami: 19%; San Francisco: 6%; LA: 4%; Atlanta: 1%; Las Vegas: 0
Hospital admissions	NEJM 323:213,1990	0.1-7.8%	Average is 1.3%
College students	NEJM 323:1538,1990	0.2%	
Childbearing women	JAMA 265:1704,1991	0.15%	Highest rates were NYC: 0.58%; Wash DC: 0.55%; NJ: 0.49%; Florida: 0.45%
STD Clinic clients	STD 19:235,1992 NEJM 326:375,1992	0.5-11%	Summary of 176,439 sera from 98 STD clinics; median - 2.3%
Applicants to military	MMWR 37:67,1988 JAIDS 3:1168,1990 JAMA 265:1709,1991	0.13%	Annual seroconversion rate is 0.04%
Blood donors		0.02%	
General population	Science 253:37,1991 MMWR 30 RR-16,1990	0.4%	Based on assumed validity of one million HIV infected persons in U.S. Annual seroconversion rate based on assumption of 60,000 new infections/year is 0.02%

TABLE 4: CARE PLAN

	All patients	CD4 300-500/cu mm	CD4 100-300/cu mm	CD4< 150
Antiretroviral		AZT[a] or ddI[b]	AZT[a] or ddI[a] AZT + ddI[b] AZT + ddC[b]	AZT[a] or ddI[a] AZT + ddI[b] AZT + ddC[b]

Opportunistic infection (Prophylaxis)	Pneumovax
	PPD + : INH[a]
	Influenza vaccine[a]
			PCP prophylaxis[a]	PCP prophylaxis[a]
				Cryptococcus[b]:
				  Ketoconazole or
				  Fluconazole
				M. avium:
				  rifabutin[a] or
				  clarithromycin
				Toxoplasmosis[a]
				  TMP-SMX or
				  dapsone plus
				  pyrimethamine

[a] Efficacy established. PCP prophylaxis advocated for patients with CD4 cell count < 200/cu mm or prior PCP.

[b] Efficacy not established; clinical trials being conducted. Benefit of ddC + AZT versus AZT alone shown for CD4 cell counts as surrogate marker (Ann Intern Med 116:13,1992); efficacy of AZT + ddI is not established.

Toxoplasmosis: TMP-SMX (4-7 DS/week) appears to be effective (Ann Intern Med 117:106,1992); for patients unable to take TMP-SMX with CD4 cell count < 100-150/cu mm plus positive toxoplasmosis serology, some advocate dapsone (50 mg/day) plus pyrimethamine (50 mg/week).

TABLE 5: ANTIRETROVIRAL AGENTS: NUCLEOSIDE ANALOGS

	AZT	ddI	ddC
Indications: FDA labeling	CD4 < 500	Advanced HIV infection + prolonged therapy with AZT	CD4 count < 300 + clinical or immunologic deterioration with AZT treatment
Usual dose	500-600 mg/day	> 60 kg: 200 mg bid < 60 kg: 125 mg bid	0.75 mg tid
Oral bioavailability	60%	Tablet: 40% Tablet is 20-25% higher than powder	85%
Serum half life	1.1 hr	1.6 hr	1.2 hr
Intracellular half life	3 hr	12 hr	3 hr
CNS penetration (% serum levels)	60%	20%	20%
Elimination	Metabolized to AZT glucuronide (GAZT)	Renal excretion - 50%	Renal excretion - 70%
Major toxicity	Marrow suppression: Anemia and/or Granulocytopenia	Pancreatitis (Peripheral neuropathy)	Peripheral neuropathy (Pancreatitis)

Table 6. MANAGEMENT OF OPPORTUNISTIC INFECTIONS IN PATIENTS WITH HIV INFECTION

	Preferred	Alternative	Comment
PROTOZOA			
Pneumocystis carinii			
Acute infection	Trimethoprim (15 mg/kg/day) + sulfamethoxazole (75 mg/kg/day) po or IV x 21 days in 3-4 daily doses	Pentamidine (4 mg/kg/day) IV (or IM) x 21 days;	Some recommend trimethoprim-sulfamethoxazole/dapsone in dose of 20 mg/kg/day (trimethoprim)
		Trimethoprim (15 mg/kg/day) po or IV + dapsone* (100 mg/day) x 21 days (100 mg/day) x 21 days	Side effects to sulfonamide (rash, fever, leukopenia, hepatitis, etc.) most common at 1-2 wks.
		Atovaquone*** 750 mg tid po with food x 21 days (mild to moderate disease)	
		Clindamycin (600 mg IV q6h or 300-450 mg po q6h) + primaquine* (15 mg based po/day) x 21 days	
		Atovaquone*** (750 mg po tid with food) x 21 days available by: 1) treatment IND for persons with mild-moderately severe PCP in patients intolerant of sulfa and 2) open label for severe PCP for persons intolerant or unresponsive to TMP-SMX + pentamidine	Patients with moderately severe or severe disease (pO₂ <70 mmHg) should receive corticosteroids (prednisone, 40 mg po bid x 5 days, then 40 mg qd x 5 days, then 20 mg/day to completion of treatment). Side effects include CNS toxicity, thrush, H. simplex infection, tuberculosis and other OIs
Prophylaxis	Trimethoprim (2.5-5 mg/kg) + sulfamethoxazole po as 1 DS qd or 3x/wk	Aerosolized pentamidine (300 mg) q month (300 mg) q month via Respirgard II nebulizer	Prophylaxis is indicated for any HIV infected patient with a history of Pneumocystis pneumonia or a CD4 count < 200/cu mm
		Dapsone* 25-100 mg po/day or 100 mg 2x/wk (usually 50 mg po/day)	
		Pyrimethamine (25 mg) + sulfadoxine (500 mg)-2x/wk (1-2 Fansidar/wk)	Serious reactions including death from Stevens-Johnson syndrome have been reported with Fansidar; efficacy not established
		Pentamidine (4 mg/kg) IM or IV q 2 wks	Efficacy not established

(continued)

	Preferred	Alternative	Comment
Toxoplasma encephalitis Acute infection	Pyrimethamine (100-200 mg loading dose, then 50-100 mg/day) po x 6 wks + folinic acid (10 mg/day) po + sulfadiazine or trisulfapyrimidines (4-8 gm/day) po for at least 6 wks	Pyrimethamine + folinic acid (prior doses) + clindamycin (600 mg) IV q6-8h for at least 6 wks	All patients who respond to primary therapy should receive life-long suppressive therapy Repeat MRI or CT scan at 2 weeks
		Atovaquone*** 750 mg 4x/day po with food	Relative merits of alternative regimens for patients who have become intolerant to or have failed pyrimethamine + sulfadiazine, are unknown
		Azithromycin*** (1800 mg po/day x 6 wks 1200 mg po/day x 6 wks, then 600 mg/day) or Atovaquone*** for patients who fail or were intolerant of standard treatment; both preferrably used in combination with pyrimethamine	Corticosteroids if significant edema/mass effect (Decadron, 4 mg po or IV q6h)
Suppressive therapy	Pyrimethamine (25-50 mg) po q d plus folinic acid (5 mg/day) or sulfadiazine or trisulfapyrimidines (2-4 gm/day) po qid	Pyrimethamine (25-50 mg) po qd plus clindamycin (300-450 mg) po q6-8h	Suppressive treatment for toxoplasmosis will also prevent PCP Possibly effective agents include atovaquone, trimethoprim-sulfa, azithromycin, clarithromycin and trimetrexate
Prophylaxis	Trimethoprim-sulfamethoxazole (1DS 4x/wk - 1 DS qd) or Dapsone* (50 mg/day) + pyrimethamine(50 mg/wk)	Pyrimethamine (25 mg) po qid (see comment)	Sometimes advocated for patients with positive toxoplasmosis serology + CD4 count <150/mm³ Pyrimethamine (25 mg 3x/wk) is ineffective; efficacy of 25 mg po qd is not established
Cryptosporidia	Symptomatic treatment with nutritional supplements and anti-diarrheal agents (Lomotil, Loperamide, paragoric, etc)	Octeotide (Sandostatin) 50-200 μg tid SC or IV at 1 mcg/hr Paromomycin 250 mg po qid	Efficacy of spiramycin, paromomycin and octreo-tide not established; other possibly effective agents: DFMO, bovine colostrum and transfer factor. Non-steroidal anti-inflammatory agents sometimes useful.
		Azithromycin*** (1200 mg po 1st day, then 600 mg/day x 27 days, then 300 mg/day)	Nutritional supplements often required; for severe cases: Vivonex, TEN or parenteral hyperalimentation

(continued)

153

	Preferred	Alternative	Comment
Isospora Acute infection	Trimethoprim (5 mg/kg) + sulfamethoxazole po bid (2 DS po bid or 1 DS tid) po x 2-4 wks	Pyrimethamine (50-75 mg po/day) + folinic acid, (5-10 mg/day) x 1 mo	Duration of high dose therapy is not well defined
Suppressive treatment	Trimethoprim (2.5-5.0 mg/kg) + sulfamethoxazole (1-2 DS/day) po	Pyrimethamine (25 mg) + sulfadoxine (500 mg) po q wk (1 Fansidar/wk); pyrimethamine, 25 mg + folinic acid 5 mg/day	Duration is not well defined
FUNGI **Candida** Thrush Initial infection	Ketoconazole** (200-400 mg) po qd; Nystatin (500,000 units) gargled 5x/day; clotrimazole oral troches (10 mg) 5x/day or fluconazole (50-100 mg) po qd	Amphotericin B (0.3-0.5 mg/kg) IV/day;	Treat until symptoms resolve (7-10 days) and then begin maintenance therapy Amphotericin B usually reserved for patients who fail with alternative regimens
Maintenance (optional or prn)	Nystatin (above doses), clotrimazole (above doses) or ketoconazole** (200 mg) po qd	Fluconazole (50-100 mg) po qd	Possible salutary advantage for fluconazole and ketoconazole for maintenance treatment is prevention of cryptococcal infection
Vaginitis	Intravaginal miconazole suppository (100 mg) or cream (2%) x 7 days; clotrimazole cream (1%) or troche (100 mg) qd x 7	Ketoconazole** (200 mg) po qd or bid x 5-7 days Fluconazole (150 mg) x 1	May require continuous treatment to prevent relapse: Ketoconazole** (200 mg) po qd or fluconazole (50-100 mg) po qd
Esophagitis Initial infection	Fluconazole (100-200 mg) po qd; up to 400 mg/day x 2-3 wks	Ketoconazole** (200-400 mg) po bid x 2-3 wks Amphotericin B (0.3-0.5 mg/kg IV/day) ± flucytosine (100 mg/kg/day) x 5-7 days	
Maintenance	Fluconazole (50-100 mg) po qd	Ketoconazole** (200 mg) po qd Nystatin (above dose) or clotrimazole (above doses)	
Cryptococcal meningitis Initial treatment	Amphotericin B (0.5-0.8 mg/kg/day IV) with or without 5-flucytosine (100-150 mg/kg/day in 4 doses) to complete 1 gm of amphotericin B (some continue amphotericin B until therapeutic response or for 10-14 days	Fluconazole (200 mg po bid) x 6-10 wks Itraconazole (200 mg) po bid (see comment)	Fluconazole is acceptable as initial treatment only for patients with normal mental status. Other favorable prognostic findings are crypt antigen < 1:32 and CSF WBC > 20/mm³

(continued)

154

	Preferred	Alternative	Comment
Initial treatment	Amphotericin B (0.7 mg/kg/day) ± 5 FC (100 mg/day po) x 2-3 wks, then fluconazole (400 mg/day) x 8-10 wks, then 200 mg/day indefinitely		Cryptococcal antigen is nearly always detected in CSF, and in blood of 95% of patients; it is less useful in monitoring response to treatment
Maintenance therapy	Fluconazole (200 mg) po qd up to 400 mg/day	Amphotericin B (1 mg/kg/wk)	Life long maintenance treatment required for all patients
Histoplasmosis			
Disseminated			
Initial treatment	Amphotericin B (0.5-1.0 mg/kg/day IV) x 4-8 wks; total dose = 1-2.5 gm		
	Itraconazole (200 mg) po bid		
Maintenance	Itraconazole (200 mg) po bid	Ketoconazole** (200 mg) po bid	
	Amphotericin B 1.0-1.5 mg/kg/wk		
Coccidioidomycosis			
Initial treatment	Amphotericin B (0.5-1.0 mg/kg IV/day x ≥ 8 wks) (2-2.5 gm total dose)	Fluconazole (200 mg) po bid	Intrathecal amphotericin B usually added for coccidioidomycosis meningitis
Maintenance	Amphotericin B (1 mg/kg/wk) or fluconazole (400 mg po qd)	Ketoconazole** (400-800 mg) po qd	
		Itraconazole (200 mg) po qd	
MYCOBACTERIA			
M. tuberculosis			
Treatment	All patients should receive <u>observed treatment</u> with <u>4 agents</u>: INH (300 mg po/day) + rifampin (600 mg po/day) + pyrazinamide (20-30 mg/kg po/day) + ethambutol (15-25 mg/kg/day) or streptomycin (1.0 gm IM/day). Treat daily x 2 weeks (above doses), then daily (above doses) or intermittent (2-3x/wk): INH (900 mg), rifampin (600 mg), PZA (50-70 mg/kg) and ethambutol (100 mg/kg/wk) or streptomycin 20-30 mg/kg) x 6 wks.	Second line drugs: Ethionamide, capreomycin, kanamycin, amikacin, cycloserine, PAS Experimental drugs: Fluoroquinolones, imipenem, clofazimine, clarithromycin	Observed treatment preferred for all patients Intermittent treatment: 2x/wk appears as effective as 3x/wk Duration of treatment: Usually 50% longer in patients with HIV infection; for sensitive strains ~ 9 mo or 6 mo post-sputum conversion INH: Should supplement with pyroxidime (50 mg/day) in AIDS patients

(continued)

155

	Preferred	Alternative	Comment
Treatment	Subsequent treatment based on sensitivity tests: Sensitivity to INH + rifampin: continue INH and rifampin alone to complete 9-12 mo (6 mo post-sputum conversion)		Aminoglycoside: Streptomycin preferred and may be given IV; capreomycin, kanamycin or amikacin may be preferred based on in vitro sensitivity tests; amikacin cost is 100x streptomycin ($60/day vs 4$/day)
	Resistant to INH or rifampin (or inability to take INH or rifampin): INH or rifampin + PAZ + ethambutol or streptomycin x18 mo or 12 mo post-sputum conversion		Suspected resistance: Give 3 drugs never seen pending in vitro sensitivity tests; never add a single drug
	Resistant to INH and rifampin: Treat with at least two drugs active in vitro x 18-24 mo		Fluoroquinolones: Ciprofloxacin (750 mg po bid) or ofloxacin (400 mg po bid) often used for resistant strains
Prophylaxis	INH (300 mg po qd) ± pyridoxine (50 mg po/day)	Rifampin (600 mg po qd)	INH prophylaxis for ≥ 1 yr is indicated for all HIV infected patients with positive PPD (≥ 5mm induration) or anergy and high risk category or simply HIV + high risk (high risk=IV drug use, homeless, migrant farm worker); for INH intolerance or INH-induced hepatitis (transaminase > 5 x normal) some advocate rifampin (600 mg/day)
			For skin test conversion following contact with multiply resistant strain: Decision for prophylaxis depends on host and in vitro sensitivity of contact strain; may use fluoroquinolones (ciprofloxacin or ofloxacin) plus pyrazinamide or ethambutol
			Pyridoxine (50 mg/day) advocated for alcoholics, pregnant patients and malnourished patients

(continued)

156

	Preferred	Alternative	Comment
M. avium-intracellulare			
Treatment	Choose 3-5 from the following: Clofazimine (100-200 mg po/day), rifampin (600 mg po/day), ethambutol (25 mg/kg po/day x 6 wks, then 15 mg/kg), ciprofloxacin (750 mg po bid), amikacin (7.5 mg/kg IM or IV q12h, then 7.5 mg/kg/day for ≤ 2 months), clarithromycin (1 gm po bid) or azithromycin (600-900 mg po qd)	Other combinations include ethionamide, rifabutin (in place of rifampin), cycloserine, pyrazinamide, imipenem	INH should be included if M. tuberculosis is considered likely, but this drug adds little with M. avium infections; role of in vitro susceptibility tests is controversial
	Clarithromycin + clofazimine or ethambutol (above doses)		
Prophylaxis	Clarithromycin (500 mg po bid) Rifabutin (300 mg po qd)		Prophylaxis sometimes advocated for patients with CD4 counts < 100 or < 150/mm³
M. kansasii	INH (300 mg po/day) + rifampin 600 mg po/day) + ethambutol (15-25 mg/day) x 12 mo ± streptomycin (1 gm IM 2x/wk) x 3 mo	Also consider ciprofloxacin (750 mg po bid) and clarithromycin (500 mg-1 gm po bid)	Usual treatment is 12 months
VIRUSES			
Herpes simplex			
Initial treatment			
Mild	Acyclovir (200 mg po 5x/day) at least 10 days (until lesions crusted)		Failure to respond: double oral dose or give IV
Severe	Acyclovir (15 mg/kg IV/day) at least 7 days	Foscarnet (40 mg/kg IV q8h) x 3 wks Topical trifluridine 1% solution q8h	If fails to respond to acyclovir give 30 mg/kg/day IV and test sensitivity of isolate to acyclovir; resistant HSV, high dose IV acyclovir (12-15 mg/kg IV q8h or by continuous infusion) or foscarnet
Maintenance	Acyclovir (400 mg po bid or 200 mg) 3-5x/day	Foscarnet (40 mg/kg IV/day)	Alternative is to treat each episode
Visceral	Acyclovir (30 mg/kg IV/day) at least 10 days	Foscarnet (60 mg/kg IV q8h) x ≥ 10 days	

157

(continued)

	Preferred	Alternative	Comment
Herpes zoster			
Dermatomal	Acyclovir (30 mg/kg IV/day) or 800 mg po 5x/day at least 7 days (until lesions crust)	Foscarnet (40 mg/kg IV q8h)	Some authorities recommend avoidance of corticosteroids; postherpetic neuralgia is less common in young patients; no maintenance therapy is recommended
			Foscarnet for preferred acyclovir-resistant cases
Disseminated ophthalmic nerve involvement or visceral	Acyclovir (30-36 mg/kg IV/day) at least 7 days	Foscarnet (40-60 mg/kg IV q8h)	No maintenance therapy recommended
Cytomegalovirus			
Retinitis			
Initial treatment	Foscarnet (60 mg/kg IV q8h) x 14-21 days		Ganciclovir and foscarnet appear comparably effective vs CMV; possible advantage of foscarnet is that it prolongs survival by an average of 3 mo; this may reflect concurrent use of AZT or synergy of foscarnet + AZT vs HIV
	Ganciclovir (5 mg/kg IV bid) x 14-21 days		Foscarnet requires infusion pump
			Alternative options with antiretroviral agents are: ganciclovir + ddI or ganciclovir + AZT with G-CSF for neutropenia
Maintenance	Foscarnet (90 mg/kg IV/day)		Maintenance therapy required life long
	Ganciclovir (5 mg/kg IV/day)		
Enteritis, colitis esophagitis, encephalitis, neuritis, pneumonitis, viremia plus fever and/or wasting, cutaneous lesions	Ganciclovir (5 mg/kg) IV bid x 14-21 days		Efficacy not clearly established for disseminated CMV other than retinitis; CMV is rare cause of pulmonary disease in AIDS patients. Ganciclovir preferred if renal failure; foscarnet preferred if neutropenia or AZT used concurrently
	Foscarnet (60 mg/kg IV q8h) x 14-21 days		Indications for maintenance therapy not established, but advocated by some authorities for CMV colitis, neuritis, encephalitis and recurrent esophagitis (continued)

158

	Preferred	Alternative	Comment
BACTERIA			
S. pneumoniae	Penicillin	Erythromycin Cephalosporins	Traditional therapy usually adequate
H. influenzae	Cefuroxime/cefamandole Ampicillin/amoxicillin	Trimethoprim-sulfamethoxazole Cephalosporins - 3rd gen	Traditional therapy usually adequate
Nocardia	Sulfadiazine (4-8 gm po or IV/day) to maintain sulfa level at 15-20 mcg/ml	Trimethoprim-sulfa (4-6 DS/day) Minocycline (100 mg po bid)	Other suggested regimens: Imipenem + amikacin Sulfonamide + amikacin or minocycline
Pseudomonas aeruginosa	Aminoglycoside + antipseudomonad penicillin (ticarcillin, piper- acillin or mezlocillin)	Aminoglycoside + antipseudomonad cephalosporin (ceftazidime or cefoperazone) or imipenem	Antibiotic selection requires in vitro sensitivity data
Rhodococcus equi	Vancomycin (2 gm IV/day) ± rifampin (600 mg po qd), cipro- floxacin (750 mg po bid) or imipenem (0.5 gm IV qid) x 2-4 wks	Erythromycin (2-4 gm IV/day)	Ciprofloxacin (750 mg po bid) may be used for long term maintenance, but resistance is likely to develop
Rochalimaea quintana (bacillary angiomatosis)	Erythromycin (250-500 mg po qid) x 2-8 wks	Doxycycline (100 mg po bid)	
Salmonella			
Acute	Ampicillin (8-12 gm IV/day x 1-4 wks) then amoxicillin (500 mg po tid) to complete 2-4 wk course	Trimethoprim (5-10 mg/kg/day) + sulfamethoxazole IV or po x 2-4 wks	Relapse common
	Ciprofloxacin (500-750 mg po bid) x 2-4 wks	Cephalosporins - 3rd gen	
Maintenance	Amoxicillin (250 mg) po bid	Ciprofloxacin (500 mg po qd or bid) Trimethoprim-sulfamethoxazole (2.5 mg/kg trimethoprim or 1 DS) po bid	Indications for maintenance therapy, specific regimens and duration not well defined
Staph aureus	Antistaphylococcal penicillin (nafcillin, oxacillin) ± gentamicin (1 mg/kg IV q8h) or rifampin (600 mg/day)	Cephalosporin: 1st gen ± gentamicin or rifampin Vancomycin (1 gm IV bid) ± gentamicin or rifampin	MRSA stains must be treated with vancomycin Oral agent: cephalexin

159

* Patients with severe forms of G6PD deficiency are at risk for hemolytic anemia when given oxident drugs such as dapsone, sulfonamides and primaquine. Some advocate screening all potential ricipients, some restrict screening to persons at greatest risk (black males, men of Mediterranean decent, from India or from the Far East, e.g., endemic malaria areas); some simply observe for evidence of hemolysis that usually occurs in first several days of treatment and often resolves with continued administration. Patients with the Mediterranean variant are at risk for severe hemolysis.

** Ketoconazole requires gastric acid for absorption; this may be enhanced by administration with orange juice, coke or 0.2 N HCl.

*** Azithromycin is FDA approved, but not for this indication. It is available from Pfizer Labs at (203) 441-5941. Clarithromycin is FDA approved, but not for this indication. It is available from Abbott at (800) 688-9118.

Table 7. TREATMENT OF MISCELLANEOUS AND NON-INFECTIOUS DISEASE COMPLICATIONS OF HIV INFECTION CLASSIFIED BY ORGAN SYSTEM*

Condition	Treatment	Comment
Cardiac		
Cardiomyopathy	Digitalis, diuretic and cautious use of vasodilators; Discontinue nucleoside (AZT, ddI or ddC) x 4 wks	Echo is best screening test. If patient does not respond to nucleoside withdrawal: Biopsy endocardium. If biopsy shows myocarditis: Solumedrol, 100-125 mg IV/day x 3 days, then prednisone 1 mg/kg/day with taper over 1 mo. If tx shows microbial agent (CMV, <u>M. avium</u>, cryptococcus): treat
Pulmonary		
Lipoid interstitial pneumonitis	AZT	Relatively rare in adult patients
	Prednisone	Indications and optimal dose of corticosteroid treatment not established; most initiate this treatment after initial observation shows progression; maintenance prednisone sometimes required
Renal		
Nephropathy (HIV-associated; Nephropathy-HIVAN)	Hemodialysis (utility of dialysis in preventing rapid progression of HIVAN is not established)	Must distinguish from: 1) heroin-associated nephropathy, which has a far better prognosis, and 2) acute tubular necrosis
Neurologic		
Peripheral neuropathy (painful peripheral neuropathy)	Nortriptyline, 10 mg hs (see comment). Capsaicin-containing ointments (Zostrix, etc) for topical application; Lidocaine 10-30% ointment for topical use.	Increase dose by 10 mg q 5 days to maximum of 50 mg hs
Myopathy	Discontinue AZT x 3 wks. Nonsteroidal anti-inflammatory agents. Prednisone, 40-60 mg/day (severe cases)	Indication for treatment is proximal muscle weakness + elevated creatine kinase. Often unclear if due to HIV or AZT so use "drug holiday"
HIV-associated dementia	AZT, 1000-1200 mg/day	Benefit of higher dose for CNS complications is not established; monitor therapy with neurocognitive tests
	ddI, 200-300 mg po bid (efficacy not established)	Nimodipine (calcium channel blocker) 30 mg q4h (experimental for this indication)
Hematologic		
Idiopathic thrombocytopenia (ITP)	Prednisone, 60-100 mg/day	Relapses common with attempts to taper or discontinue steroids
	AZT, 1000-1200 mg/day	Utility of usual doses of AZT not established; initial reports showing benefit employed 1200 mg/day

(continued)

Condition	Treatment	Comment
ITP - continued	IV gamma globulin (1 gm/kg) x 3 (days, 1, 2 & 15), then every 2-3 wks	Failure to respond common with repeated courses
	Splenectomy	Not advocated by many authorities
	Splenic irradiation	Experience limited
Anemia	Transfusions and/or erythropoietin (r-HuEPO) 50-100 U/kg 2x/wk SC; increase dose 25 U/kg if response is inadequate at 4-8 wks and again at 4-8 wk intervals; maximal dose is 300 U/kg titrate maintenance dose	Discontinue AZT for hemoglobin < 7.5 gm%. EPO recommended only if baseline EPO level is < 500 U/mL
Neutropenia	Neupogen (C-CSF) or Prokine (GM-CSF) 1 μg/kg/day SC; usual maintenance dose is 0.13 μg/kg/day (0.1-1.0 μg/kg/day)	Usual cause is AZT, ganciclovir or HIV per se. Low doses (1 mcg/kg/day) of G-CSF and GM-CSF usually adequate and higher doses are often poorly tolerated; monitor with CBC and diff 2x/wk and titrate up to 10 μg/kg; reduce dose 50% q week for maintenance to keep ANC > 750-1500/ml
Tumors		
Kaposi's sarcoma	Topical liquid nitrogen	Restrict to few lesions that are small
	Intralesional vinblastin (0.01-0.02 mg/lesion) q 2wks x ≤ 3	Restrict to few lesions
	Alpha interferon, (9-20 mil units/d ± maintenance	Documented benefit of alpha interferon only for patients with CD4 count > 200/mm³; neutropenia common with AZT: Use G-CSF or substitute ddI
	Radiation	Skin - well tolerated; oral lesion - mucositis common
	Laser	Laser, radiation or vinblastine injection preferred for oral lesions
	Chemotherapy; adriamycin, bleomycin and either vincristine or vinblastine; etoposide (VP-16) monotherapy	Preferred for patients with widespread skin involvement (> 25 lesions), edema and/or symptomatic visceral organ involvement (especially lung KS)
Lymphoma	Regimens containing cyclophosphamide, adriamycin, vincristine and corticosteroids ± cranial radiation	
	CNS lymphoma - cranial radiation ± chemotherapy	

(continued)

162

Condition	Treatment	Comment
Dermalogic		
Bacillary angiomatosis	Erythromycin, 250-500 mg po qid x 2-8 wks	Alternative: Doxycycline, 100 mg bid
Molluscum contagiosum	Freeze; surgical extirpation	
Dermatophytic fungi	Skin - Topical miconazole or clotrimazole. Refractory cases-- griseofulvin, 330-660 mg po/day or ketoconazole, 200 mg po/day x 1-3 mo. Nails - griseofulvin, 660 mg/day x 6-15 mo	Ointments (miconazole and clotrimazole) are non-prescription
Seborrhea	Skin - Steroid cream (hydrocortisone 1%) or topical ketoconazole; scalp - shampoos containing zirconium sulfide, salicylic acid or coal tar	
Gastrointestinal		
Anorexia	Megace, 80 mg po qid	May use up to 800 mg/day
Nausea/vomiting	Compazine, 5-10 mg po q6-8h; Tigan, 250 mg po q6-8h; Dramamine, 50 mg po q6-8h; Ativan 0.025-0.05 mg/kg IV or IM; Haloperidol, 1-5 mg bid po or IM, Ondansetron (Zofran) 0.2 mg/kg IV or IM	Phenothiazines (Compazine, etc.), haloperidol, benzamides (Tigan, Reglan, etc.) may cause dystonia Must consider medications as cause
Mouth		
Aphthous ulcers	Mouth rinses with Miles solution, Dyclone, Benadryl or viscous Lidocaine (2%) Intralesional or topical corticosteroids; Prednisone, 40 mg po/day x 1-2 weeks, then taper (severe or refractory cases)	Miles solution - 60 mg hydrocortisone, 20 cc mycostatin, 2 gm tetracycline and 120 cc viscous Lidocaine
Oral hairy leukoplakia	Acyclovir, 800 mg po 5 x/day x 2-3 wks	Most lesions are asymptomatic and do not require treatment Relapses are common when acyclovir is discontinued and may require acyclovir maintenance therapy
Gingivitis/periodontitis	Metronidazole, 250 mg po tid or 500 mg po bid x 7-14 days and chlorhexidine gluconate (0.12% as Peridex) for oral rinse bid	

163

(continued)

Condition	Treatment	Comment
Esophagus		
Candida	See Table 6 (pg 154)	
Cytomegalovirus	Ganciclovir, 5 mg/kg IV bid x 14-21 days or foscarnet 60 mg/kg IV q8h x 14-21 days	For patients with complete response, discontinue after induction therapy and use maintenance only if there is relapse
Herpes simplex	Acyclovir, 400-1000 mg po 5x/day or 5 mg/kg IV tid x 7-10 days	
Aphthous ulcer	Prednisone, 40 mg/day po x 2 wks, then slow taper	
Diarrhea		
Specific microbial agent	See Table 6 (pg 154)	
Bacterial overgrowth	Doxycycline (100 mg po bid), metronidazole (750 mg po bid) amoxicillin-clavulanate (500 mg po qid)	Diagnosis requires quantitative culture of small bowel aspirate or hydrogen breath test
Symptomatic treatment	Lomotil/loperamide/paregoric, etc.	Utility of bismuth salts (Pepto-Bismol), indomethacin and octreotide not known
Wasting	Polymeric formulas: Ensure, Sustical, Enrich, Magnacal, etc.	Polymeric formulas: Non-prescription, about $1.50/can; 10 cans/day required for total caloric needs
	Elemental formulas: Vivonex TEN	Elemental diet for severe malabsorption states usually cryptosporidia or severe CMV infection; parenteral hyperalimentation and feeding gastrostomy rarely used
Psychiatric and sleep disorders		
Anxiety	Lorazepan (Ativan) 0.5-1 mg bid	Benzodiazepine agonist, Class IV; limit to 2-3 days
	Buspirone (BuSpar) 5 mg tid	Nonbenzodiazepine-nonbarbiturate; dependence liability negligible; increase dose 5 mg q 2-4 day to effective daily dose of 15-30 mg
Depression	Fluoxetine (Prozac) 20 mg qd	Major side effects are nausea, nervousness, insomnia, weight loss, dry mouth, constipation; insomnia may be treated with Desyrel, 25-50 mg hs
	Nortriptyline 10 mg - 25 mg hs, then increase	Tricyclic, increase dose after 25 mg 3-4 x/day; if > 100 mg/day follow serum levels with 50-150 mg/ml
Delirium	Haldol (0.5-1 mg) hs	

(continued)

164

Condition	Treatment	Comment
Insomnia	Diphenhydramine (Benedryl), 25 mg hs	Non-prescription
	Trazodone (Desyrel), 25-50 mg po hs	Preferably for < 1 week
	Chloral hydrate, 500 mg po hs	Class IV; preferably < 1 week
Apathy	Ritalin 5-10 mg tid	Not effective with severe dementia; seizure potential
Pain	ASA, acetaminophen, 325-650 mg q4h	Acute pain is best relieved with opioides. Chronic pain is best treated with nonopioid initially (ASA, acetaminophen, ibuprofen, nortriptyline)
	Non-steroidal anti-inflammatory agents (Motrin, 200-400 mg q6h; Naprosyn, 250-375 mg bid)	
	Codeine, 30-60 mg q4-6h po SC or IM	Dependence liability for opioids
	Meperidine, 50-150 mg q3-4h po, SC, IM, IV	Side effects of opioides: Sedation, constipation, respiratory depression, nausea and vomiting
	Methadone, 2.5-10 mg q6-8h po, SC, IM	
	Dilaudid, 2-8 mg q6-8h po, SC, IM Morphine, 5-20 mg SC, IM or rectal	
Terminal Illness	Morphine or other opioides orally or parenterally; MS Contin (continuous release morphine) po 15, 30, 60 or 100 mg: usual dose is 15-60 mg po q12h	Tolerance will develop within 1 week for opioides; PCA pump is consequently preferred for some patients to reduce cumulative dose
	Patient controlled analgesia (PCA) for morphine	
	Methadone (above doses)	

Table 8. Occupational exposure to HIV (MMWR 39:1,1990)

<u>Definition</u>

<u>Exposure</u>: Needlestick or cut with sharp object, contact with mucous membranes or contact with skin (especially if chapped, abraded or dermatitis, contact is prolonged and/or involves extensive area with blood or tissue).

<u>Body fluid of source</u>: (1) Blood or body fluid, (2) other body fluids to which universal precautions apply: cerebrospinal fluid, synovial fluid, pleural fluid, peritoneal fluid, pericardial fluid and amniotic fluid, or (3) laboratory specimens containing HIV. (All seroconversions in non-laboratory health care workers have involved blood or bloody fluid). Saliva, urine and stool are not considered potential sources of HIV.

<u>Source</u>: Source must be evaluated for hepatitis B virus and HIV. If source has AIDS, is known to be seropositive or refuses testing, the worker is evaluated clinically and serologically for HIV. Some states allow testing source without consent.

<u>Serology</u>: Worker is tested serologically at 0, 6 weeks (optional), 12 weeks and 6 months post-exposure. The worker is advised to report any acute illness, especially if it resembles acute HIV infection (fever, rash, myalgia, lymphadenopathy, dysphagia, hepatosplenomegaly and leukopenia with atypical lymphocytes). Most health care workers who have acquired HIV from needlestick injuriers have noted this infectious mononucleosis-like illness at 1-3 wks post-exposure.

<u>Precautions</u>: During the follow-up, especially the first 6-12 weeks, the worker should refrain from donating blood or sperm and should abstain from sexual intercourse or use appropriate measures to prevent HIV transmission.

<u>Prophylactic AZT: Relevant issues</u>

1. The <u>risk</u> of HIV transmission with the usual type of needlestick injury from an HIV infected source is about 0.4% (1/250).

2. Data from <u>animal studies</u> are inadequate to support or refute the potential efficacy of AZT; studies in the SCID-hu mouse model showed delayed viremia without prevention of infection (McCune et al, Science 247:564,1990. Pretreatment with AZT before SIV challenge failed to prevent transmission.

3. Four anecdotal cases of patients with blood exposures showed AZT initiated within 45 minutes and 6 hrs did not prevent seroconversion (Lange JM et al, NEJM 322:1375, 1990; Looke DFM et al, Lancet 335:1280, 1990

4. <u>Side effects</u> of AZT in health care workers receiving 1200 mg/day for 6 weeks showed 29% had anemia (Hgb 9.5-12 gm/dL) and 14% discontinued the drug due to reversible subjective complaints (headache, nausea, myalgias) (MMWR 39:1,1990). Teratogenic and carcinogenic potential in humans are unknown, although prolonged administration of AZT to rats and mice resulted in vaginal carcinomas in 8% at 22 months (MMWR 31:1,1990). Men and women receiving AZT should avoid conception.

(continued)

AZT Prophylaxis: Protocol of the NIH, CDC and San Francisco General Hospital

Criteria for inclusion

1. Exposure to the following body fluids: blood, semen, vaginal secretions and bloody body fluids; tissue that has not been inactivated or fluids or tissue containing HIV in research labs.

2. Type of exposure: Occupational contact with specimens above by percutaneous inoculation, e.g., needlestick or cut with sharp object, contact with mucous membranes or non-intact skin.

3. Patient source: Patient source has AIDS or ARC, positive HIV serology or positive HIV culture. Some include patients with unknown serostatus and high risk: IV drug abuse, gay male, hemophiliac or regular sexual partner of person with HIV infection.

4. Women must not be pregnant or breast feeding.

5. Must agree to use effective method of birth control during treatment and 4 weeks thereafter.

6. Treatment must be initiated within 72 hrs of exposure. (Rapid initiation within minutes or a few hours is highly desired if prevention of transmission is the major goal; it is possible that AZT will modify the course of HIV infection if given in the first weeks of infection that are associated with high grade viremia. (NEJM 324:954,1991)

7. Informed consent that includes counseling concerning methods to minimize risk to sexual contacts, lack of documented efficacy of this treatment, the possibility that treatment will delay seroconversion, side effects of AZT including possible teratogenic and carcinogenic effects and costs of treatment (wholesale price of about $1.44/100 mg tab).

   Regimen: 200 mg 6x/day for 3 days (1200 mg/day); then 100 mg or 200 mg 5x/day for 25 days.

Monitoring

1. HIV serology at 0 (baseline), 6 wks, 3 mo, 6 mo and 12 mo. (The serology at 12 mo is desired to detect delayed seroconversion that may result from AZT treatment.)

2. CBC and SMA-12 at 2, 4 and 6 wks.

SEPSIS AND SEPSIS SYNDROME

A. Definitions (R. Bone, Ann Intern Med 115:457, 1991)[*]

Disorder	Requirements for Clinical Diagnosis
Bacteremia[T]	Positive blood cultures
Sepsis	Clinical evidence suggestive of infection *plus* signs of a systemic response to the infection (all of the following): • Tachypnea (respiration >20 breaths/min [if patient is mechanically ventilated >10L/min]) • Tachycardia (heart rate >90 beats/min) • Hyperthermia or hypothermia (core or rectal temperature >38.4°C [101°F] or <35.6°C [96.1°F])
The sepsis syndrome (may also be considered *incipient septic shock* in patients who later become hypotensive)	Clinical diagnosis of sepsis outlined above, *plus* evidence of altered organ perfusion (one or more of the following): • PaO$_2$/FIo$_2$ no higher than 280 (in the absence of other pulmonary or cardiovascular disease) • Lactate level above the upper limit of normal • Oliguria (documented urine output < 0.5 mL/kg body weight for at least 1 hour in patients with catheters in place) • Acute alteration in mental status Positive blood cultures are not required[TT]
Early septic shock	Clinical diagnosis of sepsis syndrome outlined above, *plus* hypotension (systolic blood pressure below 90 mm Hg or a 40 mm Hg decrease below baseline systolic blood pressure) that lasts for less than 1 hour and is responsive to conventional therapy (intravenous fluid administration or pharmacologic intervention)
Refractory septic shock	Clinical diagnosis of sepsis syndrome outlined above, *plus* hypotension (systolic blood pressure below 90 mm Hg or a 40 mm Hg decrease below baseline systolic blood pressure) that lasts for more than 1 hour despite adequate volume resuscitation and that requires vasopressors or higher doses of dopamine (> 6 μ/kg per hour)

[*] Adapted from Kreger BE et al, Amer J Med 68:344, 1980.

[T] The related term *septicemia* is imprecise and should be abandoned.

[TT] The sepsis syndrome may result from infection with gram-positive or gram-negative bacteria, pathogenic viruses, fungi, or rickettsia; however, an identical physiologic response may result from such noninfectious processes as severe trauma or pancreatitis. Blood cultures may or may not be positive.

B. Antibiotic selection (Medical Letter 34:49, 1992)

1. <u>Initial treatment</u>: Aminoglycoside (gentamicin, tobramycin, netilmicin or amikacin) <u>plus</u> one of the following:

    - Third generation cephalosporin (cefotaxime, ceftizoxime, cefoperazone, ceftriaxone or ceftazidine) <u>or</u>
    - Antipseudomonad penicillin (ticarcillin, piperacillin or mezlocillin) <u>or</u>
    - Ticarcillin-clavulanic acid <u>or</u>
    - Imipenem

2. <u>Suspected methicillin resistant S. aureus</u>: Add vancomycin ± rifampin

3. <u>Intra-abdominal sepsis</u>: Any of the following:

    - Metronidazole or clindamycin <u>plus</u> Aminogylcoside
    - Ticarcillin-clavulanic acid ± aminoglycoside
    - Ampicillin-sulbactam ± aminoglycoside
    - Imipenem ± aminoglycoside
    - Cefoxitin ± aminoglycoside
    - Cefotetan ± aminoglycoside

4. <u>Biliary tract</u>: Cephalosporin ± aminoglycoside ± anti-anaerobic agent (such as metronidazole)

5. <u>Neutropenia</u>: Aminoglycoside <u>plus</u> one of the following:

    - Ticarcillin, ticarcillin-clavulanic acid, mezlocillin, piperacillin, ceftazidine or imipenem
    - With or without vancomycin (see JID 163:951, 1991)

GUIDELINES FOR USE OF SYSTEMIC GLUCOCORTICOSTEROIDS
IN MANAGEMENT OF SELECTED INFECTIONS
(Adapted from Infectious Diseases Society of America, J Infect Dis 165:1-13, 1992)

1. Immunosuppression is related to several variables

   a. Dose: Usually > 0.3 mg/kg/day, especially if > 1 mg/kg/day (prednisone)
   b. Duration: < 5 days has minimal effect
   c. Concurrent drugs: Cytotoxic agents

2. Recommendations

Condition	Recommend*	Comment
Systemic		
Gram-negative sepsis and shock	E/I	Exceptions: Adrenal insufficiency and typhoid fever with shock. Four clinical trials showed no benefit in septic shock (NEJM 317:653, 1987; 317:659, 1987)
Toxic shock syndrome	C/III	Possible benefit if given in first few days (JAMA 252: 3399, 1984)
Typhoid fever	C/I	Controlled trial showed survival benefit with chloramphenicol + Decadron (3 mg/kg) vs chloro alone (NEJM 310:82, 1984). Recommended for critically ill patients with delirium, obtundation, coma or shock
Tetanus	B/I	Single study showed benefit (Clin Ther 10:276, 1988)
Tuberculosis		
Pericarditis	A/I	Survival benefit: 40-80 mg prednisone/d with taper over weeks (JAMA 266:99, 1991)
Meningitis	B/I	Recommended when elevated intracranial pressure, focal neurologic deficits, altered consciousness; prednisone, 60 mg/d with taper at 1-2 wks over 4-6 weeks (Ped Infect Dis 10:179, 1991)
Debilitated patients	C/III	Severely debilitated patients show rapid symptomatic improvement; prednisone, 20-30 mg/d
Severe hypoxia	C/III	Improve severe hypoxemia: prednisone, 60-80 mg/d
Pleurisy	C/III	Data supporting recommendations categorized as C/III poor
Peritonitis	C/III	Supporting data are poor (NEJM 28:1091, 1969)
Herpes zoster		
Routine use (all pts)	E/I	Recommended only for patients >40 yrs to reduce post-herpetic neuralgia: prednisone, 50-60 mg/day x 1 wk with taper to none by week 3 (Lancet 2:126, 1987)
Old patients	C/III	

(continued)

Condition	Recommend*	Comment
Viral infections		
marrow suppression	C/III	Refers to marrow cytopenia or hypoplasia with parvovirus B19, EBV, HSV, VZV, CMV and HCV
EBV (infectious mono-nucleosis) routine use	D/II	Reduces fever and pharyngitis, but reluctance to use in self-limited disease unless tonsil hypertrophy with impending airway closure, prolonged course with high fever or persistent morbidity: Prednisone, 80 mg/day x 2-3 days with taper to none after week 2 (JAMA 256: 1051, 1986)
Airway obstruction	B/II	
Hepatitis, myocarditis, encephalitis	C/III	
Hantaan virus	E/I	JID 162:1213, 1990
Trichinosis	C/III	JAMA 230:537, 1974
CNS infections		
Bacterial meningitis	C/II	Efficacy shown in children with H. influenzae meningitis for reduction in hearing loss: Dexamethasone, 0.6 mg/kg/day x 4 days (NEJM 319:964, 1988) Data in adults with meningitis due to other organisms is sparce, but some recommend this for adults who are severely ill with mental status changes (Ann Intern Med 112:610, 1990)
Brain abscess	C-D/III	Recommended only when elevated intracranial pressure must be reduced (Neurosurgery 23:451, 1988)
Neurocysticercosis	C-D/III	Recommended for elevated intracranial pressure; this treatment may also reduce reaction to dying larvae caused by praziquantel (Rev Infect Dis 9:961, 1987)
Neuroborreliosis	D/III	No evidence of efficacy with facial nerve palsy (Laryngoscope 95:1341, 1985)
Cerebral malaria	E/I	(JID 150:325, 1988)
Airway infections		
P. carinii pneumonia	A/I	Three controlled trials show reduced risk of death and respiratory failure (NEJM 318:988, 1988; 323:1444, 1990; 323:1451, 1990). Recommended with pO_2 < 70 mm Hg or A-a gradient >35 mm Hg (NEJM 323: 1500, 1987)
Chronic bronchitis	C/III	Controlled trial showed no clear benefit (Ann Intern Med 106:196, 1987)
Acute epiglottitis	C/III	Consider when obstruction is likely (primarily children)

(continued)

Condition	Recommend*	Comment
Allergic broncho-pulmonary aspergillosis	B/II	Response is impressive: Prednisone, 45-60 mg/day (Arch Intern Med 146:1799, 1986). Inhaled steroids also effective (Allergy 43:24, 1988)
Heart		
Viral pericarditis	C/III	Symptomatic response impressive: Prednisone, 40-60 mg/day x 3-5 days, then taper over 3-4 wks. However, non-steroidals also effective, constrictive pericarditis is not prevented and concern that myocarditis may worsen
Viral myocarditis	C/III	Clinical trials variable. Steroids in coxsackievirus myocarditis in experimental animals cause increased myocardial necrosis and increased viral replication
Liver		
Acute viral hepatitis	E/I	Controlled trials show adverse outcome with prolongation of illness, more relapses and more chronic hepatitis (NEJM 294:681, 1976)
Chronic hepatitis HBV	E/I	Controlled trials show adverse outcome (Lancet 2:1136, 1989; NEJM 304:380, 1981; Ann Intern Med 109:89, 1988)
Chronic hepatitis HCV	E/III	(Ann Intern Med 112:921, 1990)
Aphthous ulcers	C/III	Anecdotal case reports indicate dramatic response in AIDS patients (Ann Intern Med 109:338, 1988)
Eye		
Endophthalmitis bacteria	C/III	Retrospective studies and experimental animal studies support efficacy (Inf Dis Clin N Amer 3:533, 1989)
Eye infections - viruses, protozoa, etc.	C/III	

*A-E: Categories for strength of recommendation
  A = good evidence for use; B = moderate evidence for use; C = poor evidence for or against use;
  D = moderate evidence against use; E = good evidence against use

I-III: Categories for quality of evidence
  I = at least one proper study; II = evidence from at least one clinical study with suboptimal design; III = evidence based on opinions of authorities

PATHOGENS ASSOCIATED WITH IMMUNODEFICIENCY STATUS

Condition	Usual conditions	Pathogens
Neutropenia (<500/ml)	Cancer chemotherapy; adverse drug reaction; leukemia	Bacteria: Aerobic GNB (coliforms and pseudomonads) Fungi: <u>Aspergillus</u>, Phycomycetes
Cell-mediated immunity	Organ transplantation: HIV infection; lymphoma (especially Hodgkin's disease); cortico-steroid therapy	Bacteria: <u>Listeria</u>, <u>Salmonella</u>, <u>Nocardia</u>, Mycobacteria (<u>M. tuberculosis</u> & M. avium), <u>Legionella</u> Viruses: CMV, H. simplex, Varicella-zoster Parasites: <u>Pneumocystis carinii</u>; <u>Toxoplasma</u>; <u>Strongyloides stercoralis</u>; Cryptosporidia Fungi: <u>Candida</u>, Phycomycetes (Mucor), <u>Cryptococcus</u>
Hypogammaglobulinemia or dysgamma-globulinemia	Multiple myeloma; congenital or acquired deficiency; chronic lymphocytic leukemia	Bacteria: S. pneumoniae, <u>H. influenzae</u> (type B) Parasites: <u>Giardia</u> Viruses: Enteroviruses
Complement deficiencies C2, 3	Congenital	Bacteria: <u>S. pneumoniae</u>, <u>H. influenzae</u>
C5		<u>S. pneumoniae</u>, <u>S. aureus</u> Enterobacteriaceae
C6-8		<u>Neisseria meningitidis</u>
Alternative pathway		<u>S. pneumoniae</u>, <u>H. influenzae</u>, Salmonella
Hyposplenism	Splenectomy; hemolytic anemia	<u>S. pneumoniae</u>, <u>H. influenzae</u>, DF-2

173

Guidelines for use of antimicrobial agents in neutropenic patients with unexplained fever (Adapted from: Working Committee, Infectious Diseases Society of America, Hughes W et al, J Infect Dis 161:381, 1990)

Regimens	Advantages	Disadvantages
Aminoglycoside (gent, tobra or amikacin) <u>plus</u> anti-pseudomonad betalactam (ticarcillin, piperacillin, azlocillin, mezlocillin, ticarcillin-clavulanate, cefoperazone or ceftazidime)	1. Potential synergy vs GNB 2. Activity vs anaerobes (except ceftazidime) 3. Minimal emergence of resistance 4. Preferred regimen when <u>P. aeruginosa</u> is suspected	1. Potential ototoxicity and nephrotoxicity (aminoglycoside) 2. Lack of activity vs some GPC (esp meth-resistant <u>S. aureus</u> and <u>S. epidermidis</u>) 3. Need to monitor amino glycoside levels
Two betalactam drugs (third generation cephalosporin such as ceftazidime or cefoperazone <u>plus</u> a ureidopenicillin such as piperacillin or mezlocillin)	1. Reduced toxicity 2. Effective in clinical trials 3. Sometimes preferred in presence of renal failure or nephrotoxic drugs	1. Selection of resistant strains 2. Possible antagonism 3. Lack of activity vs some GPC
Single drug (ceftazidime, imipenem or cefoperazone)	1. Reduced toxicity 2. As effective as multiple drug regimens in most trials 3. Easily used in combination with other nephrotoxic drugs or in patients with renal failure	1. Reduced activity vs many GPC and some GNB 2. Must monitor closely for non-response, emergence of resistance and secondary infections 3. Ceftazidime has minimal activity vs anaerobes 4. Preferred for patients with brief and mild neutropenia (500-1000/μl)
Vancomycin <u>plus</u> aminoglycoside <u>plus</u> antipseudomonad betalactam (see agents above)	1. Broadest spectrum including GPC 2. Preferred regimen if meth-resistant <u>S. aureus</u> suspected: line infection, colonized, hospital-acquired infection	1. Some believe decision to treat GPC can await culture results 2. Potential ototoxicity (vancomycin + ceftazidime is another option) 3. Cost

Guide to initial management of febrile neutropenic patients: Reprinted from Hughes WT et al, J Infect Dis 161:381, 1990 (with permission)

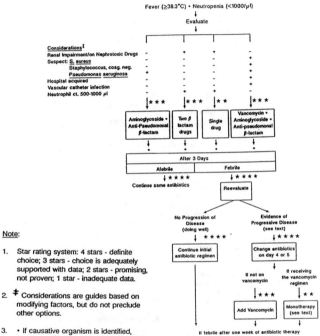

Fever (≥38.3°C) • Neutropenia (<1000/μl)

Evaluate

Considerations‡
Renal Impairment/on Nephrotoxic Drugs
Suspect: S. aureus
        Staphylococcus, coag. neg.
        Pseudomonas aeruginosa
Hospital acquired
Vascular catheter infection
Neutrophil ct. 500-1000 μl

Aminoglycoside + Anti-Pseudomonal β-lactam | Two β lactam drugs | Single drug | Vancomycin + Aminoglycoside + Anti-pseudomonal β-lactam

After 3 Days

Afebrile | Febrile

Continue same antibiotics | Reevaluate

No Progression of Disease (doing well) | Evidence of Progressive Disease (see text)

Continue initial antibiotic regimen | Change antibiotics on day 4 or 5

If not on vancomycin | If receiving the vancomycin regimen

Add Vancomycin | Monotherapy (see text)

If febrile after one week of antibiotic therapy

START AMPHOTERICIN B

Note:

1. Star rating system: 4 stars - definite choice; 3 stars - choice is adequately supported with data; 2 stars - promising, not proven; 1 star - inadequate data.

2. ‡ Considerations are guides based on modifying factors, but do not preclude other options.

3. • If causative organism is identified, modify to optimal susceptibility, but maintain broad spectrum coverage.

Common infections by time after marrow transplantation*

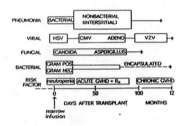

* Meyers JD: Infections in marrow transplant
   recipients. In Mandell J, et al. Principles
   and Practice of Infectious Diseases, Churchill
   Livingstone, NY, 3rd edition, 1990, pp 2291.

TOXIC SHOCK SYNDROME: Case definition of Centers for Disease Control (MMWR 29:229,1980)

1. Fever: Temperature ≥ 38.9°C (102°F).
2. Rash: Diffuse macular erythroderma.
3. Desquamation: 1-2 wks after onset, especially palms and soles.
4. Hypotension: Systolic < 90 mmHg for adults or < 5th percentile by
    age for children, or orthostatic syncope.
5. Involvement of three or more of the following organs
    GI: Vomiting or diarrhea at onset
    Muscular: Severe myalgia or creatine phosphokinase > 2x normal
    Mucous membrane: Vaginal, oropharyngeal or conjunctival hyperemia
    Renal: BUN or creatinine ≥ 2x normal or ≥ 5 WBC/HPF in absence of UTI
    Hepatic: Bilirubin or transaminase levels ≥ 2x normal
    Hematological: Platelets < 100,000/mm³
    CNS: Disoriented or altered consciousness without focal neurologic signs
        when fever and neurologic signs are absent
6. Negative results for the following (if obtained): Cultures of blood, throat
    and cerebrospinal fluid; negative serology for Rocky Mountain spotted
    fever, leptospirosis or measles.

ANAEROBIC BACTERIAL INFECTIONS

1. Activity of antibiotics versus Bacteroides fragilis (Data for 557 strains
    collected from 8 U.S. medical centers in 1986, Cuchural GJ Jr et al:
    Antimicrob Ag Chemother 34:479,1990)

Agent	Resistant	Agent	Resistant
Metronidazole	0	Piperacillin	16%
Chloramphenicol	0	Moxalactam	23%/17%
Imipenem	0.2%	Cefotetan	36%/22%
Ticarcillin-		Ceftizoxime	33%/20%
clavulanate	1.7%	Cefotaxime	53%/33%
Clindamycin	6.0%	Cefoperazone	66%/27%
Cefoxitin	11%/2%*	Ceftazadime	87%/74%

* Two figures provided indicating arbitrary breakpoints in susceptibility testing; first figure
indicates % resistant at 16 mcg/ml, 2nd figure indicates % resistant at 32 mcg/ml.

2. In vitro susceptibility of various anaerobes (from Finegold SM and
    Wexler HM: Antimicrob Ag Chemother, 32:611,1988)

	Chloro	Clinda	Erythro	Metro	Pen	Tetra	Vanco
Microaerophilic and anaerobic GPC	3*	2-3	2-3	2	4	2	3
B. fragilis group	3	2-3	1-2	3	1	1-2	1
Bacteroides sp (other)	3	3	2-3	3	2-3	2	1
Fusobacteria	3	2-3	1	3	3-4	2-3	1
C. perfringens	3	3	3	3	3	2	3
Clostridia (other)	3	2	2-3	3	3	2	2-3
Actinomyces	3	3	3	1-2	4	2-3	2-3

* 1 = poor activity; 2 = moderate activity, 3= good activity; 4 = drug of choice.

3. Susceptibility of Anaerobic bacteria. National Committee for Clinical Laboratory Standards,
    Working Group on Anaerobic Susceptibility Testing (J Clin Micro 26:1253, 1988)

Essentially always active
Metronidazole (except some nonsporulating GPB)
Chloramphenicol
Imipenem
Betalactam-betalactamase inhibitor combinations

Unpredictable activity
Cephalosporins (other)
Penicillins (other - esp
antistaphylococcal agents)
Trimethoprim-sulfamethoxazole
Vacomycin
Erythromycin

Usually active
Clindamycin
Cefoxitin
Cefotetan
Antipseudomonad penicillins
Moxalactam

Virtually never active
Aztreonam
Aminoglycoside
Quinolones

FEVER OF UNKNOWN ORIGIN

A. Definition (Petersdorf RG & Beeson PB, Medicine 40:1,1961)

1) Illness ≥ 3 weeks.
2) Documented fever ≥ 101°F (38.3°C).
3) Negative diagnostic evaluation with 1 week in hospital.

B. Causes (Adapted from: Larson E et al, Medicine 61:269,1982)*

Infections	32	Neoplastic diseases	33
Abdominal abscesses	11	Lymphoma	6
Mycobacteria	5	Hodgkin's	4
Endocarditis	0	Leukemia	5
HIV infection**	0	Lymphomatoid granulomatosis	2
Cytomegalovirus	4	Malignant histocytosis	4
Miscellaneous***	12	Pre-leukemia	1
Collagen disease	8	Solid tumor****	11
Still's disease	4	Miscellaneous	10
Polyarteritis nodosa	2	Hematoma	3
Rheumatic fever	1	Pulmonary emboli	1
Polymyalgia rheumatica	0	Familial Mediterranean	
Rheumatic fever	1	fever	1
Systemic lupus	0	Myxoma	1
Granulomatous disease	9	Periodic fever	0
Granulomatous hepatitis	4	Factitious fever	3
Sarcoidosis	2	Non-specific pericarditis	1
Giant cell arteritis	1	Undiagnosed	13
Crohn's disease	2		

*   This represents an updated version (105 cases; 1970-1980) of the classical report by Petersdorf and Beeson (100 cases, 1952-1957); more recent developments include AIDS and extensive use of scans.
**   The Seattle study predated AIDS, but HIV infection would now constitute an important diagnostic consideration.
*** Includes sinusitis, dental infections, osteomyelitis, amebiasis, candidiasis, urinary tract infection.
**** All were solid tumors in the abdomen including hepatoma (2) and hypernephroma (2).

LYME DISEASE: CASE DEFINITION OF THE CENTERS FOR DISEASE CONTROL (reprinted with permission from: Rahn DW and Malawista SE, Ann Intern Med 114:473, 1991 and MMWR 40:417, 1991)

Lyme Disease National Surveillance Case Definition

Lyme disease is a systemic, tick-borne disease with protean manifestations, including dermatologic, rheumatologic, neurologic, and cardiac abnormalities. The best clinical marker for the disease is the initial skin lesion, erythema migrans, that occurs in 60% to 80% of patients.

Case definition for the national surveillance of Lyme disease:

1. A person with erythema migrans; or
2. A person with at least one late manifestation and laboratory confirmation of infection.

General definitions:

1. Erythema migrans: For purposes of surveillance, erythema migrans is a skin lesion that typically begins as a red macule or papule and expands over a period of days or weeks to form a large round lesion, often with partial central clearing. To be considered erythema migrans, a solitary lesion must measure at least 5 cm. Secondary lesions may also occur. Annular erythematous lesions developing within several hours of a tick bite represent hypersensitivity reactions and do not qualify as erythema migrans. In most patients, the expanding erythema migrans lesion is accompanied by other acute symptoms, particularly fatigue, fever, headache, mildly stiff neck, arthralgias, and myalgias. These symptoms are typically intermittent. The diagnosis of erythema migrans must be made by a physician. Laboratory confirmation is recommended for patients with no known exposure.

2. Late manifestations: These manifestations include any of the following *when an alternate explanation is not found*:

   a. Musculoskeletal system: Recurrent, brief attacks (lasting weeks or months) of objective joint swelling in one or a few joints. Manifestations that are not considered to be criteria for diagnosis include chronic progressive arthritis that is not preceded by brief attacks and chronic symmetric polyarthritis. Additionally, arthralgias, myalgias, or fibromyalgia syndromes alone are not accepted as criteria for musculoskeletal involvement.

   b. Nervous system: Lymphocytic meningitis, cranial neuritis, particularly facial palsy (may be bilateral), radiculo-

   neuropathy or, rarely, encephalomyelitis alone or in combination. Encephalomyelitis must be confirmed with evidence of antibody production against *Borrelia burgdorferi* in the cerebrospinal fluid, shown by a higher titer of antibody in the cerebrospinal fluid than in the serum. Headache, fatigue, paresthesias, or mildly stiff neck alone are not accepted as criteria for neurologic involvement.

   c. Cardiovascular system: Acute-onset, high-grade (second- or third-degree) atrioventricular conduction defects that resolve in days to weeks and are sometimes associated with myocarditis. Palpitations, bradycardia, bundle-branch block, or myocarditis alone are not accepted as criteria for cardiovascular involvement

3. Exposure: Exposure is defined as having been in wooded, brushy, or grassy areas (potential tick habitats) in an endemic county no more than 30 days before the onset of erythema migrans. A history of tick bite is not required.

4. Endemic county: A county in which at least two definite cases have been previously acquired or in which a tick vector has been shown to be infected with *B. burgdorferi*.

5. Laboratory confirmation: Laboratory confirmation of infection with *B. burgdorferi* is established when a laboratory isolates the spirochete from tissue or blood fluid, detects diagnostic levels of immunoglobulin M or immunoglobulin G antibodies to the spirochete in the serum or the cerebrospinal fluid or detects an important change in antibody levels in paired acute and convalescent serum samples. States may determine the criteria for laboratory confirmation and diagnostic levels of antibody. Syphilis and other known biologic causes of false-positive serologic test results should be excluded, when laboratory confirmation is based on serologic testing along.

---

* This epidemiologic case definition is intended for surveillance purposes only.

TREATMENT OF LYME DISEASE
Recommendations of Rahn DH and Malawista SE, Yale University School of Medicine,
Ann Intern Med 114:472, 1991 and Medical Letter consultants 34:17, 1992

Recommendations for Antibiotic Treatment*

Tick bite: Doxycycline 100 mg orally twice daily for 14 days is cost-effective in preventing
Lyme disease if the prevalence of *B. burgdorferi* in ticks exceeds 10%. Rates for I.
<u>dammini</u> ticks in New England and Mid-Atlantic states are 0.1-1% for larvae, 25% for
nymphs and 50% for adult ticks. Rates for *I. pacificus* in Western states are 1-3%
(NEJM 327:534, 1992).

Early Lyme disease+
    Doxycycline, 100 mg bid or tid for 10 to 30 days
    Amoxicillin, 250-500 mg three times daily for 10 to 30 days
    Erythromycin, 250 mg four times daily for 10 to 30 days
        (less effective than doxycycline or amoxicillin)
    Cefuroxime axetil, 500 mg bid x 10 to 30 days (Ann Intern Med 117:273, 1992)

Lyme carditis
    Ceftriaxone, 2 g daily intravenously for 14 to 21 days
    Penicillin G, 20 million units intravenously for 14 to 21 days
    Doxycycline, 100 mg orally twice daily for 14 to 30 days
    Amoxicillin, 500 mg orally three times daily for 14 to 30 days

Neurologic manifestations
    Facial nerve paralysis
        For an isolated finding, oral regimens for early disease,
            use for at least 21 to 30 days
        For a finding associated with other neurologic manifestations,
            intravenous therapy (see below)
    Lyme meningitis, radiculoneuropathy, peripheral neuropathy and encephalitis
        Ceftriaxone, 2 g daily by single dose for 14 to 21 days
        Penicillin G, 20 million units daily in divided doses for 14 to 21 days

Lyme arthritis
    Doxycycline, 100 mg orally twice daily for 30 days
    Amoxicillin and probenecid, 500 mg each orally four times daily for 30 days
    Penicillin G, 20 million units intravenously in divided doses daily for 14 to 21 days
    Ceftriaxone, 2 g intravenously daily for 14 days

In pregnant women
    For localized early Lyme disease, amoxicillin, 500 mg three times daily for 21 days
    For disseminated early Lyme disease or any manifestation of late disease, penicillin G,
        20 million units daily for 14 to 21 days
    For asymptomatic seropositivity, no treatment necessary

*   These guidelines are to be modified by new findings and should always be applied with
    close attention to the clinical course of individual patients. Most authorities use the
    longest duration of treatment suggested.
+   Shorter courses are reserved for disease that is limited to a single skin lesion only.

INFECTIONS OF THE EPIDERMIS, DERMIS AND SUBCUTANEOUS TISSUE

Condition	Agent	Laboratory diagnosis	Treatment
Superficial erythematous lesions			
Abscess	S. aureus	Culture and Gram stain Anaerobes	Drainage
Acne rosacea	?	Appearance	Doxycycline* Metronidazole (0.75% topical) Accutane
Acne vulgaris	Propioni- bacterium acnes	Appearance	Tetracycline* Topical clindamycin
Cellulitis: Diffuse spreading infection of deep dermis	Gr A strep; S. aureus (Vibrio sp. & Aeromonas sp. with fresh or salt water exposure)	Culture advanced edge of inflammation (rarely positive), 3-mm dermal punch, ulcerated portal of entry, blood Serial DNase titer (gr A strep)	Penicillinase-resistant penicillin*, vancomycin, clindamycin, cephalosporin- 1st gen, erythromycin
Erysipelas: Superficial infection with raised edge	Gr A strep	Culture: as above Serial DNase titer	Penicillin*, clindamycin, cephalosporin - 1st gen
Lymphangitis	Gr A strep	As above	As above
Folliculitis Infected hair follicle(s)	S. aureus (P. aeruginosa whirlpools, hot tubs, etc)	Culture and gram stain (usually unnecessary)	Local compresses or topical antibiotics. Fever, cellulitis or mid-face involvement - treat as furunculosis
Furunculosis carbuncle: Abscess that starts in hair follicle; carbuncle is deeper and more extensive	S. aureus	Culture and Gram stain	Drainage ± penicillinase-resistant penicillin*, clindamycin, vancomycin, cephalosporin - 1st gen, erythromycin, amoxicillin- clavulanate

(continued)

Condition	Agent	Laboratory diagnosis	Treatment
Recurrent furunculosis			Bathe with hexachlorophene May be controlled with chronic clindamycin, 150 mg qd x 3 mo.* Nasal carriers of staph - mupirocin to ant. nares or rifampin, 300 mg bid x 5 days
Paronychia: Infection of nail fold	<u>S. aureus</u> <u>Candida</u>	Culture and Gram stain	
Impetigo: Infection of epidermis	Gr A strep (<u>S. aureus</u>)	Culture and Gram stain	Penicillin V*, penicillin G benzathine, erythromycin or mupirocin; cloxacillin, cephalexin or amoxicillin + clavulanate
Whitlow: Infection of distal phalanx finger	<u>S. aureus</u> H. simplex	Culture and Gram stain; viral culture, Tzank prep or FA stain for H. simplex	Penicillinase- resistant penicillin*, clindamycin, cephalosporin - 1st gen.
Fungal infections: Keratinized tissue-skin, nails, hair (see pg 118)	<u>Candida</u>-red, moist, satellite lesions, esp skin folds	Scrapings for KOH prep, culture on Sabouraud medium	<u>Skin</u>: Topical anti-fungal agent: Miconazole, clothrimazole, econazole, naftifine or ciclopirox
	Dermatophytes-<u>Epidermophy-ton</u>, <u>Tricho-phyton</u>, <u>Micro-sporum</u>, "ring worm"	Scrapings for KOH prep and culture; Wood's light	<u>Skin</u>: Topical agents (as above) or oral ketoconazole <u>Nail</u>: Griseofulvin or ketoconazole <u>Scalp</u>: Selenium sulfide shampoo + griseofulvin
	Tinea versicolar-<u>Malassezia furfur</u>; red or hypopigmented macules		<u>Skin</u>: Topical agents (as above), oral ketoconazole or topical selenium sulfide
<u>Bites</u> Dog & cat	<u>P. multocida</u> Dysgonic fermenter type 2 (DF$_2$) <u>S. aureus</u>, anaerobes	Culture and Gram stain	Ampicillin + clavulanate (Augmentin)*, penicillin V ± cephalexin; tetracycline

(continued)

Condition	Agent	Laboratory diagnosis	Treatment
Human including clenched-fist injury	Oral flora (strep, anaerobes, etc) <u>S. aureus</u>, <u>Eikenella corrodens</u>	Culture and Gram stain	Amoxicillin-clavulanic acid (Augmentin)*, penicillin V ± cephalexin
Rat	<u>Strepto-bacillus moniliformis</u>	<u>S. moniliformis</u>: Giemsa stain of blood or pus; culture; serology	Penicillin*, tetracycline
	<u>Spirillum minus</u>	<u>S. minus</u>: Giemsa stain of blood or exudate	Penicillin*, tetracycline
<u>Cat scratch disease</u>	<u>Rochalimaea henselae</u> or <u>Afifpia felix</u>	Warthin-Starry stain of biopsy	Efficacy not established Sulfa-trimethoprim(?) Ciprofloxacin (?) Amoxicillin-clavulanate(?)
<u>Burns</u>	<u>S. aureus</u>, GNB <u>Candida albicans</u> <u>Aspergillus</u>, Herpes simplex, Gr A strep	Quantitative culture and stain of biopsy	Removal of eschar Topical sulfa (silver sulfadiazine or mafenide) Empiric antibiotics - Aminoglycoside + nafcillin, anti-pseudomonad, penicillin, ticarcillin clavulanate, vancomycin or cephalosporin
<u>Sinus tract</u> Osteomyelitis	<u>S. aureus</u>, S. epid., GNB, anaerobes	Culture of sinus tract drainage does not reliably reflect agent(s) of osetomyelitis	Antibiotics optimally based on bone biopsy
Lymphadenitis	<u>S. aureus</u> Mycobacteria (scrofula)	Culture and Gram stain AFB smear and culture	Anti-staphylococcal agent TB-Antituberculous drugs M. scrofulaceum-excision
Actinomycosis	<u>A. israelii</u> <u>A. naeslundii</u> <u>A. odontolyticus</u> <u>Arachnia proprionica</u>	FA stain, anaerobic culture	Penicillin G*, amoxicillin, clindamycin, tetracycline

(continued)

Condition	Agent	Laboratory diagnosis	Treatment
Madura foot	Nocardia	AFB stain, culture for Nocardia	Sulfonamides
	Fungi - Petriellidium boydii, Madurella mycetomatis, Phialophora verrucosa	KOH, culture on Sabouraud medium	
Nodules/ulcers			
Sporotrichoid (cutaneous inoculation with lymphatic spread)	Sporothrix schenckii (thorns)	Histology (PAS, GMS), culture on Sabouraud medium	Oral KI
	M. marinum (tidal water, swimming pool or tropical fish tank)	Histology, AFB stain & culture (at 30-32°C)	Rifampin + ethambutol Minocycline TMP-SMX
	Nocardia	Histology, AFB stain, culture for Nocardia	Sulfonamide
Nodules/ulcers (from hematogenous dissemination)	Blastomycosis Endemic area	Culture biopsy on Sabouraud medium	Ketoconazole, amphotericin B
	Cryptococcus Defective cell mediated immunity	Blood for cryptococcal antigen and culture; histopathology and culture of biopsy	Amphotericin B, fluconazole
	Candida - Defective cell-mediated immunity	Blood culture; histopathology and culture of biopsy	Amphotericin B
Diabetic foot ulcer and decubitus ulcer	Mixed aerobes-anaerobes S. aureus Gr A strep	Culture and Gram stain of wound edge or dermal punch biopsy	Local care - debridement, bedrest Antibiotics - for fever, extensive cellulitis, regional adenopathy or osteomyelitis Agents - parenteral agents as for intra-abdominal sepsis Oral regimen - ciprofloxacin + metronidazole or clindamycin

* Preferred regimen

Deep and Serious Soft Tissue Infections
(from Bartlett JG, Cecil Textbook of Medicine, W.B. Saunders Co, 1992, pg 1679)

	Gas-Forming Cellulitis	Synergistic Necrotizing Cellulitis	Gas Gangrene	"Streptococcal" Myonecrosis	Necrotizing Fasciitis	Infected Vascular Gangrene	Streptococcal
Predisposing conditions	Traumatic	Diabetes, prior local lesions, perirectal lesions	Traumatic or surgical wound	Trauma, surgery	Diabetes, trauma, surgery, perineal infection	Arterial insufficiency	Traumatic or surgical wound
Incubation period	> 3 days	3-14 days	1-4 days	3-4 days	1-4 days	> 5 days	6 hours-2 days
Etiologic organism(s)	Clostridia, others	Mixed aerobic-anaerobic flora	Clostridia, esp. C. perfringens	Anaerobic streptococci	Mixed aerobic anaerobic flora	Mixed aerobic-anaerobic flora	S. pyogenes
Systemic toxicity	Minimal	Moderate to severe	Severe	Minimal until late in course	Moderate to severe	Minimal	Severe
Course	Gradual	Acute	Acute	Subacute	Acute to subacute	Subacute	Acute
Wound findings							
Local pain	Minimal	Moderate to severe	Severe	Late only	Minimal to moderate	Variable	Severe
Skin appearance	Swollen, minimal discoloration	Erythematous or gangrene	Tense and blanched, yellow-bronze, necrosis with hemorrhagic bullae	Erythema or yellow-bronze	Blanched, erythema, necrosis with hemorrhagic bullae	Erythema or necrosis	Erythema, necrosis
Gas	Abundant	Variable	Usually present	Variable	Variable	Variable	No
Muscle involvement	No	Variable	Myonecrosis	Myonecrosis	No	Myonecrosis limited to area of vascular insufficiency	No
Discharge	Thin, dark, sweetish or foul odor	Dark pus or "dishwater," putrid	Serosanguineous, sweet or foul odor	Seropurulent	Seropurulent or "dishwater," putrid	Minimal	None or serosanguineous
Gram stain	PMNs, Gram-positive bacilli	PMNs, mixed flora	Sparse PMNs, Gram-positive bacilli	PMNs, Gram-positive cocci	PMNs, mixed flora	PMNs, mixed flora	PMNs, Gram-positive cocci in chains
Surgical therapy	Debridement	Wide filleting incisions	Extensive excision, amputation	Excision of necrotic muscle	Wide filleting incisions	Amputation	Debridement of necrotic tissue

185

BONE AND JOINT INFECTIONS

I. Osteomyelitis

A. Classification

	Hematogenous	Contiguous infection	Vascular insufficiency
Age	1-20 yrs	> 50 yrs	> 50 yrs
Bones	Long bones	Femur, tibia	Feet
	Vertebrae	Skull, mandible	
Associated conditions	Trauma	Surgery	Diabetes
	Bacteremia	Soft tissue	Neuropathy
	(any source)	infection	Vascular disease
Bacteriology	S. aureus	Mixed	Mixed
	Gram-neg rods	S. aureus	S. aureus
		Gram-neg rods	Streptococci
		Anaerobes	Gram-neg rods

B. Special conditions

	Bones	Bacteriology
Sickle cell disease	Multiple	<u>Salmonella</u>
IV drug abuse	Clavicle	<u>S. aureus</u>
	Vertebrae	<u>Pseudomonas</u>
Penetrating injury	Foot	<u>Pseudomonas</u>
Hemodialysis	Ribs	<u>S. aureus</u>
	Thoracic vertebrae	<u>S. aureus</u>
Chronic		
Brodie's abscess	Distal tibia	<u>S. aureus</u>
Tuberculosis	Spine (Potts')	<u>M. tuberculosis</u>
	Hip, knee	
Prosthetic joint	Site of prosthesis	<u>S. aureus</u>
		<u>S. epidermidis</u>

C. Treatment

<u>Acute</u>: Antibiotics x 4-6 weeks (S. aureus - nafcillin or oxacillin ± rifampin) + drainage of purulent collections.

<u>Chronic</u>: Antibiotics, intravenous x 4-6 weeks, then oral x 2 mo. (S. aureus - nafcillin IV ± rifampin <u>or</u> cloxacillin, 5 gm/day po + probenecid, 2 gm/day) + surgical debridement (Black J et al, J Infect Dis 155:968,1987).

<u>Empiric treatment</u>:

1. Settings in which <u>S</u>. <u>aureus</u> is anticipated pathogen

   <u>Preferred</u>: Nafcillin or oxacillin with or without an aminoglycoside, vancomycin with or without aminoglycoside, clindamycin with or without aminoglycoside

2. Patient with hemoglobinopathy

   <u>Preferred</u>: Nafcillin (or oxacillin) <u>plus</u> ampicillin

   <u>Alternatives</u>: Nafcillin (or oxacillin) plus cefotaxime (or ceftriaxone) <u>or</u> nafcillin (or oxacillin) plus chloramphenicol <u>or</u> cefazolin (or cephalothin or cephapirin) plus chloramphenicol

3. Osteomyelitis with vascular insufficiency, decubitus ulcer, diabetic foot
   ulcer, etc.
   Preferred: Aminoglycoside plus clindamycin, cefoxitin, imipenem, betalactam-
   betalactamase inhibitor or anti-pseudomonad penicillin
   Alternatives: Aztreonam plus clindamycin; beta-betalactamase inhibitor
   (alone); imipenem (alone); quinolone plus metronidazole or
   quinolone plus clindamycin
   Oral regimens: Quinolone with or without metronidazole or clindamycin;
   cefixime plus clindamycin; amoxicillin-clavulanate

II. Septic arthritis

A. Acute monarticular arthritis

1. Differential diagnosis: Septic arthritis, rheumatoid arthritis, gout and
   chondrocalcinosis (pseudogout)

2. Septic arthritis in adults

a. Agent	Treatment (alternatives)	Comment
S. aureus	Penicillinase resistant penicillin (cephalosporin, vancomycin, clindamycin) x 3 weeks	Accounts for 50-80% of non-gonococcal arthritis cases Cephalosporin-1st generation preferred
N. gonorrhoeae	Ceftriaxone 1 gm IV daily x 24-48 hrs, then oral agent (cefuroxime axetil, ciprofloxacin or amoxicillin + clavulanic acid or cefixime) to complete ≥ 7 day course	Most common cause of monarticular arthritis in young sexually active adults Skin lesions rarely present and blood cultures usually neg with gonococcal monarticular arthritis; joint fluid often culture positive
Streptococci	Penicillin (cephalosporin-1st gen, vancomycin, clindamycin) x 2 wks	Accounts for 10-20% of non-gonococcal septic arthritis cases
Gram-negative bacilli	Based on in vitro sensitivity tests Treat x 3 wks	Accounts for 10-20% of non-gonococcal septic arthritis cases Most commonly in chronically debilitated host, immuno-suppressed, prior joint disease Heroin addicts prone to sacroiliac or sternoclavicular septic arthritis due to pseudomonas aeruginosa

b. Empiric treatment (negative joint fluid gram stain and pending culture)

   (1) Sexually active adolesents and adults ages 15-40 yrs: Treat for disseminated
       gonococcal infection with ceftriaxone followed by oral agent to complete
       1 wk course of treatment (see pg 215). Some authorities add nafcillin or
       oxacillin for S. aureus.

187

(2) Older adults (> 40 yrs)

Preferred: Penicillinase-resistant penicillin (nafcillin with or without an aminoglycoside or penicillinase-resistant penicillin with or without a third generation cephalosporin.

Alternative: Cephalosporin (1st generation) with or without an aminoglycoside or vancomycin with or without an aminoglycoside or imipenem with or without an aminoglycoside.

3. Prosthetic joint:

a. Bacteriology: S. aureus (20-30%), S. epidermidis (20-30%), streptococci (15-25%), gram-negative bacilli (15-25%), anaerobes (5-10%).

b. Management: Surgical drainage, antimicrobials ≥ 6 wks, retention of prosthesis: 20-30% success

Removal of prosthesis, bactericidal antibiotics x 6 wks, then reimplantation: 90-95% success

Removal of prosthesis and reimplantation of prosthesis with antibiotic impregnated cement plus course of bactericidal antibiotics: 70-80% success

c. Empiric treatment: Vancomycin plus aminoglycoside, 3rd generation cephalosporin or imipenem

B. Chronic Monarticular Arthritis

1. Bacteria: Brucella, Nocardia

2. Mycobacteria: M. tuberculosis, M. kansasii, M. marinum. M. avium-intracellulare, M. fortuitum (See pp 133-134).

3. Fungi: Sporothrix schenckii, Coccidioides immitis, Blastomyces dermatitidis, Pseudoallescheria boydii (See pp 111-117).

C. Polyarticular Arthritis

1. Bacteria: Neisseria gonorrhoeae (usually accompanied by skin lesions, positive cultures of blood and/or genital tract, negative joint cultures); N. meningitidis; Borrelia burgdorferi (Lyme disease, see pp 171-172); pyogenic (10% of cases of septic arthritis have two or more joints involved).

2. Viral: Hepatitis B (positive serum HBsAg, seen in pre-icteric phase, ascribed to immune-complexes, hands most frequently involved); rubella (usually small joints of hand, women >men, simultaneous rash, also seen with rubella vaccine in up to 40% of susceptible postpubertal women); parvovirus B19 (hand/wrists and/or knees; adults > children; women > men); mumps (0.5% of mumps cases, large and small joints, accompanies parotitis, men > women).

3. Miscellaneous: Acute rheumatic fever (Jones' criteria including evidence of preceding streptococcal infection); Reiter's syndrome (conjunctivitis and urethritis, associated infections - Shigella, Salmonella, Campylobacter, Yersinia).

OCULAR AND PERIOCULAR INFECTIONS

Condition	Microbiology	Treatment	Comment
Conjunctivitis	S. pneumoniae	Topical sulfaceta-mide, bacitracin, erythromycin	Hyperemia ± discharge photophobia, pain vision intact
	N. gonorrhoeae	Ceftriaxone, 250 mg x 1	Most are self-limited Pharyngoconjunctival
	C. trachomatis	Erythromycin x 3 wks	fever - Adenovirus 3 & 7 Epidemic keratoconjunc-
	Adenovirus	None	tivitis - Adenovirus 8
	Allergic or immune-mediated	Topical prednisone	Lab - conjunctival scraping: bacteria -
	Unknown (empiric)	Topical sulfaceta-mide or neomycin-bacitracin- poly-myxin or bacitracin-polymyxin	PMNs, viral - mononuclear; herpetic - multinucleated cells; chlamydia-mixed; allergic-eosinophils
Keratitis	S. aureus; S. pneumoniae; P. aeruginosa; Moraxella; Serratia	Usually hospitalize for treatment to prevent perfora-tion Antibiotics-systemic, sub-conjunctival and/or topical ± corticosteroids	Pain; no discharge; decreased vision Lab-conjunctival scrapings for stain (Gram, Giemsa, PAS & methenamine silver) + culture for bacteria and fungi Systemic antibiotics for deep corneal ulcers with
	Herpes simplex	Trifluridine/vidarabine and/or corticosteroids	bacterial infection Supportive care with cytoplegics, use of
	Herpes zoster	Acyclovir	corticosteroids
	Fungal-Fusarium solani, Aspergillus, Candida	Topical natamycin, miconazole or flucytosine ± systemic anti-fungal	controversial For topical antibiotics use solutions
	Acanthamoeba	Topical propamadine isethionate, dibromopropamadine isethionate + neomycin; usually requires corneal transplant	
Endophthalmitis	Bacteria Post-ocular surgery - S. aureus, Pseudomonas, S. epidermidis, P. acnes	IV antibiotics ± intravitreal antibiotics, corticosteroids, vitrectomy	Lab-Aspiration of aqueous and vitreous cavity for stain (Gram, Giemsa, PAS, methenamine silver) and culture for bacteria and fungi (continued)

Condition	Microbiology	Treatment	Comment
Endophthalmitis (continued)	Penetrating trauma - <u>Bacillus</u> sp. Hematogenous - <u>S. pneumoniae</u>, <u>N. meningitidis</u> (others)		
	<u>Fungal</u> Post-ocular surgery <u>Neurospora</u>, <u>Candida</u>, <u>Scedosporium</u>, <u>Paecilomyces</u>	IV amphotericin + topical natamycin ± corticosteroids vitrectomy	
	Hematogenous - <u>Candida</u>, <u>Aspergillus</u>	IV amphotericin B	
	Histoplasmosis	Systemic cortico-steroids	
	<u>Parasitic</u> Toxoplasmosis	Systemic + local corticosteroids ± pyrimethamine and sulfadiazine	
	Toxocara	Systemic or intra-ocular cortico-steroids	
	<u>Virus</u>: Herpes simplex, H. zoster	Topical atropine + corticosteroids, Acyclovir (?)	Recurrence rate of H. simplex: 30-40%
Periorbital **Lid** Blepharitis	<u>S. aureus</u> - Seborrhea	Topical bacitracin or erythromycin + topical corticosteroid	
Hordeolum	<u>S. aureus</u>	Topical bacitracin or erythromycin + warm compresses	
Chalazion	Chronic granuloma	Observation or curettage	
Lacrimal apparatus Canaliculitis	Anaerobes	Topical penicillin + antibiotic irrigation	
Dacryocys-titis	Acute - <u>S. aureus</u>	Systemic antistaphy-lococcal agent; then digital message + antibiotic drops	
	Chronic - <u>S. pneumoniae</u> <u>S. aureus</u>, <u>Pseudomonas</u>, mixed	Systemic antibiotics; digital message	

(continued)

Condition	Microbiology	Treatment	Comment
Orbital	S. aureus (S. pneumoniae, S. pyogenes)	IV antibiotics- Cephalosporin, Cefuroxime or 3rd gen.	Over 80% have associated sinusitis Treat sinusitis
	Fungi - Phycomycosis, Aspergillus, Bipolaris, Curvularia, Drechslera	Amphotericin B+ surgery	

INFECTIONS OF THE CENTRAL NERVOUS SYSTEM

I. **Cerebrospinal Fluid**

A. Normal findings
1. Opening pressure: 5-15 mm Hg or 65-195 mm H_2O

2. Leukocyte count: <10 mononuclear cells/mm³ (5-10/ml suspect); 1 PMN (5%)

   Bloody tap: Usually 1 WBC/700 RBC with normal peripheral RBC and WBC counts; if abnormal: true CSF WBC = WBC (CSF) - WBC (blood) x RBC (CSF)/RBC (blood)
   Note: WBCs begin to disintegrate after 90 minutes

3. Protein: 15-45 mg/dl (higher in elderly)
   Formula: 23.8 x 0.39 x age ± 15 mg/100 ml or (more simply) less than patient's age (> 35 yrs)
   Traumatic tap: 1 mg/1000 RBCs

4. Glucose: 40-80 mg% or CSF/blood glucose ratio > 0.6 (with high serum glucose usual ratio is 0.3)

B. Abnormal CSF with non-infectious causes

1. Traumatic tap: Increased protein; RBCs; WBC count and differential proportionate to RBCs in peripheral blood; clear and colorless supernatant of centrifuged CSF.

2. Chemical meningitis (injection of anesthetics, chemotherapeutic agents, air, radiographic dyes): Increased protein, lymphocytes (occasionally PMNs).

3. Cerebral contusion, subarachnoid hemorrhage, intracerebral bleed: RBCs, increased protein (1 mg/1000 RBCs), disproportionately increased PMNs (peak at 72-96 hrs); decreased glucose in 15-20%).

4. Vasculitis (SLE, etc): Increased protein (50-100 mg/dl), increased WBCs (usually mononuclear cells, occasionally PMNs); normal glucose.

5. Postictal (repeated generalized seizures): RBCs (0-500/mm³), WBCs (10-100/mm³ with variable % PMNs with peak at 1 day), protein normal or slight increase.

6. Tumors (esp. glioblastomas, leukemia, lymphoma, breast cancer, pancreatic cancer): Low glucose, increased protein, moderate PMNs.

7. Neurosurgery: Blood; increased protein; WBCs (disproportionate to RBCs with predominance of mononuclear cells) up to 2 weeks post-op.

8. Sarcoidosis: Increased protein; WBCs (up to 100/mm³ predominately mononuclear cells); low glucose in 10%.

(continued)

C. **Doses of Drugs for CNS Infections***

1. Aminoglycosides and vancomycin

Agent	Systemic	Intrathecal/intraventricular
Gentamicin	1.7-2.0 mg/kg q8h (see pg 33, 34)	4-8 mg q24h
Tobramycin	1.7-2.0 mg/kg q8h (see pg 33, 34)	4-8 mg q24h
Amikacin	5.0-7.5 mg/kg q8h (see pg 33, 34)	10-20 mg q24h
Vancomycin	1 gm q12h	5-20 mg q24h

2. Cephalosporins

> Cefuroxime: 9 gm/day in 3 doses
> Cefotaxime: 12 gm/day in 6 doses**
> Ceftizoxime: 9 gm/day in 3 doses**
> Ceftriaxone: 4-6 gm/day in 2 doses**
> Ceftazidime: 6-12 gm/day in 3 doses**

3. Chloramphenicol: 4-6 gm/day in 4 doses**

4. Penicillins

> Ampicillin: 12 gm/day in 6 doses**
>
> Antipseudomonad penicillins
> > Ticarcillin: 18-24 gm/day in 6 doses (40-60 mg/kg q 4 h)
> > Mezlocillin: 18-24 gm/day in 6 doses (40-60 mg/kg q 4 h)
> > Azlocillin: 18-24 gm/day in 6 doses (40-60 mg/kg q 4 h)
> > Pipericillin: 18-24 gm/day in 6 doses (40-60 mg/kg q 4 h)
>
> Antistaphylococcal penicillins
> > Nafcillin: 9-12 gm/day in 6 doses
> > Oxacillin: 9-12 gm/day in 6 doses
>
> Penicillin G: 20-24 million units/day in 6 doses**

5. Trimethoprim-sulfamethoxazole: 15-20 mg/kg/day (trimethoprim) in 4 doses

> Metronidazole: 2 gm/day in 2-4 doses
> Vancomycin: 2 gm/day in 2 doses**

---

*   Assume adult patient with normal renal function.
** Recommendation of Tunkel AR et al, Ann Intern Med 112:610, 1990.

II. MENINGITIS (Medical Letter 34:49, 1992)

A. Likely pathogens and treatment

Setting	Likely agent	Empiric treatment* Preferred	Empiric treatment* Alternative	Comment
Adult Immunocompetent, community-acquired	S. pneumoniae N. meningitidis	Cefotaxime Ceftriaxone	Penicillin G Chloramphenicol Ceftizoxime Ceftazidime Ampicillin	Chloramphenicol is not effective against some GNB and some S. pneumoniae. GNB are rare except in newborns, adults >60 yrs, post-neurosurgery or immunosuppressed patients. In children, early use of decadron decreased incidence of hearing loss with H. influenzae meningitis (NEJM 324: 525, 1991); some recommend this for adults with pyogenic meningitis and mental status changes (JID 165:1, 1992)
Penicillin allergy	Same	Chloramphenicol		Cephalosporins can usually be used with penicillin allergy unless reaction was IgE mediated. Vancomycin may not reach effective CSF levels: combine with rifampin for resistant S. pneumoniae
Immunosuppressed Defective humoral immunity, asplenia, complement defect	S. pneumoniae N. meningitidis	As above	As above	
Defective cell-mediated immunity	Listeria Cryptococcus	Ampicillin ± aminoglycoside	Trimethoprim-sulfamethoxazole	Cephalosporins not active vs Listeria. Negative cryptococcal antigen assay of blood and CSF virtually excludes this diagnosis

194

(continued)

The table has two sections. First table:

Setting	Likely agent	Empiric treatment* Preferred	Empiric treatment* Alternative	Comment
Post-neurosurgical procedure	Enterobacteriaceae Pseudomonas sp. <u>Staph. aureus</u>	Aminoglycoside + antipseudomonad penicillin (or ceftazidime) + antistaph penicillin (or vancomycin)		In vitro sensitivity tests required, bactericidal activity preferred Infections that are refractory or involve resistant GNB may require intrathecal or intraventricular aminoglycosides
Cranial or spinal trauma Early (0-3 days)	<u>S. pneumoniae</u>	Penicillin or ampicillin	Chloramphenicol	Occasional cases with <u>H. influenzae</u> or <u>Strep pyogenes</u>
Late (over 3 days)	Enterobacteriaceae <u>Pseudomonas</u> <u>S. aureus</u> <u>S. pneumoniae</u>	Treat as recommended for postsurgical complication		
Ventricular shunt	<u>S. epidermidis</u>	Vancomycin ± rifampin	Anti-staphylococcal penicillin	In vitro sensitivity tests required Necessity to remove shunt is highly variable; most advocate antibiotics via shunt

* Antibiotic recommendations assuming clinical (± initial CSF analysis) evidence supporting this diagnosis with no direct clues to the etiologic agent.

B. Treatment by organism (See Tunkel A et al. Ann Intern Med 112:610,1990)

Organism	Preferred drug	Alternative	Comment
Strep pneumoniae	Penicillin G or ampicillin Cefotaxime Ceftriaxone	Chloramphenicol Cefuroxime Ceftizoxime	Test susceptibility to penicillin Resistant strains: chloramphenicol or vancomycin + rifampin Treat ≥ 10 days
Neisseria meningitidis	Penicillin G or ampicillin	(As above)	Intimate contacts should receive rifampin. Treat ≥ 7 days *(continued)*

Organism	Preferred drug	Alternative	Comment
Haemophilus influenzae	Ampicillin (Ampicillin-sensitive strains)	Chloramphenicol Cefotaxime Ceftizoxime Ceftriaxone Ceftazidime	If children < 4 yrs in household, contacts should receive rifampin prophylaxis (type B only) Treat ≥ 10 days Cefuroxime found inferior to ceftriaxone (NEJM 322:141,1990)
Listeria monocytogenes	Ampicillin ± gentamicin	Trimethoprim-sulfamethoxazole	Cephalosporins are not effective Treat 14-21 days
E. coli and other coliforms	Cefotaxime Ceftizoxime Ceftriaxone Ceftazidime	Aminoglycoside ± antipseudomonad penicillin or ampicillin Sulfa-trimethoprim Aztreonam* Quinolone*	In vitro sensitivity tests required; MBC data preferred Chloramphenicol lacks bactericidal activity vs GNB - not recommended Aminoglycoside is given systemically ± intrathecally Treat ≥ 21 days Ceftazidime should be reserved for suspected or established P. aeruginosa
Pseudomonas aeruginosa	Aminoglycoside + ceftazidime	Aminoglycoside + antipseudomonad penicillin (ticarcillin, mezlocillin, piperacillin, Aminoglycoside + aztreonam,* imipenem,* quinolones*	Sulfa-trimethoprim-Acinetobacter, Ps. cepacia and Flavobacterium Aminoglycoside is given systemically ± intratheally
Staph aureus	Antistaphylococcal penicillin ± rifampin	Vancomycin + rifampin Trimethoprim-sulfa + rifampin or ciprofloxacin	Vancomycin + rifampin for methicillin-resistant S. aureus
Staph epidermidis	Vancomycin + rifampin	Teicoplanin	

* Effectiveness in meningitis is not known

C. **Differential diagnosis of chronic meningitis*** (Adapted from Harris AA, Levin S: Infect Dis Clin Prat 1:158, 1992)

Infectious disease		Neoplastic	Miscellaneous
Bacteria	Fungi	Leukemia	Systemic lupus**
M. tuberculosis	Cryptococcus	Lymphoma	Wegener's granulomatosis**
Atypical mycobacteria	Coccidioides**	Metastatic	CNS vasculitis
Treponema pallidum**	Histoplasia**	Breast	Granulomatous vasculitis
Borellia burgdorferi**	Blastomyces	Lung	Sarcoidosis
Leptospira	Sporotrichum	Thyroid	Behçet's disease
Brucella**	Pseudoallescheria	Renal	Vogt-Koyanagi's and
Listeria	Alternaria	Melanoma	Harada's syndromes
Actinomyces/Arachnia	Fusaria	Primary CNS	Benign lymphacytic
Nocardia	Aspergillus	Astrocytoma	meningitis
Parasites	Zygomycetes	Glioblastoma	
Toxoplasma gondii	Cladosporium	Ependymoma	
Cysticercus	Viruses	Pinealoma	
Angiostrongylus	HIV**	Medulloblastoma	
Spinigerum	Echovirus		
Schistosoma			

* Defined as illness present for ≥ 4 wks with or without therapy; CSF analysis usually shows lymphocytic pleocytosis. Analysis of 83 previously healthy persons in New Zealand showed 40% had tuberculosis, 7% had cryptococcosis, 8% had malignancy and 34% were enigmatic (Q J Med 63:283, 1987)

** Evaluation: Culture, serum serology,** CT scan or MRI (brain abscess, cysticercosis, toxoplasmosis), cytology CSF (lymphoma, metastatic ca, eosinophilic (parasitic, cocardioidomycosis), CSF serology or antigen (cryptococcosis, coccidioidomycosis, syphilis, histoplasmosis), blind meningeal biopsy (rarely positive), empiric treatment (TB, then penicillin, then amphotericin B., then ? corticosteroids)

D. **Aseptic Meningitis: Infectious and Non-infectious Causes***
(from American Academy of Pediatrics, Pediatrics 78 (Supplement):970, 1986)

Infectious Agents and Diseases
    Bacteria: Partially treated meningitis, Mycobacterium tuberculosis, parameningeal focus (brain abscess, epidural abscess), acute or subacute bacterial endocarditis
    Viruses: Enteroviruses, mumps, lymphocytic choriomeningitis, Epstein-Barr, arboviruses (Eastern equine, Western equine, St. Louis), cytomegalovirus, varicella-zoster, herpes simplex, human immuno-deficiency virus
    Rickettsiae: Rocky Mountain spotted fever
    Spirochetes: Syphilis, leptospirosis, Lyme disease
    Mycoplasma: M. pneumoniae, M. hominis (neonates)
    Fungi: Candida albicans, Coccidioides immitis, Cryptococcus neoformans
    Protozoa: Toxoplasma gondii, malaria, amebas, visceral larval migrans (Taenia canis)
    Nematode: Rat lung worm larvae (eosinophilic meningitis)
    Cestodes: Cysticercosis
Non-infectious Diseases
    Malignancy: Primary medulloblastoma, metastatic leukemia, Hodgkin's disease
    Collagen-vascular disease: Lupus erythematosus
    Trauma: Subarachnoid bleed, traumatic lumbar puncture, neurosurgery
    Granulomatous disease: Sarcoidosis
    Direct toxin: Intrathecal injections of contrast medium, spinal anesthesia

Poison: Lead, mercury
Autoimmune disease: Guillain-Barré syndrome
Unknown: Multiple sclerosis, Mollaret's meningitis, Behçet's syndrome,
Vogt-Koyanagi's syndrome, Harada's syndrome, Kawasaki disease

---

* Aseptic meningitis is defined as meningitis in the absence of evidence of
a bacterial pathogen detectable in CSF by usual laboratory techniques.

E. **Empiric treatment meningitis** (assumes no LP or negative LP for likely pathogens)
    (Medical Letter 34:49, 1992)

    Age   3 mo-18 yrs: Cefotaxime or ceftriaxone
          18-50 yrs: Cefotaxime or ceftriazone; alternatives
                are ampicillin or penicillin G
          > 50 yrs: Ampicillin plus cefotaxime or ceftriaxone

III. **Brain abscess**

Associated condition	Likely pathogens	Treatment
Sinusitis	Anaerobic, micro-aerophilic and aerobic streptococci, <u>Bacteroides</u> sp.	Metronidazole + penicillin or chloramphenicol + penicillin
Otitis	<u>Bacteroides</u> <u>fragilis</u>, <u>Bacteroides</u> sp., streptococci, <u>Enterobacteriaceae</u>	Metronidazole + penicillin or chloramphenicol + penicillin
Trauma, post-neurosurgery	<u>Staph.</u> <u>aureus</u>	Penicillinase-resistant penicillin Vancomycin ± rifampin
	<u>Enterobacteriaceae</u>	Cefotaxime, ceftriaxone, ceftizoxime, ceftazidime Aminoglycoside + cephalosporin
	<u>Pseudomonas</u> <u>aeruginosa</u>	Aminoglycoside + ceftazidime or an anti-pseudomonad penicillin
Endocarditis	<u>Staph.</u> <u>aureus</u>	Penicillinase-resistant penicillin or vancomycin
	<u>Streptococcus</u> sp.	Penicillin or penicillin + aminoglycoside
Cyanotic heart disease	<u>Streptococcus</u> sp.	Penicillin or metronidazole + penicillin

UPPER RESPIRATORY TRACT INFECTIONS

Condition	Usual pathogens	Preferred treatment	Alternatives	Comment
Ear & Mastoids				
Acute otitis media	S. pneumoniae H. influenzae M. catarrhalis	Amoxicillin	Trimethoprim- sulfamethoxazole Amoxicillin + clavulanate Erythromycin + sulfoxazole Cefuroxime axetil Cefixime, Loracarbef Cefaclor, Cefprozil Cefpodoxime Tetracycline Parenteral: Cephalo- sporin-3rd gen	Tympanocentesis rarely indicated Less frequent pathogens: S. aureus, Strep. pyogenes. Oral or nasal decongestants ± antihistamine
Chronic suppurative otitis media	Pseudomonas Staph. aureus	Neomycin/polymyxin/ hydrocortisone otic drops	Chloramphenicol otic drops	Persistent effusion: myringotomy
Malignant otitis externa	P. aeruginosa	Tobramycin or amikacin + ticarcillin, mezlocillin or piperacillin Ciprofloxacin ± rifampin	Tobramycin or amikacin + cefoperazone, ceftazidime, aztreonam, imipenem, or ciprofloxacin	Surgical drainage and/or debridement sometimes required Treat 4-8 weeks Oral regimen - See Rubin J. Arch Otolaryngol Head Neck Surg 115:1063,1989
Acute diffuse otitis externa ("swimmer's ear")	P. aeruginosa Coliforms Staph. aureus	Topical neomycin + polymyxin otic drops	Boric or acetic acid (2%) drops Topical chloram- phenicol	Initially cleanse with 3% saline or 70-95% alcohol + acetic acid Systemic antibiotics for significant tissue infection
Otomycosis	Aspergillus niger	Boric or acetic acid drops	M-cresyl acetic otic drops	

(continued)

Condition	Usual pathogens	Preferred treatment	Alternatives	Comment
Acute mastoiditis	<u>S. pneumoniae</u> <u>H. influenzae</u>	Cefuroxime, trimethoprim-sulfamethoxazole, cephalosporin-3rd gen	Amoxicillin or ampicillin Amoxicillin + clavulanate	Surgery required for abscess in mastoid bone S. aureus is occasional pathogen, esp. in subacute cases
Chronic mastoiditis	Anaerobes Pseudomonas sp. Coliforms Staph. aureus	None		Surgery often required Pre-op: Tobramycin + ticarcillin or piperacillin
Sinusitis				
Acute sinusitis	<u>H. influenzae</u> <u>S. pneumoniae</u> <u>M. catarrhalis</u>	Amoxicillin	Trimethoprim-sulfamethoxazole Cefaclor, cefuroxime axetil, cefpodoxime Loracarbef, cefprozil Amoxicillin + clavulanate	Nasal decongestant Sinus lavage for refractory cases
Chronic sinusitis	Anaerobes S. aureus	Penicillin or amoxicillin	Amoxicillin + clavulanate Clindamycin	Usually reserve antibiotic treatment for acute flares Surgery may be required
Nosocomial sinusitis	<u>Pseudomonas</u> Coliforms	Aminoglycoside + anti-pseudomonad penicillin or aminoglycoside + cephalosporin-3rd gen (ceftazidime)	Imipenem, cephalosporin - 3rd gen	Complication of nasal intubation
Pharynx				
Pharyngitis	<u>Strep. pyogenes</u> (<u>Corynebacterium</u> <u>hemolyticum</u>, <u>C.</u> <u>diphtheriae</u>, <u>N.</u> <u>gonorrhoeae</u>, <u>Mycoplasma</u>, <u>C.</u> <u>pneumoniae</u>, viruses including EBV)	Penicillin po (strep only) x 10 days or benzathine penicillin IM x 1 Cefpodoxime Cefuroxime axetil	Erythromycin x 10 days Cephalosporin x 10 day Clarithromycin x 10 days Azithromycin x 5 days	If compliance questionable use benzathine pen Gx1 1M Penicillin sometimes preferred due to established efficacy in preventing rheumatic fever although

(continued)

Condition	Usual pathogens	Preferred treatment	Alternatives	Comment
Pharyngitis (continued)				some report higher strep eradication rates with some cephalosporins Erythromycin: About 5% of Gr A strep are resistant
Gonococcal pharyngitis	N. gonorrhoeae	Ceftriaxone (250 mg x 1)	Ciprofloxacin (500 mg x 1)	Most cases are asymptomatic
Peritonsillar or tonsillar abscess	Strep. progenes Peptostreptococci	Penicillin G	Clindamycin	Drainage necessary
Membranous pharyngitis	C. diphtheriae Epstein-Barr virus Vincent's angina (anaerobes)	Penicillin or erythromycin (diphtheria) Penicillin/clindamycin (anaerobes)		Diphtheria: Antitoxin
Epiglottitis	H. influenzae	Cefotaxime, ceftizoxime, ceftriaxone, ceftazidime	Cefuroxime Chloramphenicol + ampicillin	Ensure patent airway (usually with endotracheal tube) Rifampin prophylaxis for household contacts < 4 yrs (x 4 days)
Laryngitis	Viruses (M. catarrhalis)			For M. catarrhalis: trimethoprim-sulfa, erythromycin, amoxicillin-clavulanate or cefaclor
Perimandibular Actinomycosis	A. israelii	Penicillin G or V	Clindamycin	Treat for 3-6 months: Tetracycline, erythromycin
Parotitis	S. aureus (anaerobes)	Penicillinase-resistant penicillin	Cephalosporin-1st gen Clindamycin, vancomycin	Surgical drainage usually required
Space infections	Anaerobes	Penicillin Clindamycin	Cefoxitin, penicillin + metronidazole	Surgical drainage required (continued)

201

Condition	Usual pathogens	Preferred treatment	Alternatives	Comment
Cervical				
Cervical adenitis				
Acute	S. aureus Strep. pyogenes Anaerobes Viral Toxoplasmosis	Penicillin (S. pyogenes, anaerobes) Penicillinase-resistant penicillin (S. aureus)	Erythromycin Clindamycin Amoxicillin + clavulanate (Bacterial infections) Oral cephalosporin (not cefixime)	
Chronic	Mycobacteria, cat scratch disease, HIV infection	TB: INH, rifampin + pyrazinamide M. scrofulaceum: excision		Non-infectious causes include tumors, lymphoma, sarcoid
Dental				
Periapical abscess Gum boil Gingivitis Pyorrhea	Anaerobes Streptococci	Penicillin Clindamycin	Metronidazole + penicillin	Metronidazole often preferred for periodontal disease, i.e., gingivitis, periodontitis
Stomatitis				
Thrush	C. albicans	Oral nystatin (swish and swallow) or clotrimazole troches	Ketoconazole po Fluconazole po	
Vincent's angina	Anaerobes	Penicillin Clindamycin	Metronidazole, tetracycline	
Aphthous stomatitis	No pathogen identified	Topical corticosteroid (Topicort gel)	Systemic corticosteroids (Prednisone, 40 mg/day, then rapid taper) Silver nitrate	
Herpetiform ulcers	H. simplex	Acyclovir		Usually reserved for immunocompromised hosts

Cost of Oral Drugs Commonly Advocated for Upper Respiratory Infections

	Wholesale price for 10 day supply*	
Penicillins		
Penicillin G: 400,000 units po qid	$ 2.80**	
Penicillin V: 500 mg po qid	$ 3.20**	($ 9.60)
Ampicillin: 500 mg po qid	$ 5.40**	($ 8.22)
Amoxicillin: 250 mg po tid	$ 2.40**	($ 6.30)
Amoxicillin + clavulanate 250 mg po tid	$51.00	--
Dicloxacillin: 500 mg po qid	$18.50**	($30.00)
Cephalosporins		
Cefaclor: 250 mg po qid	$73.20	--
Cephalexin: 250 mg po qid	$ 6.00**	($46.00)
Cephradine: 250 mg po qid	$11.36**	($32.80)
Cefuroxime axetil: 250 mg po bid	$55.80	--
Cefprozil: 250 mg po bid	$52.60	
Clindamycin: 300 mg po tid	$64.11	--
Trimethoprim-sulfamethoxazole: 1 DS bid	$ 1.35**	($19.80)
Metronidazole: 500 mg po bid	$ 1.50**	($41.80)
Erythromycin: 500 mg po qid	$ 8.60**	($ 9.60)
Tetracycline: 500 mg po qid	$ 2.07**	($ 4.50)
Doxycycline: 100 mg po bid	$ 2.13**	($63.00)
Azithromycin: 6 250 mg tabs	$48.72	
Clarithromycin: 250 mg bid	$50.00	

* Approximate wholesale prices according to Medi-Span, Hospital Formulary Pricing Guide, Indianapolis, May, 1992. (Prices to patient will be higher.)

** Price provided is for generic product; price in parentheses is for a representative brand product when both brand and generic products are available.

A. Specimens and Tests for Detection of Lower Respiratory Pathogens. (Reprinted with permission from: Bartlett JG et al: Cumitech 7A, Sept 1987, pg 3)

Organism	Specimen	Test			
		Microscopy	Culture	Serology	Other
Bacteria					
Aerobic and facultatively anaerobic	Expectorated sputum, blood, TTA, empyema fluid, lung biopsy	Gram stain	X		
Anaerobic	TTA, empyema fluid	Gram stain	X		
Legionella sp.	Sputum, lung biopsy, pleural fluid, TTA, serum	FA	X	IFA, EIA	Urinary antigen[b]
Nocardia sp.	Expectorated sputum, TTA, bronchial washing, BAL fluid, tissue, abscess	Gram and/or modified carbol fuchsin stain	X		
Chlamydia sp.	Nasopharyngeal swab, lung aspirate or biopsy, serum		X[a]	CF for *C. psittaci*	PCR for *C. pneumoniae*[b] (experimental)
Mycoplasma sp.	Expectorated sputum, nasopharyngeal swab, serum		X[a]	CF,EIA or MI; cold agglutinins	
Mycobacteria	Expectorated or induced sputum, TTA, bronchial washing, BAL fluid,	Fluorochrome stain or carbol fuchsin	X		PPD
Fungi					
Deep-seated					
Blastomyces sp.	Expectorated or induced sputum, TTA, bronchial washing or biopsy, BAL fluid, tissue, serum	KOH with phase contrast; GMS stain	X	CF, ID	
Coccidioides sp.			X	CF, ID, LA	
Histoplasma sp.			X	CF, ID	Antigen assay BAL[b]
Opportunistic					
Aspergillus sp.	Lung biopsy	H&E, GMS stain	X	ID	CT scan[b]
Candida sp.	Lung biopsy	H&E, GMS stain	X		
Cryptococcus sp.	Expectorated sputum, serum, transbronch bx or BAL	H&E, GMS stain Calcofluor white	X	LA	Serum or BAL antigen assay[b]
Zygomycetes	Expectorated sputum, tissue	H&E, GMS stain	X		
Viruses: Influenza Paraflu, RSV, CMV	Nasal washings, naso-pharyngeal aspirate or swab, BAL fluid, lung biopsy, serum	FA: influenza and RSV	X	CF, EIA, LA, FA	CMV: shell viral culture, FA stain of BAL or bx[b]
Pneumocystis sp.	Induced sputum or bronchial brushings, washings, BAL fluid	Toluidine blue, Giemsa, or GMS stain			

Abbreviations: CF, complement fixation; MI, metabolic inhibition; PPD, purified protein derivative; ID, immunodiffusion; LA, latex agglutination; H & E, hematoxylin and eosin; CIE, counterimmunoelectrophoresis; EIA, enzyme immunoassay; FA, fluorescent antibody stain; IFA, indirect fluorescent antibody.

a Few clinical microbiology labs offer these cultures and those that do infrequently recover the indicated organisms.

b Added by author.

B. PREFERRED ANTIBIOTICS FOR PNEUMONITIS

Agent	Preferred antimicrobial	Alternatives	Comment
Bacteria			
S. pneumoniae	Penicillin G or V	Ampicillin/amoxicillin Cephalosporins (1st gen) Erythromycin Clindamycin Chloramphenicol Ofloxacin	Quinolones (ciprofloxacin) and some 3rd gen cephalosporins (ceftriaxone) are relatively inactive Penicillin resistance (high level): 2.6% in U.S. (1990-1991), 20-40% in Spain, S. Africa, Mexico, Alaska and East Europe.
Enterobacteriaceae (coliforms)	Cephalosporin (3rd gen) ± aminoglycoside	Aminoglycoside Aztreonam Antipseudomonad penicillin, Imipenem or betalactam- betalactamase inhibitor Fluoroquinolone	In vitro sensitivity tests required Aminoglycoside + second agent may be required for multiply resistant GNB
Pseudomonas aeruginosa	Aminoglycoside + anti-pseudomonad penicillin, or ceftazidime	Ciprofloxacin ± aminoglycoside Imipenem + aminoglycoside Aztreonam + aminoglycoside	In vitro sensitivity tests required Aminoglycoside combinations required for serious infections
Moraxella catarrhalis (Branhamella catarrhalis)	Trimethoprim-sulfa Erythromycin	Tetracycline Amoxicillin + clavulanate Cephalosporins Fluoroquinolones	70-80% of strains produce betalactamase
S. aureus Methicillin-sensitive	Penicillinase-resistant penicillin (nafcillin, oxacillin) ± gentamicin or rifampin	Cephalosporin - 1st gen Vancomycin Clindamycin	May add aminoglycoside or rifampin for serious or refractory infections
Methicillin-resistant	Vancomycin ± gentamicin or rifampin	Teicoplanin, fluoroquinolone Sulfa-trimethoprim	

(continued)

Agent	Preferred antimicrobial	Alternatives	Comment
H. influenzae	Ampicillin/amoxicillin (susceptible strains) Cephalosporin (3rd gen)	Cefuroxime Sulfa-trimethoprim Tetracycline Chloramphenicol Betalactam-beta-lactamase inhibitor Fluoroquinolones	15-30% of strains are ampicillin resistant
Anaerobes	Clindamycin	Penicillin Metronidazole + penicillin Betalactam-beta-lactamase inhibitor Cefoxitin	Penicillins other than anti-staphylococcal agents are equally effective compared to penicillin G Cephalosporins (esp cefoxitin) are probably effective, but published experience is limited Metronidazole should not be used alone
Mycoplasma pneumoniae	Tetracycline Erythromycin		Treat for 1-2 weeks
Chlamydia pneumoniae (TWAR agent)	Tetracycline or erythromycin		Treat for 10-14 days
Chlamydia psittaci	Tetracycline		Treat at least 10-14 days
Legionella	Erythromycin ± rifampin	Sulfa-trimethoprim + rifampin Doxycycline + rifampin Ciprofloxacin + rifampin Azithromycin or clarithromycin + rifampin	Treat for 3 weeks. Erythromycin is the only agent with established merit in clinical trials
Nocardia	Sulfonamide	Doxycycline Sulfa-trimethoprim Sulfa + minocycline or amikacin Imipenem ± amikacin	Usual sulfa is sulfadiazine Treat 3-6 months

(continued)

Agent	Preferred antimicrobial	Alternatives	Comment
Coxiella burnetii (Q fever)	Tetracycline	Chloramphenicol	

Mycobacteria: See section on Mycobacterial Infection:

Fungi: See section on Fungal Infections

Viruses: See section on Viral Infections

Parasites: See section on PCP Treatment

Pneumonia with no identified pathogen according to expectorated sputum stain and culture: community-acquired cases in immunocompetent adults

Agent	Preferred antimicrobial	Alternatives	Comment
Mycoplasma pneumoniae Chlamydia trachomatis Legionella sp. Anaerobes Viral (esp influenza) S. pneumoniae H. influenzae (S. aureus, GNB, Moraxella)	Outpatient: Erythromycin Hospital patient: Erythromycin + cefuroxime or 3rd generation cephalosporin	Outpatient: Cephalosporin, betalactam-betalactamase inhibitor, clarithromycin azithromycin, ofloxacin, tetracycline, sulfa-trimethoprim. Hospitalized patient: cefuroxime, cephalosporin-3rd gen; erythromycin ± sulfa-trimethoprim	Some cases are due to failure to detect fastidious bacteria such as S. pneumoniae and H. influenzae or lack of an adequate specimen Other possible agents: C. psittaci, C. psittaci, Coxiella (Q fever), Nocardia, Actinomyces
Pneumonia, nosocomial Gram-negative bacilli (esp P. aeruginosa, Klebsiella sp. and Enterobacter), S. aureus and anaerobes	Aminoglycoside + ceftazidime or antipseudomonad penicillin ± vancomycin	Aminoglycoside + 3rd gen cephalosporin, imipenem aztreonam or betalactam-betalactamase inhibitor ± vancomycin. Antipseudomonad penicillin + 3rd gen cephalosporin. Monotherapy: Imipenem, betalactam-betalactamase inhibitor or ceftazidime.	GNB and S. aureus causing pneumonitis or tracheo-bronchitis (intubation, tracheostomy) should be easily detected with gram stain and culture of respiratory sections Sporadic and nosocomial outbreaks may be due to Legionella sp. and C. pneumoniae has been implicated in 5-10% of cases; consider erythromycin in enigmatic cases

(continued)

207

C. **Lung abscess**

Agent	Preferred antimicrobial	Alternatives	Comment
Anaerobic bacteria	Clindamycin	Metronidazole + penicillin Penicillin/amoxicillin	Many antibiotics would probably work; suggestions are based on published reports with successful results in large numbers of patients

D. **Bronchitis**

Without chronic lung disease, intubation or tracheostomy

Agent	Preferred antimicrobial	Alternatives	Comment
Viral	None		Some cases due to <u>Mycoplasma pneumoniae</u> or <u>Chlamydia pneumoniae</u>: Tetracycline or erythromycin
Chronic bronchitis: exacerbation <u>S. pneumoniae</u> <u>H. influenzae</u>	Amoxicillin Tetracycline Sulfa-trimethoprim	Cefaclor, cefuroxime, cefpodoxime Cefixime, cefprozil, Loracarbef Amoxicillin + clavulanate Ciprofloxacin	

Tracheobronchitis: intubation or tracheostomy - see nosocomial pneumonia

ENDOCARDITIS

I.   ANTICIPATED AGENTS
     A. Non-addicts, native value
         Streptococcus sp: 55-65%
             Viridans strep (*S. sanguis, S. mutans, S. milleri, S. mitor*, etc): 35-40%
             Other (Microaerophilic, anaerobic and non-enterococcal gr D-
                 S. bovis): 10-15%
         Enterococcus faecalis: 10-15%
         Staphylococcal aureus: 15-20%
         HACEK (Hemophilus sp., Actinobacillus actinomycetemcomitans,
             Cardiobacterium hominis, Eikenella corrodens, Kingella kingii): 5-10%
     B. Prosthetic valve
             S. epidermidis > 50% occurring within 2 months post-op
             Others: S. aureus, GNB, diphtheroids and Candida
     C. Narcotic addicts
         S. aureus: 50%
         Streptococci: 20%
         GNB, especially Ps. aeruginosa: 20%
         Fungi, especially Candida sp: 10%

II. TREATMENT OF ENDOCARDITIS

     A. **Medical Management (Committee on Rheumatic Fever, Endocarditis and Kawasaki Disease of the American Heart Association's Council on Cardiovascular Disease in the Young: Antimicrobial Treatment of Infective Endocarditis due to Viridans, Streptococci,Enterococci and Staphylococci. JAMA 261:1471, 1989)**

         1. Streptococci

             a) Penicillin-sensitive streptococci (minimum inhibitory concentration < 0.1 μg/mL)

                 (1) Penicillin only: Aqueous penicillin G, 10-20 million units/day IV x 4 weeks. (Preferred regimen for patients with a relative contraindication to streptomycin including age > 65 years, renal impairment or prior 8th cranial nerve damage.)

                 (2) Penicillin + streptomycin x 4 weeks: Procaine penicillin G, 1.2 million units IM q 6 h or aqueous penicillin G, 10-20 million units/day x 4 weeks plus streptomycin, 7.5 mg/kg IM (up to 500 mg) q 12 h or gentamicin, 1 mg/kg IM or IV (up to 80 mg) q 8 h for first 2 weeks. (The disadvantage of the procaine penicillin + streptomycin is the necessity of 140 IM injections.)

                 (3) Two week course: Procaine penicillin G, 1.2 million units q 6 h IM or aqueous penicillin G, 10-20 million units plus streptomycin, 7.5 mg/kg IM (up to 500 mg) q 12 h. (Advocated as most cost-effective regimen by Mayo Clinic group for uncomplicated cases with relapse rates of < 1%.)

(4) <u>Penicillin allergy:</u> Vancomycin, 30 mg/kg/day IV x 4 weeks in 2-4 doses not to exceed 2 gm/day unless serum levels are monitored.

(5) <u>Penicillin allergy, cephalosporins:</u> Cephalothin, 2 gm q 4h x 4 wks or cefazolin, 1 gm IM or IV q 8 h x 4 wks. (Avoid in patients with immediate hypersensitivity to penicillin.)

Note

- Aqueous penicillin G should be given in 6 equally divided daily doses or by continuous infusion; disadvantage of procaine penicillin is the large number of IM injections.

- Streptococcus bovis and tolerant streptococci with MIC < 0.1 μg/mL may receive any of these regimens.

- Nutritionally deficient streptococci with MIC < 0.1 ug/mL should receive regimen #2 with IV penicillin; if susceptibility cannot be reliably determined treat for MIC > 0.1 mg/mL and < 0.5 μg/mL.

- Prosthetic valve endocarditis: Regimen #2 with IV penicillin for 6 weeks and aminoglycoside (streptomycin or gentamicin) for at least 2 weeks.

- Streptococci with MICs > 1000 mg/mL to streptomycin should be treated with gentamicin in aminoglycoside containing regimens. Gentamicin and streptomycin are considered equally effective for strains sensitive to both. An advantage of gentamicin is the ability to administer IV as well as IM.

- Cephalosporin regimens: Other cephalosporins may be effective, but clinical experience for agents other than cephalothin and cefazolin is limited.

- Two week treatment regimen is <u>not</u> recommended for complicated cases, e.g., shock, extracardiac foci of infection or intra-cardiac abscess.

- Desired peak serum levels if obtained: Streptomycin - 20 μg/mL, gentamicin - 3 μg/mL, vancomycin - 20-35 μg/mL (qid), or 30-45 μg/mL (bid).

b) Viridans streptococci and <u>Streptococcus bovis</u> relatively resistant to penicillin G (minimum inhibitory concentration > 0.1 μg/mL and < 0.5 μg/mL).

(1) Aqueous penicillin G, 20 million units/day IV x 4 weeks <u>plus</u> streptomycin, 7.5 mg/kg IM (up to 500 mg) q 12 h or gentamicin, 1.0 mg/kg (up to 80 mg) q 8 h x 2 wks.

    (2)   <u>Penicillin allergy</u>: Vancomycin, 30 mg/kg/day x 4 wks
          in 2-4 daily doses.

    (3)   <u>Penicillin allergy, cephalosporins</u>: Cephalothin, 2 gm IV
          q 4 h or cefazolin, 1 gm IM or IV q 8 h x 4 wks.

c)   Penicillin-resistant streptococci including enterococci and
     strains with minimum inhibitory concentrations of > 0.5 μg/ml.

    (1)   <u>Penicillin + aminoglycoside</u>:

Aq pen G 20-30		Strep, 7.5 mg/kg IM q12h
units/day IV <u>or</u>	plus	<u>or</u>
Ampicillin, 12 mg/		Gent, 1 mg/kg IM or IV
day IV		

    (2)   <u>Penicillin allergy</u>: <u>Vancomycin + aminoglycoside</u>

Vanco, 30 mg/kg/		Streptomycin, 7.5 mg/kg IM q12h
day IV in 2-4	plus	<u>or</u>
doses		Gent, 1 mg/kg IM or IV q8h

Note

- Choice of aminoglycoside is usually determined by <u>in vitro</u> sensitivity
  testing. Gentamicin and streptomycin are considered equally effective
  for treatment of strains susceptible at 2000 μg/mL; high level
  resistance is more likely with streptomycin so that gentamicin is
  preferred when <u>in vitro</u> testing cannot be done. Other aminoglycosides
  should not be used.

- Occasional strains produce beta-lactamase and should be treated with
  vancomycin.

- Patients with symptoms for over 3 months before treatment and those
  with prosthetic valve endocarditis should receive combined treatment
  for 6 wks.

- Serum levels of aminoglycosides should be monitored. Desirable peak
  levels are: Streptomycin - 20 μg/mL and gentamicin - 3 μg/mL.

2.   <u>Staphylococcus aureus</u> or <u>S</u>. <u>epidermidis</u>

   a.   No prosthetic device - methicillin-sensitive

     (1)   Nafcillin or oxacillin, 2 gm IV q 4 h x 4-6 wks $\pm$
           gentamicin, 1 mg/kg IV or IM q 8 h x 3-5 days.

     (2)   <u>Penicillin allergy, cephalosporin</u>: Cephalothin, 2 gm IV q 4 h <u>or</u>
           cefazolin, 2 gm IV q 8 h x 4-6 wks $\pm$ gentamicin, 1 mg/kg
           IV or IM q 8 h x 3-5 days (should not be used with
           immediate type penicillin hypersensitivity).

(3) <u>Penicillin allergy</u>: Vancomycin, 30 mg/kg/day in 2-4 doses (not to exceed 2 gm/day unless serum levels monitored) x 4-6 wks.

(4) <u>Methicillin-resistant strain</u>: Vancomycin, 30 mg/kg/day in 2-4 doses (not to exceed 2 gm/day unless serum levels monitored) x 4-6 wks.

B. Prosthetic valve or prosthetic material

1. Methicillin-sensitive strains: Nafcillin, 2 gm IV q 4 h x $\geq$ 6 wks <u>plus</u> rifampin, 300 mg po q 8 h x $\geq$ 6 wks <u>plus</u> gentamicin, 1 mg/kg IV or IM (not to exceed 80 mg) x 2 wks.

2. Methicillin-resistant strains: Vancomycin, 30 mg/kg/day in 2-4 doses (not to exceed 2 gm/day unless serum levels monitored) x $\geq$ 6 wks <u>plus</u> rifampin, 300 mg po q 8 h x $\geq$ 6 wks <u>plus</u> gentamicin, 1 mg/kg IV or IM (not to exceed 80 mg) x 2 wks.

Note

- Methicillin-resistant staphylococci should be considered resistant to cephalosporins.

- Tolerance has no important effect on antibiotic selection.

- The occasional strains of staphylococci that are sensitive to penicillin G at $\leq$ 0.1 μg/mL may be treated with regimens advocated for penicillin-sensitive streptococci.

- For native valve endocarditis, the addition of gentamicin to nafcillin or oxacillin causes a more rapid clearing of bacteremia, but has no impact on cure rates; use of gentamicin (or rifampin) with either methicillin-sensitive or methicillin-resistant strains is arbitrary. With vancomycin regimens, there is evidence for synergistic nephrotoxic effects and no enhanced efficacy; addition of aminoglycosides should be restricted to cases involving aminoglycoside-sensitive strains and duration limited to 3-5 days.

- Coagulase-negative strains infecting prosthetic valves should be considered methicillin-resistant unless sensitivity is conclusively demonstrated.

- Aminoglycoside selection for coagulase- negative strains should be selected on the basis of <u>in vitro</u> sensitivity tests; if not active, these agents should be omitted.

C. Empiric treatment for acute endocarditis (Recommendations of AMA's Drug Evaluations, AMA, Chicago, II/INF - 2:10, 1991)

1. Native valve
   a) Nafcillin or oxacillin: 2 gm IV q 4h plus Gentamicin (normal renal function): 1 mg/kg IV q 8h (adjust to keep peak serum level of about 3 mcg/ml) plus Aqueous penicillin G: 20 million units/day IV or ampicillin: 12 gm/day IV

   b) Vancomycin: 30 mg/kg/day IV (up to 2 gm/day) Gentamicin (above doses)

2. Prosthetic valve
   a) Vancomycin (above doses) plus Gentamicin (above doses) plus Ampicillin (above doses)

   b) Vancomycin (above doses) plus Gentamicin (above doses) plus Cephalosporin - 3rd generation: cefotaxime - 12 gm/day, ceftizoxime - 12 gm/day or ceftriaxone - 4 gm/day

III. **Indications for Cardiac Surgery in Patients with Endocarditis (Alsip SG, et al: Amer J Med 78(suppl 6B):138,1985)**

1. Indications for urgent cardiac surgery

   Hemodynamic compromise
     Severe heart failure (esp with aortic insufficiency)
     Vascular obstruction
   Uncontrolled infection
     Fungal endocarditis
     Persistent bacteremia (or persistent signs of sepsis)
     Lack of effective antimicrobial agents
   Unstable prosthetic valve

2. Relative indications for cardiac surgery

   a. Native valve
     Bacterial agent other than susceptible streptococci (such as S. aureus or gram-neg bacilli)
     Relapse (esp if non-streptococcal agent)
     Evidence of intracardiac extension
       Rupture of sinus of Valsalva or ventricular septum
       Ruptured chordae tendineae or papillary muscle
       Heart block (new conduction disturbance)
       Abscess shown by echo or catheterization
     Two or more emboli
     Vegetations demonstrated by echo (especially large vegetation or aortic valve vegetations)
     Mitral valve preclosure by echo (correlates with severe acute aortic insufficiency)

b. Prosthetic valve

Early post-operative endocarditis (< 8 wks)
Nonstreptococcal late endocarditis
Periprosthetic leak
Two or more emboli
Relapse
Evidence of intracardiac extension (see above)
Miscellaneous: Heart failure, aortic valve involvement, new or increased regurgitant murmur or mechanical valve versus bioprosthesis

3. <u>Point system</u>: Urgent surgery should be strongly considered with 5 accumulated points (Cobbs CG and Gnann JW: Indications for surgery in infective endocarditis. <u>In</u> Sande MA, Kaye D (Eds), Contemporary Issues in Infectious Disease. Churchill Livingstone, New York, 1984, pp 201-212).

	Native valve	Prosthetic valve
Heart failure		
Severe	5	5
Moderate	3	5
Mild	1	2
Fungal etiology	5	5
Persistent bacteremia	5	5
Organism other than susceptible strep	1	2
Relapse	2	3
One major embolus	2	2
Two or more systemic emboli	4	4
Vegetations by echocardiography	1	1
Ruptured chordae tendinae or papillary mm	3	-
Ruptured sinus of Valsalva	4	4
Ruptured ventricular septum	4	4
Heart block	3	3
Early mitral valve closure by echo	2	
Unstable prosthesis	-	5
Early prosthetic valve endocarditis	-	2
Periprosthetic leak	-	2

INTRA-ABDOMINAL SEPSIS: ANTIBIOTIC SELECTION

I. **Peritonitis**

    A. Polymicrobial infection

        1. Combination treatment*

        An aminoglycoside vs. coliforms**

        a. Gentamicin, 2.0 mg/kg, then 1.7 mg/kg IV q 8 h (usually preferred) <u>or</u>

        b. Tobramycin, 2.0 mg/kg, then 1.7 mg/kg IV q 8 h <u>or</u>

        c. Amikacin, 7.5 mg/kg, then 5.0 mg/kg IV q 8 h <u>or</u>

        Plus an agent vs. anaerobes

        a. Clindamycin, 600 mg IV q 8 h <u>or</u>

        b. Cefoxitin, 2 gm IV q 6 h <u>or</u>

        c. Metronidazole, 500 mg IV q 8 h

---

*   Some authorities add an agent for the enterococcus:
Ampicillin, 1-2 gm IV q 6 h.

** Aztreonam, 1-1.5 gm IV q6-8h, may be used in place of
aminoglycoside in combination with metronidazole or
clindamycin.

        2. Single drug treatment

        a. Cefoxitin, 2 gm IV q 6 h (not advocated as single agent if infection was acquired during hospitalization or if there has been antibiotic administration during prior 2 weeks). Alternatives to cefoxitin are: cefotetan, 1 gm IV q 12 h or cefmetazole, 2 gm q6-12h.

        b. Imipenem, 500 mg IV q 6-8 h (See Solomkin J et al. Ann Surg 212:581,1990).

        c. Ticarcillin, 3 gm + clavulanic acid, 100 mg (Timentin) IV q 4-6 h

        d. Ampicillin, 2 gm + sulbactam, 1 gm (Unasyn) IV q 6 h

    B. Monomicrobial infections

        1. Spontaneous peritonitis or "primary peritonitis"

        a. Gentamicin or tobramycin, 2 mg/kg IV, then 1.7 mg/kg q 8 h <u>plus</u> a betalactam: Cefoxitin, 2 gm IV q 6 h; cefotaxime, 1.5-2 gm IV q 6 h; ampicillin, 2 gm IV q 6 h; or piperacillin, 4-5 gm IV q 6 h

        b. Cefotaxime, 1.5-2 gm IV q 6 h $\pm$ ampicillin, 2 gm IV q 6 h

2. Peritonitis associated with peritoneal dialysis

   a. Vancomycin, 1 gm IV (single dose)

   b. Antibiotics added to dialysate based on in vitro sensitivity:
      Nafcillin, 10 mg/L; ampicillin, 20 mg/L; ticarcillin, 100
      100 mg/L; penicillin G, 1,000-2,000 units/L; cephalothin,
      20 mg/L; gentamicin or tobramycin, 5 mg/L; amikacin,
      25 mg/L; clindamycin, 10 mg/L

3. Candida peritonitis (diagnostic criteria and indications to
   treat in absence of peritoneal dialysis are nebulous)

   a. Amphotericin B, 200-1000 mg (total dose) 1 mg IV over 6 hrs,
      then increase by 5-10 mg/day to maintenance dose of 20-30
      mg/day

   b. Peritoneal dialysis: Systemic amphotericin B (above regimen)
      plus addition to dialysate, 2-5 μg/ml

4. Tuberculous
   INH, 300 mg/day po, plus rifampin, 600 mg/day po, plus
   pyrazinamide, 15-30 mg/kg/day po x 2 months, then INH plus
   rifampin x 7-22 months

II. Localized Infections

A. Intra-abdominal abscess(es) (not further defined): Use regimens
   recommended for polymicrobial infections with peritonitis.

B. Liver abscess

   1. Amebic

      a. Preferred: Metronidazole, 750 mg po or IV tid x 10 days plus
         diloxanide furate, 500 mg po tid x 10 day or paromomycin, 500 mg
         po bid x 7 days.

      b. Alternative: Emetine, 1 mg/kg/day IM x 5 days (or dehydro-
         emetine, 1-1.5 mg/kg day x 5 days) followed by chloroquine,
         500 mg po bid x 2 days, then 250 mg po bid x 3 weeks plus
         iodoquinol, 650 mg po tid x 20 days

   2. Pyogenic

      a. Gentamicin or tobramycin, 2.0 mg/kg IV, then 1.7 mg/kg IV
         q 8 h plus metronidazole, 500 mg IV q 8 h; clindamycin,
         600 mg IV q 8 h, or cefoxitin, 2 gm IV q 6 h plus ampicillin,
         2 gm IV q 6 h or penicillin G, 2 million units IV q 6 h

      b. Gentamicin or tobramycin (above doses) plus clindamycin (above
         doses), cefoxitin (above doses) or piperacillin 4-5 gm IV q 6 h

C. Biliary tract infections

    1. Cholecystitis

        a. Combination treatment: Gentamicin or tobramycin, 2.0 mg/kg IV, then 1.7 mg/kg IV q 8 h <u>plus</u> ampicillin, 2 gm IV q 6 h, piperacillin, 2-5 gm IV q 6 h, or cefoperazone, 1-2 gm IV q 12 h*

        b. Single agent: Cefoperazone, 1-2 gm IV q 12 h*. Ampicillin + sulbactam, 1-2 gm IV q 6 h; ticarcillin-clavulanate, 2-3 gm IV q 6 h; for mild infections the usual recommendation is cefazolin, 1-2 gm IM or IV q 8 h, or ampicillin 1-2 gm IV q 6 h.

---

* Other cephalosporins (2nd and 3rd generation) are probably equally effective. Some authorities add ampicillin (1-2 gm IV q 6 h) to cephalosporin containing regimens.

    2. Ascending cholangitis, empyema of the gallbladder, or emphysematous cholecystitis: Treat with regimens advocated for peritonitis or intra-abdominal abscess.

D. <u>Appendicitis</u> (adult doses) (Role of antibiotics in nonperforative appendicitis is unclear.)

    1. Combination treatment: Gentamicin <u>or</u> tobramycin, 2.0 mg/kg IV, then 1.7 mg/kg q 8 h <u>plus</u> clindamycin, 600 mg IV q 8 h, cefoxitin, 2 gm IV q 6 h <u>or</u> metronidazole, 500 mg IV q 6 h

    2. Single agent: Cefoxitin, 2 gm IV q 6 h

E. <u>Diverticulitis</u> (Role of antibiotics in uncomplicated diverticulitis is unclear.)

    1. Ambulatory patient

        a. Ampicillin, 500 mg po qid
        b. Tetracycline, 500 mg po qid
        c. Amoxicillin plus clavulanic acid (Augmentin), 500 mg po qid
        d. Cephalexin, 500 mg po qid <u>plus</u> metronidazole, 500 mg po qid

    2. Hospitalized patients: Use regimens advocated for peritonitis or intra-abdominal abscess.

HEPATITIS

A. Types, clinical features and prognosis (MMWR 34:313,1985; MMWR 37:341, 1988; MMWR 39:1, 1990 and MMWR 40RR 12:1, 1991)

Type	Source	Incubation period	Diagnosis of acute viral hepatitis*	Prognosis
A (HAV)	Person-to-person fecal-oral Contaminated food & water (epidemic) Seroprevalence: Anti-HAV in adults U.S.: 40-50%	15-50 days Avg: 28 days	IgM-anti-HAV	Self limited: > 99% Fulminant & fatal: 0.6% No carrier state or chronic infection Severity increases with age
B (HBV)	Sexual contact or contaminated needles from HBsAg carrier (transmission via blood transfusions is rare due to HBsAg screening) Efficacy of transmission increased if source is HBeAg positive Seroprevalence (any marker, U.S.) (see pg 83) General population: 3-14% blacks: 14%; whites: 3% IV drug abuse: 60-80% Gay men: 35-80% Hemodialysis patients: 20-80% Health care workers (unvaccinated, frequent blood exp): 15-30% (unvaccinated, no frequent blood exp): 3-10%	45-160 days Avg: 120 days	HBsAg and/or IgM anti-HBc	Fulminant & fatal: 1.4% Carrier state, (defined as HBsAg-pos, twice separated by 6 months or HBsAg pos and IgM anti-HBc neg): 6-10% of adults; 25-50% of children < 5 yrs (this means 6-10% of adults with any marker will be HBsAg pos) Chronic carriers: 25% develop chronic active hepatitis that progresses to cirrhosis in 15-30%, fatal cirrhosis in 1%/yr and/or fatal hepatocellular carcinoma in 0.25%/yr Perinatal with HBsAg-pos and HBeAg-pos mother: 70-90% acquire perinatal HBV infection and 85-90% of these will become chronic carriers; > 25% of these carriers will develop cirrhosis or hepatocellular carcinoma Risk of transmission with needlestick from HBsAg-pos source: 6-30%

(continued)

Type	Source	Incubation period	Diagnosis of acute viral hepatitis[*]	Prognosis
C (HCV) (parenterally transmitted non-A,non-B) also causes sporadic NANB hepatitis	Contaminated transfused blood: 10%; IVDA-40%; heterosexual contact-10%; unknown-40% Seroprevalence rates (U.S.) Blood donors: 0.5-0.6% General population: 2% Hemophiliacs: 60-90% IV drug abuse: 60-90% Dialysis patients: 15-20% Gay men: 8%; Cryptogenic cirrhosis: 50-70% Chronic NANB hepatitis: 90-96%	14-84 days	Neg IgM anti-HAV, neg HBsAg and/or IgM anti-HBC; anti-HCV now available, but requires mean of 6 mo. to seroconvert with acute hepatitis; only about 30% of positive serologic tests in blood donors are true positives False positives with hyperglobulinemia including 5-6% with autoimmune chronic active hepatitis Preferred diagnostic tests are "2nd gen" such as RIBA-2 and PCR for HCV RNA (increased sensitivy, increased specificity and more rapid seroconversion)	Fulminant & fatal: rare Chronic hepatitis: 50%; cirrhosis: 10% (20% of those with chronic hepatitis); relationship to hepatocellular carcinoma is probable
Delta	Defective virus that requires presence of active HBV, e.g., co-infection with HBV or superinfection in HBsAg carrier; main source is blood (IV drug abuse, hemophilia) Seroprevalence in HBsAg carriers: IV drug abusers: 10-40% Hemophiliacs: 50-80% Hemodialysis patients: 20%	Superinfection: 30-60 days Co-infection: same as HBV	HBsAg + anti-HDV, but in delta hepatitis anti-HDV appears late and is short lived Co-infection: IgM anti-HBc + anti-HDV Superinfection: persistent HBs + anti-HDV in high titer (> 1:100)	Acute co-infection with HBV: 1-10% acute fatality; < 5% chronic hepatitis Acute superinfection: 5-20% acute fatility >75% develop chronic hepatitis with 70-80% developing cirrhosis Epidemics in underdeveloped countries: fulminant fatal hepatitis in 10-20% of children Chronic delta hepatitis: Worsens prognosis of chronic HBV infection

219

(continued)

Type	Source	Incubation period	Diagnosis of acute viral hepatitis*	Prognosis
Delta	Endemic areas (Mediterranean Basin, Middle East, Amazon Basin): 20-40% Medical care workers and gay men: low			
E (HEV) (enterally transmitted non-A,non-B or epidemic (NANB)	Epidemic fecal-oral (Burma, Borneo, Somalia, Pakistan, China, Soviet Union, throughout Africa)	20-60 days (mean 40 days)	As above but neg anti-HCV at 1 yr No chronic infection	Mortality < 2% except for pregnant women with mortality of 10-20% Usually mild disease predominately in adults > 15 yrs; chronic liver disease has not been reported

* Symptoms or signs of viral hepatitis, serum aminotransferase > 2.5 x upper limit of normal, and absence of other causes of liver injury.

Centers for Disease Control Hepatitis Hotline: Automated telephone information system concerning modes of transmission, prevention, serologic diagnosis, statistics and infection control (404) 332-4555.

B. Hepatitis nomenclature (MMWR 39:6,1990)

	Abbreviation	Term	Definition/Comments
Hepatitis A	HAV	Hepatitis A virus	Etiologic agent of "infectious" hepatitis; a picornavirus; single serotype.
	Anti-HAV	Antibody to HAV	Detectable at onset of symptoms; lifetime persistence.
	IgM anti-HAV	IgM class antibody to HAV	Indicates recent infection with hepatitis A; detectable for 4-6 months after infection.
Hepatitis B	HBV	Hepatitis B virus	Etiologic agent of "serum" hepatitis; also known as Dane particle.
	HBsAg	Hepatitis B surface antigen	Surface antigen(s) of HBV detectable in large quantity in serum; several subtypes identified.
	HBeAg	Hepatitis B e antigen	Soluble antigen; correlates with HBV replication, high titer HBV in serum, and infectivity of serum.
	HBcAg	Hepatitis B core antigen	No commercial test available
	Anti-HBs	Antibody to HBsAg	Indicates past infection with and immunity to HBV, passive antibody from HBIG, or immune response from HB vaccine.
	Anti-HBe	Antibody to HBeAg	Presence in serum of HBsAg carrier indicates lower titer of HBV.
	Anti-HBc	Antibody to HBcAg	Indicates prior infection with HBV at some undefined time.
	IgM anti-HBc	IgM class antibody to HBcAg	Indicates recent infection with HBV; detectable for 4-6 mo after infection
Delta hepatitis	HDV	Hepatitis D virus	Etiologic agent of delta hepatitis; can cause infection only in presence of HBV.
	HDAg	Delta antigen	Detectable in early acute delta infection.
	Anti-HDV	Antibody to delta antigen	Indicates present or past infection with delta virus.
Hepatitis C	HCV	Hepatitis C	Formerly parenterally transmitted non-A, non-B hepatitis (PT-NANB); shares epidemiologic features with hepatitis B.
	Anti-HCV	Antibody to HCV	Indicates past infection with HCV; usually means persistent HCV infection.
Hepatitis E	HEV	Hepatitis E	Formerly enterically transmitted non-A, non-B hepatitis (ET-NANB); shares epidemiologic features with hepatitis A.
Immune globulins	IG	Immune globulin (previously ISG, immune serum globulin, or gamma globulin)	Contains antibodies to HAV, low-titer antibodies to HBV.
	HBIG	Hepatitis B immune globulin	Contains high-titer antibodies to HBV.

INFECTIOUS DIARRHEA

A. ANTIMICROBIAL TREATMENT

Microbial Agent	Preferred	Alternative	Comment
Bacteria			
Aeromonas hydrophilia	Sulfa-trimethoprim 1 DS bid x 5 days Ciprofloxacin, 500 mg po bid x 5 days	Tetracycline, 500 mg po qid x 5 days Gentamicin, 1.7 mg/kg IV q8h x 5 days	Efficacy of treatment not established and should be reserved for patients with severe disease, immunosuppression, extraintestinal infection or prolonged diarrhea.
Campylobacter jejuni	Erythromycin, 250-500 mg po qid x 7 days Ciprofloxacin, 500 mg po bid x 7 days	Doxycycline, 100 mg po bid x 7 days Furazolidone, 100 mg po qid x 7 days	May not alter course unless given early or for severe Sx. Indications include: acutely ill, persistent fever, bloody diarrhea, > 8 stools/day, dehydration symptoms < 4 days or to prevent transmission. Resistance to erythromycin has been described. Clinical course not altered when treatment started > 4 days after onset of symptoms.
Clostridium difficile	Vancomycin, 125 mg po q6h x 10-14 days Metronidazole, 250 mg po qid x 10-14 days	Bacitracin, 25,000 units po qid x 10-14 days Cholestyramine, 4 gm packet tid	Vancomycin is preferred for severe disease. Discontinuation of implicated antibiotic is often adequate. Some strains are highly resistant to bacitracin. Relapses: Vancomycin or metronidazole x 10-14 days, _then_ cholestyramine (4 gm po tid), vancomycin (125 mg po tid) or lactobacilli (1 gm qid) x 21 days _or_ vancomycin + rifampin (600 mg/day). When oral treatment is not possible: metronidazole, 500 mg q8h IV.

(continued)

Microbial Agent	Preferred	Alternative	Comment
E. coli Enterotoxigenic E. coli (ETEC) Enteroadherent E. coli (EAEC)	Sulfa-trimethoprim 1 DS po bid x 3 days Ciprofloxacin, 500 mg po bid x 3 days Ofloxacin 300 mg po bid x 3 days	Trimethoprim, 200 mg po bid x 3 days Doxycycline, 100 mg po bid x 3 days Bismuth subsalicylate 60 ml quid x 5 days	Laboratory confirmation for E. coli - associated diarrhea is usually not available except for EHEC. Efficacy not established except for enterotoxin producing strains, e.g., ETEC (traveler's diarrhea). Many ETEC strains are now resistant to doxycycline and TMP-SMX
Enterohemorrhagic E. coli (EHEC)	Ciprofloxacin, 500-750 mg po bid x 5-7 days		Efficacy not established. Sulfa-trimethoprim may increase toxin production.
Enteroinvasive E. coli (EIEC)	Ampicillin, 500 mg po or 1 gm IV qid x 5 days Sulfa-trimethoprim 1 DS po bid x 5 days	Ciprofloxacin, 500 mg po bid x 5 days	Associated with hemolytic-uremic syndrome and TTP. Laboratory detection: stool culture for E. coli serotype 0157:H7 or analysis for Shiga toxin
Enteropathogenic E. coli (EPEC)	Sulfa-trimethoprim 1 DS po bid x 3-5 days	Neomycin, 100 mg/kg/day po x 3-5 days Furazolidone, 100 mg po qid x 3-5 days	Presentation is dysentery as with Shigella
Food poisoning Clostridium perfringens, Staph. aureus, Bacillus cereus, Listeria	None		Self-limited and toxin mediated: antimicrobial treatment is not indicated.
Plesiomonas shigelloides	Sulfa-trimethoprim, 1 DS po bid x 5 days Ciprofloxacin, 500 mg po bid x 5 days	Tetracycline, 500 mg po qid x 5 days	Efficacy of treatment is not established and should be reserved for patients with extraintestinal infection, prolonged diarrhea or immunosuppression.

(continued)

223

Microbial Agent	Preferred	Alternative	Comment

Salmonella
Typhoid fever
  S. typhi
Non-typhoid
  Salmonella
Enteric fever (non-typhoid Salmonella)
Metastatic infection
Chronic bacteremia
Enterocolitis in compromised host
	Sulfa-trimethoprim 1-2 DS po bid x 14 days
	Ampicillin, 2-6 gm po or IV/day x 14 days
	Amoxicillin, 2-4 gm po/day x 14 days
	Chloramphenicol, 3-4 gm/day IV or po x 14 days
	Cefotaxime, 4-8 gm/day IV x 14 days
	Cefoperazone, 1 gm bid IV IV x 14 days
	Ceftriaxone, 1 gm IV bid x 14 days
		Ciprofloxacin, 500 mg po qid x 14 days	Antibiotic treatment is contraindicated in patients with uncomplicated enterocolitis; indications are typhoid fever, chronic bacteremia, metastatic infection or enterocolitis in compromised host (AIDS, sickle cell hemoglobinopathy, lymphoma, etc).
			AIDS patients may require long term suppressive treatment with ampicillin or ciprofloxacin.
			Patients with typhoid fever or enteric fever should receive antibiotics in high doses initially; with severe toxicity give dexamethasone (3 mg/kg x 1, then 1 mg/kg q6h x 48 hr) or prednisone (60 mg/day 20 mg/day over 3 days).

Carrier	Ampicillin, 4-6 gm/day or amoxicillin, 6 gm/day + probenecid, 2 gm/day x 6 weeks	Ciprofloxacin, 500-750 mg po bid x 6 wks Rifampin, 300 mg bid + sulfa-trimethoprim, 1 DS bid x 6 wks	Cholecystectomy for cholelithiasis and carriers who relapse.
Shigella	Ciprofloxacin, 500 mg po bid or norfloxacin, 400 mg po bid x 3-5 days Sulfa-trimethoprim 1 DS po bid x 3-5 days	Ampicillin, 500 mg po or 1 gm IV qid x 3-5 days Nalidixic acid, 1 gm po qid x 5-7 days Cefoperazone, 1-2 gm IV q12h x 5-7 days	Preferred agents for empiric treatment are sulfa-trimethoprim or ciprofloxacin/norfloxacin. Ampicillin-resistant strains are common; for ampicillin-susceptible strains, amoxicillin should not be used. Sulfa-trimethoprim resistance is increasing and is common in strains from underdeveloped areas.

(continued)

Microbial Agent	Preferred	Alternative	Comment
Vibrio cholerae	Tetracycline, 500 mg po qid x 3-5 days Doxycycline, 300 mg po x 1	Sulfa-trimethoprim, 1 DS po bid x 3 days Furazolidine, 100 mg po qid x 3 days Erythromycin, 250 mg po qid x 3 days	Efficacy of treatment is not established and should be reserved for severe disease.
Vibrio sp. (V. parahaemolyticus, V. fluvialis, V. mimicus, V. hollisae, V. furnissii, V. vulnificus)	Tetracycline (as above - see comments)	Ciprofloxacin, 500 mg po bid x 5 days	
Yersinia enterocolitica	Sulfa-trimethoprim 1 DS po bid x 7 days Gentamicin, 1.7 mg/kg IV q8h x 7 days	Ciprofloxacin, 500-750 po bid x 7 days Doxycycline, 100 mg po bid x 7 days Chloramphenicol, 3-4 gm/day po or IV x 7 days	Efficacy of treatment for enterocolitis or mesenteric adenitis is not established, especially when instituted late; major indications are prolonged diarrhea or generalized infection.
Parasites Cryptosporidia	Symptomatic treatment: Loparamide, lomotil etc. plus nutritional support Compromised host: Consider octretide (5-80 µg tid SC) paromomycin (500 mg po qid) or azithromycin (1500 mg/day, then 600 mg/day x 27 day, then 100 mg/day)		Consider treatment only for chronic diarrhea in compromised host. No antimicrobial agent has established efficacy
Balantidium coli	Tetracycline, 500 mg po qid x 10 days	Iodoquinol, 650 mg tid x 21 days Metronidazole, 500 mg po tid x 10 days	No antimicrobial agent has established efficacy

(continued)

225

Microbial Agent	Preferred	Alternative	Comment
Blastocystis hominis (see comments)	Metronidazole, 1.5-2.0 gm/day x 7 days		Role as enteric pathogen is not clear.
Entamoeba histolytica Acute dysentery	Metronidazole, 750 mg po tid x 5-10 days <u>then</u> diloxanide furoate, 500 mg po tid x 10 days or iodoquinol 650 mg po tid x 21 days	Dehydroemetine, 1-1.5 mg/kg/day IM x 5 days, then diloxanide furoate	Alternatives to diloxanide furoate as oral luminal-acting drug are: iodoquinol, 650 mg po tid x 21 days, and paromomycin, 500 mg po tid x 7 days. Metronidazole may be given IV for severely ill patients (7.5 mg/kg q6h). Diloxanide furoate is available from the CDC.
Mild disease	Metronidazole, 500 mg po tid x 5-10 days, then diloxanide furoate (as above)	Paromomycin, 500 mg po tid x 7 days Metronidazole, 2.4 gm/day x 2-3 days, then diloxanide furoate Metronidazole, 50 mg/kg x 1, then diloxanide furoate	
Cyst passer	Iodoquinol, 650 mg po tid x 21 days Diloxanide furoate, 500 mg po tid x 10 days Paromomycin, 500 mg po tid x 7 days	Metronidazole, 500-750 mg po tid x 10 days	Need to treat is arbitrary, but luminal amebicides (diloxanide furoate, paromomycin or iodoquinol) are preferred. Diloxanide furoate is available from CDC 404-639-3670
Giardia lamblia	Quinacrine, 100 mg po tid x 5-7 days	Metronidazole, 250 mg po tid x 7 days Furazolidone, 8 mg/kg/day po day po x 10 days Tinidazole, 2 gm single dose	Metronidazole is less effective than quinacrine, but better tolerated. Pregnancy: Consider paromomycin, 25-30 mg/kg/day x 5-10 days.
Isospora belli	Sulfa-trimethoprim 2 DS po bid x 2-4 wks	Pyrimethamine, 25 mg + folonic acid, 5-10 mg/day x 1 month	Patients with AIDS and other immuno-suppressive disorders usually require prolonged maintenance treatment.

226

B. FECAL LEUKOCYTE EXAM

Often present	Variable	Not present
Campylobacter jejuni	Salmonella	Vibrio cholerae
Shigella	Yersinia	Enteroadherent
Enteroinvasive E. coli	Vibrio parahaemolyticus	E. coli
Exacerbations of	C. difficile	Enterotoxigenic
inflammatory bowel	Aeromonas	E. coli
disease	Plesiomonas	Food poisoning
	Enterohemorrhagic	S. aureus
	E. coli	B. cereus
		C. perfringens
		Viral gastroenteritis
		Adenovirus
		Rotavirus
		Norwalk agent
		Calicivirus
		Parasitic infection
		Giardia
		E. histolytica*
		Cryptosporidia
		Isospora
		Small bowel overgrowth
		"AIDS enteropathy"

* Frequently associated with blood.

C. EMPIRIC TREATMENT:

1. Indications (AMA's Drug Evaluation, AMA, Chicago, Vol 2, 1:20, 1991):
   Fever and acute moderate-to-severe diarrhea with dysentery (gross
   blood and mucus in stools) and/or PMN's in stool by direct exam.

2. Patients with acute, severe diarrhea (adults with $\geq$ 4 watery stools/day, $\leq$ 7 days)
   may be treated empirically with ciprofloxacin (500 mg po bid x 5 days) or
   norfloxacin (400 mg po bid x 5 days). (See Arch Intern Med 150:541, 1990
   and Ann Intern Med 117:202, 1992)

   Alternative regimen: Trimethoprim-sulfamethoxazole, 1 DS bid with or without
   erythromycin 250-500 mg po bid.

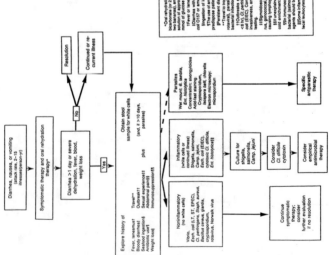

Approach to Infectious Diarrhea
(Reprinted from: Guerrant RL and Bobak DA
N Engl J Med 325:327, 1991 with permission)

URINARY TRACT INFECTIONS

I. Classification based on guidelines established by the Infectious Diseases Society of America and the FDA (Previewed in Clin Infect Dis 14, Suppl 2, S246, 1992)

Category	Criteria for stated category		Treatment
	Clinical	Laboratory*	
Acute, uncomplicated UTI in women	Dysuria, urgency, frequency; no sx in last 4 wks; no fever or flank pain	> 10 WBC/mm^3 > 10^2 cfu/ml in MSU	All drugs active vs GNB show cure rates > 80% Single dose: TMP-SMX favored Advantages: Inexpensive, high response rates, few side effects (principally GI and Candida vaginitis) Disadvantages: Higher relapse rates due to persistence of uropathogenic E. coli in vagina and GI tract Three day treatment: Generally preferred
Acute, uncomplicated pyelonephritis	Fever chills, flank pain No urologic abnormalities	> 10 WBC/mm^3 > 10^5 cfu/ml in MSU	Mild sx: Oral TMP-SMX or fluoroquinolone x 2wk Seriously ill: Parenteral therapy until afebrile 24-48 hrs followed by oral agent x 2wks
Complicated UTI men or obstruction	Any combination of symptoms in above categories	> 10 WBC/mm^3 > 10^5 cfu/ml in MSU	UTI in men: Assure tissue invasion-renal or prostate Agents: TMP-SMX, carbenicillin, trimethoprim or fluoroquinolone Duration: 2-6 wks Obstruction: Anticipate 90% bacteriologic response rates with high frequency of relapse (same strain) or reinfection (new strain) Agents: Fluoroquinolone, 3rd generation cephalosporins
Asymptomatic**	No urinary symptoms	> 10 WBC/mm^3 > 10^5 cfu/ml x 2 separated by 24 hrs	Indications for treatment: Pregnant women, diabetic patients, immunocompromised patients and children**

* WBC = white blood cells (unspun urine); MSU = midstream urine culture

** Added by author

229

II. Definitions of bacteriuric syndromes (Reprinted with permission from: Wilhelm MP and Edson RS, Mayo Clin Proc 62:1027,1987)*

Syndrome	Definition
Lower urinary tract infection	Lower urinary tract symptoms [T] + urine culture with $\geq 10^2$ bacteria/ml
Acute cystitis	Lower urinary tract symptoms + urine culture with $\geq 10^5$ bacteria/ml
Acute urethral syndrome	Lower urinary tract symptoms + 10^2 to 10^5 bacteria/ml or venereally transmitted agent (for example *Neisseria gonorrhoeae, Chlamydia trachomatis, Herpes simplex*) or no identifiable pathogen
Acute pyelonephritis	Upper urinary tract symptoms [TT] + urine with $\geq 10^5$ bacteria/ml
Asymptomatic bacteriuria	No symptoms + urine culture with $\geq 10^5$ bacteria/ml
Recurrent bacteriuria	Recurrent lower urinary tract symptoms [§] + urine culture with $\geq 10^2$ bacteria/ml
Relapse	Recurrent infection with same bacterial strain
Reinfection	Recurrent infection with different bacterial strain
Complicated bacteriuria	Urine culture with $\geq 10^5$ bacteria/ml with associated structural abnormality of the urinary tract [§] (for example, involvement with stones or catheter)

* All syndromes usually associated with pyuria (≥ 8 leukocytes/mm³ unspun urine.)
[T] Dysuria, urgency, frequency, suprapubic pain.
[TT] Fever, rigors, flank pain, nausea, prostration.
[§] May be asymptomatic.

III. Recommendations of J. Johnson and W.E. Stamm (Urinary Tract Infections in Women: Diagnosis and Treatment. Ann Intern Med 111:906,1989)

Cystitis: Single dose (only for uncomplicated cases)
Trimethoprim, 400 mg*
Sulfa-trimethoprim, 320/1600 mg (2 DS)*
Nitrofurantoin, 200 mg*
Amoxicillin, 3 gm
Amoxicillin plus clavulanate, 500 mg

Ampicillin, 3 gm
Cephalexin, 2 gm
Sulfisoxazole, 2 gm
Ciprofloxacin, 250 mg
Norfloxacin, 400 mg

Cystitis: Multidose regimens (3-7 days)
Trimethoprim, 100 mg q12h*
Sulfa-trimethoprim, 160/800 mg q12h*
Nitrofurantoin, 100 mg q6h*
Amoxicillin, 500 mg q8h
Amoxicillin + clavulanate, 500 mg q8h

Cephalexin, 500 mg q 6 h
Ciprofloxacin, 250 mg q12h
Norfloxacin, 400 mg q12h
Sulfisoxazole, 500 mg q6h
Tetracycline, 500 mg q6h

Pyelonephritis, oral therapy for mild pyelonephritis (treat $\geq$ 14 days)
Trimethoprim, 100 mg q12h*
Sulfa-trimethoprim, 160/800 q12h*
Cephalexin, 500 mg q6h
Amoxicillin, 500 mg q8h

Amoxicillin + clavulanate, 500 mg q8h
Ciprofloxacin, 250 mg q12h
Norfloxacin, 400 mg q12h

Pyelonephritis, parenteral therapy (Intravenous administration until afebrile and improved, then oral therapy to complete total of 14 days)
Gentamicin, 1.5 mg/kg q8h*
Ceftriaxone, 1 gm q12h*
Sulfa-trimethoprim, 160/800 mg q12h*
Ampicillin, 1 gm (or higher) q8h

Ampicillin plus gentamicin (above doses) q8h
Cefazolin, 1 gm (or higher) q8h
Mezlocillin, 1 gm (or higher) q6h

* Preferred regimens

IV. **Recommendations for upper and lower urinary tract infections**
(AMA's Drug Evaluations, AMA, Chicago, Vol 2, Section 12, 1:33, 1991)

A. ASYMPTOMATIC BACTERIURIA

Indications for treatment: Pregnant women, diabetic patients, immunocompromised
patients and children.
Regimens: Based on susceptibility tests; see cystitis for regimens.

B. ACUTE URETHRAL SYNDROME

Definition: Symptoms of acute cystitis (dysuria, frequency, urgency) without significant
bacteriuria; most have pyuria.
Causes: Low concentrations of usual UTI pathogens or C. trachomatis (STD);
vaginitis, N. gonorrhoeae and H. simplex may also cause symptoms of the acute
urethral syndrome; patients with sterile urine and no pyuria have no
demonstrable infection.
Empiric treatment: Doxycycline, 100 mg bid x 10 days
Alternative: Diagnostic evaluation and treatment for specific agents (findings
suggesting E. coli UTI include abrupt onset of sx, symptoms < 4 days,
hematuria, suprapubic pain, prior UTI and no recent change in sex partner;
findings suggesting C. trachomatis are gradual onset of symptoms, symptoms
over 7 days, no hematuria, no suprapubic pain and recent changes in sex
partners).

C. CYSTITIS

1. Short course: Single dose therapy is considered inferior to 3 day courses and
should be reserved for women who are not pregnant, have no evidence of
pyelonephritis, have symptoms < 7 days and are available for follow-up.

Preferred regimens:	Single dose	3 days
TMP-SMX	2 DS	1 DS bid
Trimethoprim	400 mg	100 mg bid
Amoxicillin	3 gm	500 mg q8h
Nitrofurantoin	200 mg	100 mg q6h

Note: 1. Usual pathogens are E. coli (80%), Staph. saprophiticus (10%) and
Enterococcus faecalis.
2. Typical symptoms and urinalysis showing pyuria are adequate to
initiate treatment; urine culture is optional.
3. Must exclude vaginitis and STDs.
4. Patients who fail to respond or relapse within 96 hrs are considered
to have silent renal infections. These patients should have urine
culture, and treatment 10-14 days or up to 6 wks.
5. "Test-of-cure" urine culture at 1 week after single dose treatment is
controversial.

2. Conventional therapy (7-14 days)
Preferred regimens: Trimethoprim-sulfamethoxazole; ampicillin/amoxicillin,
sulfasoxazole or nitrofurantoin.

    <u>Alternatives</u>: Trimethoprim, tetracycline, oral cephalosporin, fluoroquinolones, amoxicillin-clavulanate.

    <u>Note</u>:   1.   Treatment is 7-14 days.

             2.   If relapse occurs, suspect pyelonephritis, treat for up to 6 wks and evaluate for underlying urinary tract abnormality.

D.   RECURRENT UTIs

    1.   <u>Relapse</u>: Post-treatment infection caused by same organism, usually within 2 wks and usually indicates renal involvement

       Recommendations: **a)** Rule out structural abnormality or chronic prostatitis and **b)** Antibiotic treatment x 6 wks.

    2.   <u>Reinfection</u>: Recurrent infections with different organisms. This mechanism accounts for > 80% of recurrent infections in women.

       Recommendations: If > 3 episodes/yr consider long-term prophylaxis with **a)** trimethoprim-sulfamethoxazole, 1/2 tab daily or 3 days/wk, **b)** nitrofurantoin macrocrystals, 50 mg daily or **c)** trimethoprim, 50 mg (1/2 100 mg tab) daily.

E.   PYELONEPHRITIS

    1.   <u>In-patient treatment</u>
       Preferred: Aminoglycoside + ampicillin.
       Alternatives: Trimethoprim-sulfamethoxazole, cephalosporins - 3rd generation, or aztreonam.
       Regimens: Parenteral treatment until afebrile 24-48 hr, total duration $\geq$ 14 days; relapse - treat up to 6 wks.

    2.   <u>Outpatient treatment</u>
       Preferred: Trimethoprim-sulfamethoxazole.
       Alternatives: Cephalosporin - oral, quinolone, amoxicillin-clavulanate.
       Duration: 14 days, relapse - treat up to 6 wks.

F.   PROSTATITIS

    1.   <u>Acute</u>
       Bacteriology: <u>E</u>. <u>coli</u> (> 80%), other GNB
       Treatment regimens
       a)   Trimethoprim-sulfamethoxazole: 160 mg/800 mg bid x 30 days.
       b)   Aminoglycoside + ampicillin: Parenteral treatment until afebrile, then oral regimen based on susceptibility test of urine isolate to complete 30 days of treatment.
       c)   Ciprofloxacin, lomefloxacin or ofloxacin x 30 days.

    2.   <u>Chronic</u>
       Bacteriology: <u>E</u>. <u>coli</u> (most common), other GNB, enterococcus, <u>Ureoplasma</u> <u>ureolyticum</u> (?)
       Treatment regimens
       a)   Trimethoprim-sulfamethoxazole: 1 DS po bid x $\geq$ 12-24 wks.
       b)   Ciprofloxacin, 500-750 mg po bid; Ofloxacin, 400 mg po bid or lomefloxacin, 400 mg po/day $\geq$ x 12.

    c) Trimethoprim, 100 mg bid x 12 wks.
    d) Doxycycline or erythromycin are suggested for nonbacterial prostatitis due
        possibly to Ureoplasma urealyticum.

G. EPIDIDYMO-ORCHITIS

    1. STD form: See Neisseria gonorrhoeae or Chlamydia trachomatis (pp 233, 236).
    2. Non-STD form: Usual pathogens, E. coli and other GNB.
       Preferred empiric treatment
       a) Aminoglycoside with or without ampicillin or
       b) Trimethoprim-sulfamethoxadole
       Alternatives:
       a) Ciprofloxacin, ofloxacin or lomefloxacin
       b) Cephalosporin - 3rd generation

V. Cost of oral drugs commonly used for urinary tract infections

Antimicrobial agent and regimen	Wholesale price for 10 day supply*	
Ampicillin: 500 mg po tid	$ 3.90**	($ 7.50)
Amoxicillin: 250 mg po tid	$ 3.23**	($8.40)
Amoxicillin + clavulanate (Augmentin): 250 mg po tid	$51.00	
Carbenicillin (Geocillin): 380 mg po qid	$64.00	
Cephradine (Anspor, Velosef): 250 mg po qid	$11.36**	($32.80)
Cephalexin (Keflex): 250 mg po qid	$ 6.00**	($46.00)
Ciprofloxacin (Cipro): 500 mg po bid	$58.40	
Doxycycline (Vibramycin): 100 mg po bid	$ 2.13**	($63.00)
Lomefloxacin (Maxquin): 400 mg po qd	$44.70	
Methenamine mandelate: 1 gm po qid	$ 2.80	
Methenamine hippurate (Hiprex): 1 gm po bid	$18.40	
Nalidixic acid (NegGram): 1 gm caplet po qid	$58.60	
Nitrofurantoin (Furadantin): 50 mg cap po qid	$24.00	
Norfloxacin (Noroxin): 400 mg po bid	$45.00	
Ofloxacin (Floxin): 400 mg po bid	$67.60	
Sulfisoxazole (Gantrisin): 1 gm po qid	$ 2.80**	($16.80)
Tetracycline: 500 mg po qid	$ 2.07**	($ 4.50)
Trimethoprim: 100 mg po bid	$ 2.86	
Trimethoprim-sulfa (Bactrim, Septra): 1 DS po bid	$ 1.35**	($19.80)

* Approximate wholesale prices according to Medi-Span, Hospital Formulary
Pricing Guide, Indianapolis, May, 1992 (prices to patient will be higher).

**Price is provided for generic product if available; price in parentheses is for
representative brand product.

(CDC recommendations adapted from MMWR 38:S8, pp 1-43, 1989)

Revised CDC guidelines are expected in late 1992; anticipated revisions added by author in consultation with J. Zenilman are indicated by single asterisk (*)

I. Gonococcal infections

    A. Treatment recommendations are influenced by:

        1) Spread of infections due to antibiotic-resistant N. gonorrhoeae including penicillinase-producing strains (PPNG), tetracycline-resistant strains (TRNG) and strains with chromosomally mediated resistance to multiple antibiotics.

        2) High frequency of chlamydial infections in patients with gonorrhea.

        3) Recognition of serious complications of chlamydial and gonococcal infection.

        4) Absence of a rapid, inexpensive and highly accurate test for chlamydial infection.

    B. All cases of gonorrhea should be diagnosed or confirmed by culture to enable antimicrobial susceptibility testing. (This recommendation is no longer necessary due to gonococcal surveillance and use of drugs effective for virtually all strains)*

    C. Treatment of uncomplicated urethral, endocervical and rectal infections

        1. Recommended: Cefixime, 400 mg po* x 1 plus doxycycline**, 100 mg po bid x 7 days or fluoroquinolone *,*** (ciprofloxacin 500 mg po x 1; ofloxacin 400 mg po x 1 or norfloxacin 800 mg po x 1) plus doxycycline, 100 mg po bid x 7 days or ceftriaxone, 125 mg IM* plus doxycycline, 100 mg po bid x 7 days.

        2. Alternative:
           a. Cefuroxime axetil, 1 gm po x 1 + probenecid, 1 gm **
           b. Cefotaxime, 1 gm IM x 1 **
           c. Ceftizoxime, 500 mg IM x 1 **
           d. Spectinomycin, 2 gm IM**

** All regimens should include a 7 day course of doxycycline (100 mg po bid x 7 days) or tetracycline (500 mg po qid x 7 days) for presumed concurrent infection with Chlamydia trachomatis. Alternative to tetracyclines for C. trachomatis is erythromycin base or stearate (500 mg po qid x 7 days), erythromycin ethylsuccinate (800 mg po qid x 7 days) or azithromycin (1 gm po x 1).*

*** Quinolones are contraindicated in pregnant women and children < 16 yrs; activity of quinolones or spectinomycin in incubating syphilis is unknown so serology for syphilis should be obtained in 1 month.

        3. Special considerations:
           a. Incubating syphilis: All patients with gonorrhea should have syphilis serology; patients treated with quinolones or spectinomycin should have repeat serology in 1 month to exclude incubating syphilis.
           b. Sex partners: All persons exposed during preceding 30 days should be examined, cultured and treated (for gonorrhea and chlamydial infection).
           c. Follow-up: Treatment failure with recommended regimen is rare so that "test-of-cure" is not essential; re-exam at 1-2 months ("re-screening") may be more cost effective.
           d. Treatment failures: Culture for N. gonorrhoeae and test for antibiotic sensitivity. Many "treatment failures" are due to chlamydial infection, reinfection or non-compliance. Treat recurrent gonococcal infection with ceftriaxone, 250 mg IM x 1 plus doxycycline, 100 mg po bid x 7 days.

e. <u>Pregnancy</u>: Cefixime, 400 mg* po or ceftriaxone, 125 mg IM x 1 <u>plus</u> erythromycin base or stearate, 500 mg po qid x 7 days. (Quinolones and tetracyclines are contraindicated.)

D. Gonococcal infection at other anatomical sites

1. <u>Rectal and pharyngeal infection</u>: Cefixime, 400 mg po x 1* <u>or</u> Ciprofloxacin, 500 mg po x 1 <u>or</u> Ceftriaxone, 250 mg IM x 1 and repeat culture 4-7 days later.

2. <u>Salpingitis</u>: See Pelvic inflammatory disease.

3. <u>Disseminated gonococcal infection (DGI)</u>
Hospitalize and treat with: Ceftriaxone*, 1 gm IV or IM q24h <u>or</u> Ceftizoxime*, 1 gm IV q8h <u>or</u> Ceftazidime*, 1 gm IV q8h
Alternative to betalactams: Spectinomycin*, 2 gm IM q12h <u>or</u> IV fluoroquinolone*
* Test for genital chlamydia or treat empirically; reliable patients with uncomplicated DGI may be discharged at 24-48 hrs after symptoms resolve and should complete 1 wk of treatment with cefixime, 400 mg po bid* <u>or</u> ciprofloxacin, 500 mg bid.

4. <u>Gonococcal endocarditis or meningitis</u>
IV therapy with effective agent such as ceftriaxone 1-2 gm q12h for 10-14 days (meningitis) or 4 weeks (endocarditis).

5. <u>Gonococcal ophthalmia</u>
Treatment of adult: Ceftriaxone, 1 gm IM x 1 <u>plus</u> ophthalmologic assessment. Antibiotic irrigation is not required.

Prevention in newborn infants (required by law in most states, must be done within 1 hr after delivery, efficacy in preventing chlamydial infections of eye is unknown):
Erythromycin 0.5% ophthalmic ointment x 1 <u>or</u>
Tetracycline 1% ophthalmic ointment x 1 <u>or</u>
Silver nitrate 1% aqueous solution

II. <u>Syphilis</u>

A. Treatment (adult, non-pregnant)

1. <u>Exposed</u>: Evaluate clinically and serologically; if exposure < 90 days treat presumptively (regimen for early syphilis).

2. <u>Early syphilis</u> including primary, secondary or latent of less than 1 year duration.

- Benzathine penicillin G, 2.4 million units IM x 1.

- Penicillin allergy: Doxycycline, 100 mg po bid x 14 days or tetracycline, 500 mg po qid x 14 days.

- Penicillin allergy and tetracycline contraindication or intolerance: **a)** erythromycin, 500 mg po qid x 15 days (this is acceptable only if compliance plus follow-up serology is assured); **b)** skin testing for penicillin allergy and desensitization if necessary; **c)** ceftriaxone, 250 mg IM x 1/day x 10 days with caution for sensitivity reaction.

3. Syphilis over 1 year (except neurosyphilis) including latent syphilis, cardiovascular syphilis or gummas.

   - Benzathine penicillin G, 2.4 million units q week x 3 successive weeks.

   - Penicillin allergy (efficacy of alternative regimens for neurosyphilis not established and CSF exam mandatory to exclude this complication): Doxycycline, 100 mg po bid or tetracycline, 500 mg po qid x 4 weeks.

4. Neurosyphilis

   - Aqueous penicillin G, 12-24 million units IV/day x 10-14 days, then benzathine penicillin G, 2.4 million units IM weekly x 3.

   - Procaine penicillin G, 2-4 million units IM daily plus probenecid, 500 mg po qid x 10-14 days; some recommend adding benzathine penicillin G, 2.4 million units IM weekly x 3.

   - Penicillin allergy: Confirm allergy and "consult expert"; desensitization required if truly allergic.

5. Pregnancy

   - Penicillin regimens as noted above.

   - Tetracyclines are contraindicated in pregnancy and erythromycins have a high failure rate in fetal infection. Patients with convincing histories of penicillin allergy should have skin testing and desensitization.

6. HIV infection

   a. All patients with syphilis should be counseled concerning risks of HIV and encouraged to have HIV serology.

   b. CSF from patients with HIV infection often shows mononuclear cells and increased protein. With a negative CSF VDRL there is no practical method to confirm or exclude neurosyphilis. Sensitivity of CSF VDRL is 60-70%.

B. CSF exam: Should be performed in patients with clinical symptoms or signs consistent with neurosyphilis and is desired in all persons with syphilis > 1 yr, although this decision should be individualized. Tests in CSF should include leukocyte count, protein and VDRL. A positive VDRL is diagnostic of neurosyphilis; negative VDRL does not exclude it. (Elderly patients with low titer serum VDRL probably do not require a LP.)*

C. Follow up

Form	Follow-up quantitative non-treponemal test*	Expectation	Additional comments
Early syphilis	3 & 6 months post-treatment	4-fold decrease by 3 mo. or by 6 mo. with early latent syphilis	If titer not decreased should do CSF exam and re-treat
Early syphilis + HIV infected	1, 2, 3, 6, 9 and 12 mo.		If titer does not decrease (4-fold) by 3 mo. for primary or by 6 mo. for secondary, or if titer increases (4-fold): re-evaluate for treatment failure versus reinfection, and examine CSF
Syphilis > 1 yr	6 and 12 months post-treatment	Titer declines more gradually	CSF exam if there are neurological signs or symptoms; treatment failure (titer increases 4-fold or initially high titer of ≥ 1:32 fails to decrease); non-penicillin therapy; HIV seropositive
Neurosyphilis	Six-month intervals at least 2 yrs (see comments)		Clinical evaluation and CSF analysis at 6 mo. intervals until cell count normal; if titer not decreased at 6 mo. or normal at 2 yrs, consider retreatment

* Nontreponemal tests = VDRL and RPR; treponemal tests = FTA-ABS, MHA-TP and HATTS

III. Chlamydia trachomatis

    A. Treatment (urethral, endocervical and rectal infection)

        - Doxycycline, 100 mg po bid x 7 days.

        - Tetracycline, 500 mg po qid x 7 days.

        - Azithromycin, 1 gm po x 1*.

    Pregnancy: Erythromycin base or stearate, 500 mg po qid x 7 days or erythromycin ethylsuccinate, 800 mg po qid x 7 days. Women who cannot tolerate this regimen should receive half the suggested daily dose qid for at least 14 days. Alternative to erythromycin is azithromycin, 1 mg x 1 (Category II for pregnancy).

    B. Sex partners: Examine for STD and treat using above regimen if contact was within 30 days.

C. Follow up: Post-treatment test-of-cure cultures are not advocated because treatment failures with recommended regimens have not been observed.

IV. Genital herpes simplex

A. Treatment

1. First episode (genital or rectal infection)

Genital: Acyclovir, 200 mg po 5 x daily for 7-10 days or until clinical resolution occurs.

Rectal: 400 mg po 5 x daily for 10 days or until clinical resolution occurs.

Hospitalized patients: 5 mg/kg IV q8h for 5-7 days or until clinical resolution occurs.

2. Recurrent episodes (most do not benefit from treatment unless recurrences are severe and acyclovir is started at the beginning of the prodrome or within 2 days of onset of lesions).

- Acyclovir, 200 mg po 5 times daily x 5 days or acyclovir, 800 mg po bid x 5 days.

3. Prophylaxis for recurrences (for patients with > 6 recurrences/yr): 200 mg po 2-5 x/day or 400 mg po bid. This suppressive regimen is contraindicated in women who become pregnant during treatment.

B. HIV disease: The need for higher therapeutic or suppressive doses is suspected, but not established.

C. Pregnancy: Safety of acyclovir is not established, but post-marketing surveillance shows probable safety; acyclovir is indicated during primary HSV infection during pregnancy* and for life-threatening maternal HSV disease. Major risk of neonatal HSV infection is primary infection in mother at the time of delivery (NEJM 326:916, 1992)*

V. Chancroid (Haemophilus ducreyi) infection: Recommended treatment varies by susceptibility of strains in different geographic areas.

Recommended: Ceftriaxone, 250 mg IM x 1 or Ciprofloxacin, 500 mg po qid x 7 days.*

Alternative regimens: Trimethoprim-sulfamethoxazole, 1 double strength tablet (160/800 mg) po bid x at least 7 days; amoxicillin, 500 mg plus clavulanic acid 125 mg po tid x 7 days or erythromycin, 500 mg po bid x 3 days

VI. Lymphogranuloma venereum treatment (genital, inguinal and anorectal)

Recommended: Doxycycline, 100 mg po bid x 21 days.

Alternatives: Tetracycline, 500 mg po qid x 21 days or Erythromycin, 500 mg po qid x 21 days or Sulfasoxazole, 500 mg qid x 21 days. (Azithromycin: efficacy is not established.)

VII. Pediculosis pubis

A. Treatment

Permethrin (1%) cream rinse applied to affected area and washed after 10 minutes or Lindane (1%) shampoo applied 4 minutes and then thoroughly washed off (not recommened for pregnant or lactating women) or Pyrethrins and piperonyl butoxide (non-prescription) applied to affected areas and washed off after 10 minutes.

B. <u>Adjunctive</u>: Retreat after 7 days if lice or eggs are detected at hair-skin junction. Clothes and bed linen of past 2 days should be washed and dried by machine (hot cycle each) or dry cleaned.

C. <u>Sex partners</u>: Treat as above.

VIII. <u>Scabies</u>

<u>Recommended</u>: Permethrin (5% cream, 30 gm) massaged and left 8-14 hrs considered preferable drug for scabies by Medical Letter Consultants (32:21-22,1990).*

<u>Alternatives</u>: Lindane (1%) 1 oz lotion or 30 gm cream applied thinly to all areas of body below neck and washed thoroughly at 8 hr. (Not recommended for pregnant or lactating women) <u>or</u> Crotamiton (10%) applied to body below neck nightly for 2 nights and washed thoroughly 24 hr after second application.

<u>Sex partners and close household contacts</u>: Treat as above.

<u>Adjunctive</u>: Clothing or bed linen contaminated by patient should be washed and dried by machine (hot cycle) or dry cleaned.

IX. <u>Warts (Condylomata acuminata)</u> (Medical Letter 117, 1991; JAMA 265:2684, 1991)

Location	Treatment	Comment
External genital and perianal	Cryotherapy, e.g., liquid nitrogen or cryoprobe Podofilox, 0.5% bid x 3d* Podophyllin, 10%-25% applied carefully to each wart, wash at 1-4 hr, and reapply weekly; limit to < 10 cm² each session. Trichloroacetic acid (TCA) applied locally and repeat weekly; powder with talc or baking soda to remove unreacted acid Alternatives: Surgical removal electrocautery, laser therapy	All treatments show high rate of recurrence Podofilox: repeat q/wk x ≤4 Podophyllin is contra-indicated in pregnancy Women with anogenital warts should have Pap smear annually Cryotherapy is preferred because it is non-toxic, does not require anesthesia and does not cause scarring Interferon is not recommended because of low efficacy, frequent toxicity and high cost
Vaginal	Cryotherapy with liquid nitrogen Alternatives: TCA (80-90%) or podophyllin (10-25%) as above; treat < 2 cm²/session	Podophyllin is contraindicated in pregnancy Cryotherapy is preferred -- cryoprobe should not be used due to risk of vaginal perforation
Cervical	(See comment)	Must rule out dysphagia so that an expert consultant is required

(continued)

Location	Treatment	Comment
Urethral and meatal	Cryotherapy with liquid nitrogen Alternative: Podophyllin (10-25% as above)	Podophyllin is contraindicated in pregnancy
Anal	Cryotherapy with liquid nitrogen Alternative: TCA, electro- cautery, or surgical excision	Podophyllin is contraindicated

Syndromes - Female

I. <u>Pelvic inflammatory disease</u> (MMWR 40, RR-5:1-25, 1991)

    A.   Agents

        1.   Gonococcal PID: <u>N</u>. <u>gonorrhoeae</u>.

        2.   Non-gonococcal PID: <u>Chlamydia</u> <u>trachomatis</u>, anaerobic bacteria $\pm$ facultative gram-negative bacilli, <u>Actinomyces</u> <u>israelii</u>, streptococci and mycoplasmas.

    B.   Diagnosis

        1.   Minimal criteria - lower abdominal adnexal and cervical motion tenderness.

        2.   Additional criteria - oral temperature > 38.3°C, abnormal cervical or vaginal discharge, elevated ESR or creatine protein, microbial evidence of cervical infection with <u>N</u>. <u>gonorrhoeae</u> or <u>C</u>. <u>trachomatis</u>.

        3.   Recommended tests - culture for <u>N</u>. <u>gonorrhoeae</u> and test for <u>C</u>. <u>trachomatis</u>.

    C.   Indications for hospitalization: **1)** diagnosis uncertain, **2)** surgical emergencies cannot be excluded (such as appendicitis or ectopic pregnancy), **3)** pelvic abscess suspected, **4)** severe illness prevents outpatient management, **5)** pregnancy, **6)** patient unable to follow or tolerate outpatient treatment, **7)** failure to respond within 72 hours to outpatient treatment, **8)** clinical follow-up at 72 hours not possible, **9)** patient is an adolescent (less reliable and greater long-term sequelae), **10)** patient with HIV infection.*

    D.   Treatment

        1.   Antibiotics: <u>Outpatient regimen</u> - Patients treated as outpatients need to be monitored closely and re-evaluated in 72 hours.

            <u>Recommended</u>: Ceftriaxone, 250 mg IM x 1 dose <u>or</u> cefoxitin, 2 gm IM plus probenecid, 1 gm concurrently <u>plus</u> azithromycin, 1 gm po x 1* <u>or</u> doxycycline, 100 mg po bid x 10-14 days <u>or</u> tetracycline, 500 mg po qid for 10-14 days. Longer treatment may be necessary to prevent late sequelae.

            <u>Alternative to tetracyclines</u>: Erythromycin, 500 mg po qid x 10-14 days.

2. Antibiotics: <u>Inpatient regimen</u>.

Initial**	Oral follow-up***
Doxycycline, 100 mg IV bid + cefoxitin, 2 gm IV qid <u>or</u> cefotetan, 2 gm IV q12h	Doxycycline, 100 mg po bid <u>or</u> Azithromycin, 1 gm po x 1*
Clindamycin, 900 mg IV qid + gentamicin, 2.0 mg/kg IV, then 1.5 mg/kg tid	Clindamycin, 450 mg po 5x/day <u>or</u> doxycycline, 100 mg po bid (doxycycline preferred if <u>C</u>. trachomatis is suspected or confirmed)

** Parenteral treatment to continue at least 48 hrs after patient clinically improves.
*** Oral regimen to be continued to complete 10-14 days of treatment.

3. Male sex partners: Examine and treat with regimen for uncomplicated gonococcal and chlamydial infection.

4. Follow up: Outpatients should be re-evaluated within 72 hrs and patients not responding should be hospitalized.

5. Intra-uterine device: Removal is recommended soon after antimicrobial treatment is started.

II. <u>Mucopurulent cervicitis</u>

   A. Diagnosis: **(1)** Mucopurulent endocervical exudate that may appear yellow or green on white cotton-tipped swab (positive swab test); **(2)** gram-stained smear of endocervical secretions shows over 10 PMN/oil immersion field; or **(3)** cervicitis documented by cervical friability (bleeding when the first swab is taken) and/or erythema or edema within a zone of cervical ectopy.

   B. Laboratory evaluation: Gram stain, culture for <u>N</u>. <u>gonorrhoeae</u>, test for <u>Chlamydia trachomatis</u> and wet mount for <u>Trichomonas</u>.

   C. Treatment

      1. Gonococcal: <u>N</u>. <u>gonorrhoeae</u> found on gram stain or culture - treat for uncomplicated gonococcal infection and presumed chlamydial infection.

      2. Non-gonococcal: <u>N</u>. <u>gonorrhoeae</u> not found on gram stain or culture - treat for <u>C</u>. trachomatis (pg 237).

III. <u>Vaginitis/vaginosis</u>

   A. Trichomoniasis (almost always a STD)

      1. Diagnosis: Wet mount or culture.

      2. Usual treatment: Metronidazole, 2 gm po as single dose
         Alternative: Metronidazole, 500 mg po bid x 7 days.

      3. Asymptomatic women: Treat as above.

4. Pregnant women: Metronidazole is contraindicated in first trimester and should be avoided throughout pregnancy. For severe symptomatic disease after first trimester, give metronidazole, 2 gm x 1.

5. Lactating women: Treat with 2 gm dose of metronidazole and suspend breast feeding x 24 hours.

6. Sex partners: Treat with 2 gm dose of metronidazole or 500 mg po bid x 7 days.

7. Treatment failures: Retreat with metronidazole, 500 mg po bid x 7 days. Persistent failures: 2 gm dose daily x 3-5 days.

B. Bacterial vaginosis (non-specific vaginitis)

1. Diagnosis: Non-irritating, malodorous, thin, white vaginal disharge with pH over 4.5, elaboration of fishy odor after 10% KOH, microscopic exam showing sparse lactobacilli and numerous cocco-bacillary forms on epithelial cells ("clue cells"). Cultures for <u>Gardnerella vaginalis</u> are not recommended. Asymptomatic infections are common; necessity to treat asymptomatic infections is controversial.

2. Treatment
   - Metronidazole, 500 mg po bid x 7 days or 2 gm po x 1.*
   - Alternative: Clindamycin, 300 mg po bid x 7 days.* Clindamycin vaginal cream (2%), 100 mg (5g) intravaginally daily x 7*.

3. Sex partners: Treatment not indicated

4. Pregnancy: Metronidazole is contraindicated; use clindamycin regimen.

C. <u>Vulvovaginal candidiasis</u> (not considered an STD)

1. Treatment

   <u>Recommended</u>: Miconazole nitrate suppository or clotrimazole (tablet, 200 mg) intra-vaginally at bedtime x 3 days; betaconazole (2% cream, 5 g) intravaginally at bedtime x 3 days; tetaconazole (80 mg suppository or 0.4% cream) intravaginally at bedtime x 3 days.

   <u>Alternatives</u>: Miconazole nitrate vaginal suppository (100 mg or 2% cream, 5 g) intravaginally at bedtime x 7 days <u>or</u> clotrimazole (vaginal tabs, 100 mg or 1% cream, 5 gm) intravaginally at bedtime x 7 days).
   <u>Systemic</u>: Fluconazole, 150 mg po x 1 <u>or</u> ketoconazole, 200 mg po bid x 5-7 days.*

2. Sex partners: Treat only for symptomatic <u>Candida balanitis</u>.

3. Pregnancy: As for non-pregnant patients.

4. Prophylaxis for recurrent candida vaginitis*: Yogurt, 8oz/d po (Ann Intern Med 116:353, 1992) <u>or</u> ketoconazole (NEJM 315:1455, 1986)

Syndromes - Male

I. <u>Urethritis</u>

    A. Categories

        1. Gonococcal

        2. Non-gonococcal: Usually caused by <u>C</u>. <u>trachomatis</u> (40-50%), other organisms (10-15%) (<u>Ureaplasma</u> <u>urealyticum</u>, <u>T</u>. <u>vaginalis</u>, herpes simplex virus); unknown cause (35-50%).

    B. Diagnosis: Gram stain and culture of urethral discharge or urethral swab obtained with calcium amalgamate swab.

        1. Gram negative intracellular diplococci or positive culture for <u>N</u>. <u>gonorrhoeae</u>: Treat for uncomplicated gonococci infection (pg 234).

        2. Gram stain shows > 5 PMN/low power field plus no intracellular gram-negative intracellular diplococci: Treat for <u>Chlamydia</u> <u>trachomatis</u> (pg 237).

        3. Stain shows < 5 PMN: Patient should return for repeat test next morning before voiding.

    C. Persistent or recurrent NGU: Consider

        1. Failure to treat sexual partner.

        2. Alternative causes of discharge.

II. <u>Epididymitis</u>

    A. <u>STD form</u>: Usually occurs in adults < 35 yrs in association with urethritis without urinary tract infection or underlying GU pathology.

        1. Usual agents: <u>C</u>. <u>trachomatis</u> and/or <u>N</u>. <u>gonorrhoeae</u>.

        2. Evaluation: Urethral smear for gram stain, culture for <u>N</u>. <u>gonorrhoeae</u> and <u>Chlamydia</u> <u>trachomatis</u> and urine culture.

        3. Treatment: Use regimens for uncomplicated <u>N</u>. <u>gonorrhoeae</u> infection.

        4. Adjuncts: Bed rest and scrotal elevation recommended until fever and local inflammation have resolved.

    B. <u>Non-STD form</u> (usually older men in association with GU pathology and/or UTI verified by positive urine gram stain and culture).

        1. Agents: Coliforms and pseudomonads (usual agents of urinary tract infections).

        2. Treatment: Based on severity of disease and urine culture results (pg 233).

        3. Adjunctive treatment as above.

DURATION OF ANTIBIOTIC TREATMENT

Location	Diagnosis	Duration (days)
Actinomycosis	Cervicofacial	4-6 wks IV, then oral x 6-12 mo
Bacteremia	Gram-negative bacteremia	10-14 days
	<u>S. aureus</u>, portal of entry known 2 wks	
	<u>S. aureus</u>, no portal of entry	4 wks
	Line sepsis: Bacteria	3-5 days (post-removal)
	<u>Candida</u>	10 days (post-removal)
	Vascular graft	4 wks (post-removal)
Bone	Osteomyelitis, acute	4-6 wks IV
	chronic	4 wks IV, then po x 2 mo
Central nervous system	Cerebral abscess	4-6 wks, then oral
	Meningitis: <u>H. influenzae</u>	10 days
	<u>Listeria</u>	14-21 days
	<u>N. meningitidis</u>	7 days
	<u>S. pneumoniae</u>	10 days
Ear	Otitis media, acute	10 days
Gastrointestinal	Diarrhea: <u>C. difficile</u>	7-14 days
	<u>C. jejuni</u>	7 days
	<u>E. histolytica</u>	5-10 days
	<u>Giardia</u>	5-7 days
	<u>Salmonella</u>	14 days
	<u>Shigella</u>	3-5 days
	Traveler's	3-5 days
	Gastritis, H. pylori	≥ 3 wks
	Sprue	6 mo
	Whipple's disease	1 yr
Heart	Endocarditis: Pen-sensitive strep	14-28 days
	Pen-resistant strep	4-6 wks
	<u>Staph. aureus</u>	4 wks
	Microbes, other	4 wks
	Prosthetic valve	≥ 6 wks
Intra-abdominal	Cholecystitis	3-7 days post-cholecystectomy
	Primary peritonitis	10-14 days
	Peritonitis/intra-abdominal abscess	7-10 days after drainage
Joint	Septic arthritis, gonococcal	7 days
	Pyogenic, non-gonococcal	3 wks
	Prosthetic joint	6 wks
Liver	Pyogenic liver abscess	4-16 wks
	Amebic	10 days

(continued)

Location	Diagnosis	Duration (days)
Lung	Pneumonia: <u>Chlamydia pneumoniae</u>	10-14 days
	<u>Legionella</u>	21 days
	<u>Mycoplasma</u>	2-3 wks
	<u>Nocardia</u>	6-12 months
	Pneumococcal	Until febrile 3-5 days
	Pneumocystis	21 days
	Staphylococcal	≥ 21 days
	Tuberculosis	6-9 mo
	Lung abscess	Until x-ray clear or until small stable residual lesion
Nocardia	Nocardiosis	6-12 months
Pharynx	Pharyngitis - Gr A strep	10 days
	Pharyngitis, gonococcal	1 dose
	Diphtheria	14 days
Prostate	Prostatitis, acute	2 wks
	chronic	3-4 mo
Sinus	Sinusitis, acute	10 days
Sexually transmitted disease	Cervicitis, gonococcal	1 dose
	Chancroid	7 days
	<u>Chlamydia</u>	7 days (Azithromycin - 1 dose)
	Disseminated gonococcal infection	7 days
	H. simplex	7-10 days
	Lymphogranuloma venereum	21 days
	Pelvic inflammatory disease	10-14 days
	Syphilis	10-21 days
	Urethritis, gonococcal	1 dose
Systemic	Brucellosis	6 wks
	Listeria: Immunosuppressed host	3-6 wks
	Lyme disease	14-21 days
	Meningococcemia	7-10 days
	Rocky Mountain spotted fever	7 days
	Salmonellosis	
	Bacteremia	10-14 days
	AIDS patients	≥ 3-4 wks
	Localized infection	4-6 wks
	Carrier state	6 wks
	Tuberculosis, pulmonary	6-9 mo
	extrapulmonary	9 mo
	Tularemia	7-14 days
Vaginitis	Bacterial vaginosis	7 days
	<u>Candida albicans</u>	3 days
	Trichomoniasis	7 days

251

252

257

258

259

THE TEAMMATES
THE TARGETS

Barry W. Enoch, Chief Gunners Mate, SEAL Team One—A teacher, a leader, a living legend among the SEALs. His actions in Vietnam earned the respect of his men . . . and put fear into his enemies. Modest in word, courageous in deed, committed in battle, he is what being a SEAL—or any other special warfare operator—is all about.

Gary "Abe" Abrahamson—Enoch's fellow squad member, they almost always marched together, developing an unspoken bond from their very first patrol. On base, he had a knack for finding trouble, but in the field he was above all else a tough warrior and a sharp operator. You could always depend on Abe and his Stoner 63 machine gun when the spit started to fly.

DUNG ISLAND

Learning from two local women that a large VC complex is located at the mouth of the Bassac River, the team plans a predawn sea launch, from the USS *Harnett County,* and raid on the camp. Through mud and reed-choked swamps, avoiding trip wires and booby traps, SEAL Team One succeeds in liberating twenty-six POWs without a single friendly casualty.

Senator Bob Kerrey—The first SEAL in Team history to receive the "Big Blue"—the Congressional Medal of Honor—for gallantry in action, he credits Barry Enoch for instilling in him the skills needed to survive. Says Kerrey: "If [Enoch] says it happened, it did. If he says someone else did all the work and deserves all the glory, he probably deserves at least half. He is a man who always did more than his share and always asked for less than he was owed."

RD2 Billy W. Machen—Killed in action, 19 August 1966, the first SEAL member to fall in Vietnam—and Barry Enoch's best friend. Opening fire in the kill zone both to warn and cover the members of his patrol, Machen saved his teammates' lives at the cost of his own. His death was a turning point for Barry Enoch—one which, in the months to come, would have a deadly effect on the enemy.

TAN AN

Slogging their way through open rice paddies, exposed to VC eyes, the team stumbles upon a large base camp concealed by nipa palm. Making contact with the 314th North Vietnamese Light Force Company, the SEALs kill one district and one province level VCI, undermining the NVA's attack plan for the upcoming Tet holiday.

Tich—Five feet, four inches tall, one hundred and forty pounds, he was a South Vietnamese jungle fighter who fought side by side with Barry Enoch. He hated the VC and NVA and vowed to continue the battle until his land was free. It was his obsession, and he would remain true to his convictions until the day he fell from a VC bullet. The memory of Tich haunts Enoch to this day.

Mike Thornton—Brash and always ready for a good time, he could walk into a room and tear the place up, but had a heart of gold for his teammates. "Big Mike" was the kind of man that you were thankful to have on your side in combat. If he felt fear, his teammates never knew it. He proved his courage when he saved the life of Medal of Honor recipient Lt. Thomas Norris, becoming only the third SEAL in history to be awarded the Congressional Medal of Honor.

TRON ISLAND

Traveling by Skimmer boat up the "Tee Tee" canal, the SEALs execute a late-afternoon, high-tide assault on a VC junk construction yard. Infiltrating the yard, Enoch and his team stun the enemy into panic and inaction. Their demolition work destroys an array of VC junks, sampans, and hootches—an operation that lifts the platoon's spirits and breaks a vital link in the enemy's chain of supply.

TEAMMATES: SEALs AT WAR

BARRY W. ENOCH
Chief Gunners Mate, U.S. Navy (Ret.)

WITH GREGORY A. WALKER

POCKET BOOKS
New York   London   Toronto   Sydney   Tokyo   Singapore

An *Original* Publication of POCKET BOOKS

POCKET BOOKS, a division of Simon & Schuster Inc.
1230 Avenue of the Americas, New York, NY 10020

Copyright © 1996 by Greg Walker and Barry Enoch

ISBN: 0-671-56830-2

First Pocket Books printing December 1996

10 9 8 7 6 5 4 3 2 1

POCKET and colophon are registered trademarks of Simon & Schuster Inc.

Cover photo courtesy of the author

Printed in the U.S.A.

IN MEMORY OF
MY FRIEND AND TEAMMATE

BILL MACHEN

It has never been the same without him.

after he'd passed away, a double-breasted beauty with pinstripes. Sue and I had never seen eye to eye about any clothing but under the circumstances I'd accepted the suit.

Acknowledgments

This book became a reality because of a newfound friend in Greg Walker who insisted my story be told. He has been a true teammate as coauthor in this work, always encouraging and guiding me from chapter to chapter. It was Greg who originally inspired me to look deep within and to bring out the sights and sounds left far behind in Vietnam. My sincere thanks goes to Lt. Comdr. Michael J. Walsh who introduced me to Greg and involved me in the manuscript review of his own book *SEAL!*

My deepest thanks to U.S. Senator Bob Kerrey, who without hesitation took the time to remember his teammates in the introduction of this book. Also, the author takes this opportunity to acknowledge the contributions of my teammates and personal friends for their perspectives and recollections. Among them are: Tom and Janet Boyhan, Gary and Celia Parrott, and Hal and Denise Kuydendall who opened their hearts and homes to me. Many thanks to John Ware who flew across the country in a snowstorm to tell me his story and to his wife, Jimmie, who sent me John's letters from Vietnam, which she has kept for twenty-five years.

Others who allowed me to sift through their personal files:

Acknowledgments

Scott Lyon, for his story on the release of POWs; Ralph Stafford, Stoner 63 weapons historian; my longtime friend Chip Maury for the use of his photographs in this book; Dennis Cummings for sending ALFA platoon's after action reports; and my deepest thanks to Tom Norris for spending time with me talking about Mike Thornton, our mutual friend and teammate.

I wish to express my most sincere thanks to my family without whom my work would be meaningless: to my wife, Eatsie, who stayed behind raising three children while I was in Vietnam, for her loyalty and love over the last forty years, and her assistance with this endeavor. To my daughter, Laura, now herself a Navy wife, and to my two sons, Ken and Mike, who encouraged me every step of the way.

I am forever indebted to a new teammate in my life, one who has kept a protective shield around this SEAL and helped me gain closure to my darkest times.

He is Jesus Christ.

SEAL Team One Personnel Killed in the Line of Duty in the Republic of Vietnam from 1966 through 1972

RD2	Billy W. Machen	KIA 19 Aug 66	Rung Sat Zone
Lt.	Daniel M. Mann	KIA 07 Apr 67	Rung Sat Zone
IC3	Donald E. Boston	KIA 07 Apr 67	Rung Sat Zone
RM3	Robert K. Neal	KIA 21 Apr 67	Rung Sat Zone
SM3	Leslie H. Funk	KIA 06 Oct 67	Rung Sat Zone
SN	Frank G. Antone	KIA 23 Dec 67	Rung Sat Zone
SN	Roy B. Kieth	KIA 11 Jan 68	Ba Xuye
BM1	Walter G. Pope	KIA 28 Apr 68	Kien Hoa
SFP2	David E. Devine	KIA 04 May 68	Kien Hoa
SK2	Donald H. Zillgitt	KIA 12 May 68	Vinh Binh
CS1	Donnie L. Patrick	KIA 14 May 68	Vinh Long
EMC	Gordon C. Brown	KIA 19 May 68	Kien Giang
SK1	Robert K. Wagner	KIA 15 Aug 68	Vinh Binh
WO1	Eugene S. Tinnin	KIA 20 Aug 68	Vinh Long
ETN3	James K. Sanders	KIA 22 Nov 68	Saigon
SM1	David A. Wilson	KIA 13 Jan 69	Vinh Long
ATN1	Kenneth E. Van Hoy	KIA 18 May 69	Kien Giang
QM2	Ronald E. Pace	KIA 18 May 69	Kien Giang
MM2	Lowell W. Meyer	KIA 18 May 69	Kien Giang
HM1	Lin A. Mahner	KIA 25 May 69	Kien Giang
Lt. (jg)	David L. Nicholas	KIA 17 Oct 69	Nam Cam
HM1	Richard O. Wolfe	KIA 30 Nov 69	Nam Cam
BM3	James R. Gore	KIA 23 Jun 70	Can Tho
MM2	Richard J. Solano	KIA 23 Jun 70	Can Tho
SM3	John S. Durlin	KIA 23 Jun 70	Can Tho
RMSN	John J. Donelly III	KIA 23 Jun 70	Can Tho
FN	Toby A. Thomas	KIA 23 Jun 70	Can Tho
EMC	Frank W. Bomar	KIA 20 Dec 70	Truc Giang
EM3	J.L. Ritter	KIA 20 Dec 70	Truc Giang
Lt.	J.F. Thames	KIA 19 Jan 71	Nam Cam
FN	Harold E. Birky	KIA 30 Jan 71	Ben Tre
Lt.	Michael R. Collins	KIA 04 Mar 71	Kien Hoa
TM1	Lester J. Moe	KIA 29 Mar 71	Kien Giang
Lt.	Melvin S. Dry	KIA 06 Jun 72	Tonkin Gulf

"Maybe Someday It Won't Hurt to Remember"

Contents

Contents

Foreword

It is a pleasure and an honor to write a few words of introduction to Barry Enoch's book about SEAL Team One. His attention to the importance of our being a team is extremely relevant and all too often overlooked. Without the TEAM there are no SEALs. None of us were SEALs; we were members of a SEAL Team.

I am probably not the only man who should give Barry credit for acquiring the skills needed to survive. He was a teacher, a leader who would follow orders, and a follower who knew how to save the rear end of many a green officer . . . and did so to everyone's benefit.

Barry Enoch is the right person to write sagely about TEAM work. He is not a braggart. If he says it happened, it did. If he says someone else did all the work and deserves all the glory, he probably deserves at least half. He is a man who always did more than his share and always asked for less than he was owed.

In December of 1965 I was practicing pharmacy in Sioux City, Iowa, when I received my invitation to take a free physical examination paid for by the United States government. I was twenty-two years old and two months beyond the safety of a college deferment. It was time to make a decision about which branch of the military I would select to do my time. I had just read Herman Wouk's *The Caine Mutiny* and had fallen in love with the excitement of the sea. So, I volunteered for the Navy.

While I was learning the skills needed to be an ensign (how to use a knife and fork) at Newport, Rhode Island, I made another decision: to volunteer for underwater demolition training, or UDT. This was another well-thought-out choice; I had become severely nauseous while touring a destroyer that was safely tied up at dockside. UDT offered thrills without having to throw up. Upon successful completion of my training class, I was selected for SEAL Team One.

Life for this young ensign became much more serious.

SEALs were serious about being a team. *Webster's* defines a team player as "one who subordinates personal aspirations and works in a coordinated effort with other members of a group in striving for a common goal." That was the expectation made of us at the beginning of training and for those who remained afterward it was our reality. I learned this from a great football coach in high school, but in football all that was at stake was a game or state championship. In the teams we knew that the lives of our teammates depended on each of us doing our job.

Barry Enoch taught us how to do our job and to respect the integrity of the team. He was a gunners mate who was qualified by skill and desire to teach us how to care for and use our ordnance. He taught us the meaning of "aimed fire" and reminded us that noise counted for nothing when your numbers were small. Either hit the target or the target hits you.

SEAL Team did have its heroes, but we could not and did not allow them to remain above the rest. A man might be faster, stronger, smarter, or braver . . . but he could not survive without the team. Glory came to the platoon not the individual. In 1969 when I was told I had been recommended for the Congressional Medal of Honor, I traveled from the Philadelphia Naval Hospital to the SEAL Team One compound in Coronado, California, to talk with teammates. I especially sought out the opinion of Barry Enoch as to whether or not I should accept something I believed I did not deserve when compared to the performance of others under similar conditions. Barry advised me to accept the MOH for everyone whose actions weren't seen, reported, or perhaps even recorded. "Take it for all of us," he said. And I did.

It's not that we were full of sentimental attachments or that we were incapable of acting alone. In fact I would be reluctant to tell the story in the preceding paragraph to teammates for fear they might hoot me out of the room. I didn't even tell them I had three sisters until I (and they) were safely out of reach. We weren't foolish with our trust. However, we did trust that the team would never leave us behind. You knew this to be fact and you counted on it as such. For this reason not one SEAL has ever been left behind for dead or as a POW. As teammates we will not allow it.

Knowing that once in my life I gave all I could for the cause of making a team better than it would have been without my commitment is as good a memory as I have of the teams today. There were disappointments, failures, and even betrayals; but never did we doubt the importance of our cause. We sometimes fought each other in bitter rivalries, but we never forgot to erase the grudge for the good of the group. Men can excel as individuals; they should not do less than that which they are capable. But, men are more as a team than they are as solitary wolves. Thanks to Barry Enoch I learned this early in my life as a proud member of SEAL Team One.

SENATOR BOB KERREY

Introduction

Naval Special Warfare Today

SEALs operate in maritime/riverine environments to conduct tasks against either tactical or strategic targets which are in the national interest. These may be conventional or unconventional in nature. Swimmer Delivery Vehicle (SDV) assets are organized and trained to conduct submerged operations in support of NavSpecWar and are a critical factor in today's SEAL capability. SEAL tasks include Reconnaissance, Direct Action, Combat Craft Operations, Unconventional Warfare, Foreign Internal Defense, and support of raiding parties.

Organization of SEAL elements is structured at the platoon level. Today each platoon is made up of sixteen enlisted men and two officers. Attachments with specialized skills pertaining to the successful conduct of a mission may be folded into the platoon if necessary. Each platoon reflects one to two SEAL qualified medical corpsmen. Platoons are trained and equipped to meet specific mission requirements. Platoons focus their training and proficiency to those identified missions and/or requirements given them. Weapons systems are likewise focused making SEAL platoons truly special application forces within the SOF community.

1

Limitations on SEAL conducted warfare include the following. Attachments cannot inhibit the mission due to any number of factors to include a lack of physical conditioning. SEAL firepower is light in nature and will only control short ranges on the battlefield. Communications are determined by the caliber of equipment issued on a mission by mission basis. Endurance and fatigue will affect the mission from one degree to another. Terrain and weather, likewise. The enemy situation per mission is also a limitation as to what a SEAL team can accomplish. Security is dependent not only upon the element of surprise but also freedom of movement. Accurate and timely intelligence has been proven time and again to either make or break SEAL missions. Today, timely preplanning and coordination with civilian and political considerations is absolutely necessary. Special Operations are dependent on political and military measures to include the proper coordination of military actions with appropriate civilian agencies. Basic language requirements to conduct missions have been a part of SEAL ops since 1963. Unlike their Army special forces brethren the SEALs seek only a rudimentary language base in order to execute their tasks "on the ground."

Command and Control of SEAL platoons are sourced by Naval Special Warfare Groups to Special Operations Forces and Navy fleet commanders. They are then op-conned—or turned over operationally—to on-scene commanders for specific mission taskings in any given theater of operations. Unified or Specific Sub Commands include Joint Task forces, Fleet, MAAG or MilGrp (country teams, foreign service), and Other Services/Non Military command and control agencies such as the CIA.

Tactical employment of SEAL teams requires qualified operators be present during the planning and preparation for a mission. Since Vietnam it has become critical not to task SEALs with missions better suited for other SOF assets if such assets are available to the SOF or fleet commander. SEALs no longer will conduct missions better executed by Army rangers or Marine recon elements. Extensive rehearsals are necessary for SEAL operations and adequate time must be provided for such practice to ensure the best possible execution of the mission.

Target areas must be suitable for the delivery and extraction of SEAL elements conducting the mission. Base areas must be suitable in terms of facilities for logistic and administrative support of SEAL operations and/or taskings. Again, the lessons learned in Vietnam proved SEALs operate best when they can prepare and rest in secure areas. Over time, to include operations in El Salvador, Grenada, Panama, and the Persian Gulf, the use of secure areas allows SEAL platoons the greatest degree of staging and mission prep.

Employment of SEALs can rely upon submarine operations in terms of delivery and recovery. Civilian authority may dictate/command of individual mission basics, with such authority coming not only from the commander in chief but from specific agencies such as the Central Intelligence Agency, which often relies upon SEAL forces to conduct clandestine and covert warfare as well as intelligence gathering operations in denied or sensitive areas.

One vital mission which has seen recent emphasis during the war in Bosnia is the extended maritime Escape and Evasion tasking. This is meant to assist the successful E&E of Navy/NATO/UN from land out to (and into) the sea. SEALs train in various location and rescue scenarios in order to assist downed pilots who might have to ditch at sea.

The delivery and recovery of SEAL team elements is dependent upon whether the mission is overt, clandestine, or covert in nature. In addition, SEALs must consider time frame, enemy situation, topography, oceanography, weather in the target area, personnel capabilities, and equipment situation when framing a mission for execution.

For example, SEAL platoons have an organic rigger who is also JumpMaster, Fast Rope Master, Helo Cast Master, and Rappel Master qualified. Like Special Forces and selected Long Range Reconnaissance Units (LRSUs) SEALs can be used in a stay-behind role to report enemy movements and positions or to conduct small unit warfare (harassment/direct action). Submarine or SDV use is preferred by SEAL teams for covert or clandestine infiltration and exfiltration from a target site.

Mission success is greatly based upon undetected entry to the target area, speedy execution of mission, rapid withdrawal from target area, and avoidance of pitched battles with enemy forces of any size. General and specific intelligence requirements assist in mission success and SEAL intelligence requirements are extensive. Photo intelligence is critical. For example, infiltration/exfiltration from coastal target areas is greatly assisted by those photos taken by submarine periscope during premission scouting efforts.

Essential Elements of Intelligence requirements include target ID and data class code. Target location, description, and construction, use of aerial photos to ID access and egress routes, seasonal changes on terrain, and target and ground photos of the target to include match-up with appropriate maps are standard SOF concerns. Environmental data, enemy order of battle, threat level assessment at the target, and evaluation of enemy forces follow Army thought processes on ground warfare. Local forces or assets (guerrillas, for example) which might be available to assist SEALs in their mission are likewise studied.

SEALs make the best use of state-of-the-art communications to accomplish their missions. Teams are capable of voice, secure voice, CW, Data, Data Burst, Semaphore, Flashing Lights, and Clandestine Light Sources. Communications can be augmented by commo specialists as attachments to SEAL elements if such specialists are required for mission accomplishment.

Today's SEALs owe their unique expertise to those teammates who came before. The importance of those early UDT/SEAL operators, the men who wrote the book on naval special warfare because there was no book to begin with, cannot be allowed to disappear with time. The recollections and admonitions of men like Barry Enoch serve to secure the bond between each generation of Navy SEAL. The price paid was in sweat, blood, and tears so today's SEALs might enjoy the fruits of success without the sourness of bitter failure.

The reader will note the author's deliberate intent to portray his teammates far more so than himself in this book. Barry Enoch is this kind of man. Still, his awards and decorations include the Navy Cross, two Silver Stars, two Bronze Stars, the Navy Commendation Medal with combat "V," the Combat Action Ribbon, the Presidential Unit

Citation Ribbon (SEAL Team One), the Navy Unit Commendation Ribbon (SEAL Team One), the Republic of Vietnam Cross of Gallantry (Silver Star) and RVN Cross of Gallantry (Bronze Star), and the much prized Naval Special Warfare breast insignia, or SEAL Trident. Chief Gunners Mate Enoch is easily one of the most humble men I've been privileged to become associated with. His values and presence reflect what being a Navy SEAL—or any other special warfare operator—is all about. He is simply a teammate, whether on point or rear security.

His story is as much about the future of the teams as it is about their past.

Gregory A. Walker, a teammate
U.S. Army Special Forces

1

Pride vs Humble Spirit

*Heroism is when the right man sees you in combat at
the wrong time doing the job you were trained to do.*

—Bud Jurick, UDT TRA, 1967

In the fall of 1969, Charlie Platoon, SEAL Team One, was
diligently preparing to deploy to South Vietnam just before
Christmas. The last two and a half years had been hard on
the team. Twenty-two SEALs had been killed in the line of
duty with many more wounded, some so seriously they'd
had to leave the Navy. Still, we were proud warriors and
certainly combat ready but I knew in my heart we needed
an extra boost moralewise. Word had come down that Lt.
(jg) Bob Kerrey was to be awarded the Medal of Honor for
his gallantry in a recent action. He would be the first SEAL
in our history to receive the "Big Blue" as it was known in
the teams. Kerrey was from SEAL Team One, a teammate,
and in him I saw our morale booster.

The award came in lieu of a firefight during which Lt. (jg)
Kerrey was seriously wounded. Intelligence had come to
him about a small force of Vietcong cadre which was
attached to an intelligence unit operating on Ham Tam
Island in Nha Trang Bay. Kerrey interviewed two *chieu hoi*
(defectors) and, based upon their stories and his own
intelligence sources, planned a mission against the VC. On
March 14, 1969, Lt. Kerrey took a seven-man SEAL squad
and two South Vietnamese frogmen (LDNN) onto the

7

island. Infiltrating by small boat after dark, the assault team free climbed a 350-foot rock wall so as to launch their raid from the least expected direction on the camp. Upon reaching the top of the cliff a quiet recon told the SEALs and their LDNNs the VC were split into two groups. Kerrey split his reinforced squad into two fire teams. The first team was supposed to cover the immediate VC in the area while Kerrey took the second group after the cadre element. As happens in combat, the enemy somehow spotted the SEALs first and the fight was on.

Lt. Kerrey was struck by grenade fragments almost immediately. The blast destroyed the lower part of his right leg. Despite being brutally wounded, the SEAL officer directed his squad's intense firepower with calmness and such accuracy that the VC were suppressed under a withering crossfire from the two fire teams. With the enemy destroyed, Kerrey's men captured several important VC cadre leaders as well as critical intelligence documents and various weapons. Kerrey had remained in charge of the operation even as the extraction helicopter was taking the team out, disregarding his injuries in favor of seeing the mission completed under his command.

I had just finished taking CHARLIE platoon for a four-mile run on the beach when someone told me, "Bob Kerrey is back." As the men began cooling down in the SEAL Team One compound I asked where he was as I wanted to pay my respects. Directed to the SEAL quarterdeck area I spotted a man in uniform on crutches and leaning against a steel post.

It was Bob Kerrey.

He had been watching the men as we'd been pounding back up the beach from our conditioning run. His face bore no expression I could recognize, and no emotion one way or the other was evident. He had lost weight and his uniform was slightly loose on his leaner than usual frame. I remember his eyes more than anything else. There was pain in them, a deep abiding pain which came up from the very depths of the man's being. This was more than the physical discomfort or pain I was very used to. The pain in Bob Kerrey's eyes that day on the quarterdeck told me the firefight with the VC might be over but the battle inside Lt. Kerrey was not.

"Hello, Mr. Kerrey," I offered quietly.

He turned toward me and an earnest smile broke through the internal war I'd just witnessed. We shook hands and I asked how he was, mentioning the leg he'd lost and asking how it had happened. Talk then turned to the Medal of Honor and I congratulated him upon being recommended for it. "Yes, thank you," he replied, "but I'm seriously considering turning it down, Chief." Upon hearing this pronouncement I was dumbstruck. It was clear something was troubling the lieutenant and I intended to find out just what it was.

As we talked alone on the quarterdeck I began to sense a very humble spirit in Bob Kerrey. He was thinking of his men and offered they had not done anything less than he during the night's battle on Ham Tam Island. Clearly, the wounded officer was uncomfortable being submitted for our nation's highest decoration for bravery under fire. "I didn't do anything differently than any other SEAL would have done under the same conditions," he said. Lt. Kerrey was a teammate, one of our teammates, as he belonged to SEAL Team One in particular. It went against his grain to be singled out like this.

"Mr. Kerrey," I said, "you must accept that medal." I told him how proud all of us were of him and that he was the first SEAL to be so highly decorated in the teams. "The medal is rightly yours," I said. "But it is also a part of all of us and that's how you should think of it." In my mind we needed this young, courageous Navy officer to represent all those SEALs who'd paid the ultimate price in Vietnam, as well as those of us going back to the war, so the nation would know of our commitment to it. At the same time we needed the spark the Medal of Honor could ignite in terms of increased pride and morale. CHARLIE Platoon was going to war and I wanted my men charged up and ready for the upcoming task.

There was another reason, as well. I sensed Mr. Kerrey was suffering from a reduced sense of self because of his wound. It had been there in his eyes as he'd watched us run up the beach. Where he might have believed his actions that night were worthy of the medal, his physical injury seemed to be getting in the way of accepting it as much for himself as for anyone else. In my mind, Bob Kerrey needed to hear he was okay from me, one of his teammates.

"Thanks, Chief, I'll give it some more thought," he finally told me. We shook hands one more time and went our separate ways.

In May of 1970 Lt. (jg) Kerrey accepted his Medal of Honor. He did so aided by an artificial leg but he was by no means crippled. Much later and long after the war was over I spoke with him by telephone. It was the night before the 1991 New Hampshire presidential primaries and now Senator Kerrey reminded me of our quarterdeck conversation. I was touched he would remember it and at the kind words he said to me. Bob Kerrey will always be a teammate, and he has not lost the humble spirit of a true warrior.

No one I ever knew who graduated from Underwater Demolition Team (UDT) training truly disliked any of their instructors regardless of the pain and misery they might have been subjected to. We all looked up to these men both during and after the difficult course, but certainly there were those outstanding individuals who had a long-term impact on you. For me, Bud Jurick is one of those men.

It was at graduation that we first saw our UDT instructors in their white, or dress, uniforms. Before this they were only seen in the olive green work uniform of a UDT instructor, their name tag and the UDT instructor patch our only indication of who and what they were. At the ceremony's end they each passed by us, shaking our hands in congratulations. When Bud Jurick reached me I realized for the first time he was a WWII veteran by the campaign ribbons above his left breast. He'd also won the Bronze Star with "V" device for valor and a Purple Heart, indicating he'd been wounded in combat. I remember wondering at the time what the story was behind the man who'd just accepted me into the brotherhood.

In 1964 I was transferred from SEAL Team One to UDT TRA to serve as an instructor myself. Bud Jurick was still there teaching land warfare to the young frogmen-to-be. Bud was a family man and didn't spend much time hanging out with the other instructors after work. Even during the duty day he was a quiet man, prone to keep to himself. I was assigned to teach weapons and demolitions out at San Clemente Island which put Jurick and me together with every class headed for the island and its rigors.

As the war in Vietnam progressed, the need for more and more SEALs grew. More classes were formed and trained, and at times Bud and I would stay behind on the island to prepare for the next week's inbound class. These were special times for me to draw closer to Jurick, whom I'd grown to respect even more. I wanted to learn from his experiences as I knew I'd be returning to the war sooner or later myself.

It was during one of these quiet weekends that Bud and I decided to recon the south end of the island at China Point. We gathered up some steaks and a grill, loaded a jeep, and headed down the road. That night while sitting at the campfire I asked Jurick for the first time about his Bronze Star. The story he told me came slowly, spoken in a deep, strong—but strangely soft—voice. I have never forgotten it.

Bud Jurick had been in the Army during WWII as a paratrooper. It was D day, the invasion of Europe by the Allies. Bud had never imagined so many airplanes, lined up in row after row on the runway where he and his comrades suited up for the jump into Normandy. They'd climbed into their aircraft only to wait in its uncomfortable confines until the order was given to take off.

The plan was for the plane to fly over its drop zone at high altitude once, then return at a much lower altitude in order for the men to jump. It was hoped this tactic would convince the Germans the planes were bombers on their way to targets far inland rather than troop carriers. Bud's company was to link up once they'd landed and to destroy a key bridge.

As their plane made its final turn and assumed drop altitude, its crew had no way of knowing they were crossing over a Nazi rest and relaxation area. Enemy ground fire greeted the aircraft as it made its approach, the paratroopers straining under their heavy loads and standing "in the door" ready to jump. Hit time and again, the men dived out into the flak below to give the aircrew a chance at surviving.

As they hit the ground the company was badly split up. Jurick's leg was injured but he still managed to link up with four other members from his company.

None of the men had a map of the area but they knew the name of the road and bridge which was their target. With enough explosives between them to do the job, they decided to head for the bridge where they figured the rest of the company would sooner or later arrive. With luck, and by reading the road signs as best they could, the tiny group reached the bridge before daylight. Placing their explosives they then waited for others from the unit to arrive. When no one else showed up, Bud and his fellow paratroopers pulled their fuses and headed back toward the front lines of the invasion, the bridge going up in smoke behind them.

There was more.

Jurick recounted there were firefights going on all around them as they leap-frogged and crawled across the battlefield. The countryside was laced with thick hedgerows which provided cover for both the Americans and the Germans. At one point, while patrolling along a dirt farm road, the men found themselves staring down the barrel of a German tank not twenty feet away! Captured, the paratroopers were taken to a farmhouse where they were kept captive.

Each night a German medic came and checked on Bud's injured leg. He spoke English and Jurick told him the Germans were losing the war. If the medic would give Bud the key to the locker holding the Americans' weapons, Jurick said, it would be better for the man when the German position was overrun and it was discovered they were holding American POWs.

The German was an old man and was afraid Bud and his friends would use their weapons on him. Jurick convinced him he only wanted the compass which was also in the locker. One night, after checking his leg, the medic put his hand on Bud's head and with the other slipped the locker's key into Jurick's shirt. Later that same night the paratroopers gathered up their equipment and weapons, slipping out of the farmhouse and successfully evading further capture until reaching American lines. For his efforts and courage Bud Jurick was awarded the Bronze Star with "V" device.

After Bud finished his story we sat at the fire in silence. I thought about how men like Jurick and others helped change the world and the generation I grew up with. What it took to do so wasn't fully appreciated even today, I thought. How much did I owe to men like Bud Jurick? I knew it was not the Bronze Star which thrilled this mentor of mine, but the relief at coming home alive which was his greatest reward. In Jurick's mind no one owed him anything, he'd simply done what he'd been called upon and trained to do.

Men such as Bob Kerrey and Bud Jurick are regarded in the teams as role models for past, present, and future frogmen or SEALs. They are not role models by their own choosing, however. Beneath the SEAL breast insignia lies a pride which is second to none, and it is eager to come out. However, beneath the rows of awards and decorations of such men is a humble common spirit which gives all credit to their teammates. The *true* SEAL operator sees himself as part of a team. He does not protray himself as standing alone or accomplishing great things by himself. Those of us who are SEALs do not perceive ourselves as others outside of the fraternity might. Personal bravery is not considered as a singular, self-serving act for one's own benefit.

When my time came to receive those medals awarded to me I was filled with mixed emotions. There was pride and there was great humility. I recalled Bob Kerrey and Bud Jurick and their actions under fire and in captivity. In my own mind, at the time, I felt undeserving of such recognition when compared to men like these. Then and now I feel differently about myself than perhaps others do about me. Even as the medals were pinned to my uniform I remembered those who were filled with courage and fell in the darkness, never to get up again.

Often, they received less for the giving of their lives than I have—who still has his.

So to those who slipped over the side into the dark waters and went before us, through the heavy surf, and crossed the bar to wait for us on the other side in gallant ranks, we remember You.

For you are what this story is all about. . . .

2

"Bear" Roots

Barry "The Bear" Enoch was already a living legend in the teams. Enoch left his mark on many a SEAL walking around today, including me. I still get regular "rudder guidance" from him.

—Lt. Comdr. Michael Walsh (ret.)

Marion is a small town in Kentucky, located in Crittenden County, which is bordered to the north by the Ohio River. On May 23, 1936, Barry Enoch was brought into a world just beginning to see a light at the end of the Great Depression's long tunnel. He would grow up on a small farm until nineteen years of age, learning to fish, trap, and hunt on land covered with woods that tapered down to a bluff and a stream called Crooked Creek.

His father worked at the Keystone Mines in Crittenden County. The Keystone was a hard rock mine that produced fluspar, which was shipped up the Ohio River by barge to the steel mills in Pittsburgh, Pa. Mrs. Enoch was happy as a housewife and mother, content with her husband and son.

Young Barry was an only child. He spent most of his early years with his dog, exploring the woods and stream of his father's farm. The woods became his private playground, filled with wildlife and other natural mysteries. When old enough by his father's standards, Barry was schooled in the use of a rifle and shotgun. Hunting became a year-round activity. The young Enoch quickly became a marksman, duck hunting along the Ohio River a favorite pastime. Years

14

later he would draw deeply from his life in the woods as a Navy SEAL in Vietnam.

In December of 1941, America went to war against Japan. The bombing of Pearl Harbor in Hawaii was the talk of the town. Work at the nearby mines was stepped up because the country's struggling war machine suddenly needed vast amounts of quality steel for its ships, planes, and guns. The war brought many things, including rationing. Barry's feet grew faster than the rest of him so his mother used her shoe ration for her son's shoes most of the war. To allow the family more sweetener the Enochs grew sugarcane to make molasses; sugar was rationed as well as shoes.

Barry remembers never hearing his mother complain. Instead, she stopped knitting afghans and began knitting olive drab sweaters for the soldiers fighting in Europe. She would write notes and hide these in the sweaters, with many soldiers writing her back to thank her for the support upon their discovery. Some became pen pals. Barry was eager for a sweater of his own but was told by his mother they were only intended for the soldiers, and that she was accountable for the yarn and its use by the government.

The Enochs received the *Courier-Journal* newspaper published out of Louisville, Kentucky. Mrs. Enoch read the war news aloud every day, with Barry listening intently. She would show him the maps on the front page, complete with great black sweeping arrows where Allied troops were advancing. Once a story was printed about a downed pilot and his crew. They were lost at sea in their rubber rafts. Every day Barry would run to the mailbox to get the paper once the story broke. The pilot's name was Eddie Rickenbacker, the famed WWI fighter ace.

It was a time when each school day began with the Pledge of Allegiance to the flag and the Lord's Prayer. Once a week the students would go to the auditorium to hear about the war and to sing songs like "America the Beautiful" and "When Johnny Comes Marching Home Again." Barry and his classmates each had a little book no larger than a checkbook, and during these assemblies they would march up on stage and buy ten-cent stamps to put in them. When the book was filled it could be turned in for a twenty-five dollar War Bond. One day, the students were let out of school to gather scrap iron for the war effort. When they were finished a pile thirty feet high covered the baseball diamond.

One morning Barry's teacher was called from the classroom just before recess. After recess the principal entered their classroom and informed the class that their teacher's brother was missing in action in the South Pacific. Barry and his classmates were told to be very quiet and to come to the principal's classroom. There they sat, two to a seat. There was only one phone in the school and it was in the principal's office, just off her classroom. Barry discovered when he put his head on his desk that he could see his teacher in the office. She was praying, then crying, then praying again beside the old black telephone. The principal would pray, then have the students do some quiet work, then put their heads on the desks, then start the routine all over again as the day went on.

It was a long day for the little boy, ending only when the phone rang to announce the teacher's brother had been found wounded in action and he would be all right. Prayer, Barry discovered, is sometimes answered quickly.

Mr. and Mrs. Enoch took Barry to visit his teacher's brother in the VA hospital much later. Standing near the bed he could see right into the wound itself, which was located in the soldier's leg. War for Barry Enoch became very, very real that night.

On Saturday nights the family would often go into town. They would sit in the car and watch the soldiers walking up and down the main street. His parents often commented on how young the men were, and Barry would ask to get a haircut "like the soldiers have." Eighteen miles from Marion at Sturgis, Kentucky, there was a glider base. Camp Breckenridge Army Base was at Morgafield. There were always a lot of soldiers in town. The railroad came through Marion and the trains were often loaded with Army tanks and big guns. Troop trains rolled through loaded with the Army. Sitting on his front porch Enoch could watch convoys of military trucks which were two to three miles long roll by. He remembers always seeing a jeep both in front and at the rear of such processions.

16

The war was the talk of every store, barbershop, and street corner. Little boys have big ears and nothing said got past Barry. The American flag was everywhere, with little flags boasting a star in the middle for every member of a family who was serving. These hung in windows facing the street all over town.

Barry Enoch wanted to grow up quickly so he could join the Army. He never heard anything but good about the "boys over there" and like his friends he wanted to serve. When the war ended, he came in from the woods to find a strange car in his parents driveway. An Army colonel was talking with his parents. One of his father's friends was sending his son to a military academy and had given the colonel the Enochs' name as they might consider the same for Barry. There were discussions about where the money would come from, and Mrs. Enoch was not at all positive about the idea to begin with. But her son waged his own campaign and after a month his parents capitulated. In September he was sent to the Columbia Military Academy, in Columbia, Tennessee, for his eighth grade school year.

The academy was made up of two-story buildings built of gray stone. Each building had walls so thick you could sit on either the inside or the outside of the windowsills. The campus was filled with things to see and do, and Barry was beside himself with pleasure. Cadets wore Confederate gray uniforms with black stripes down the outside of the pants legs. They had a dress blouse with large white belts that crossed in front and back. Their undress uniform replaced the blouse with a gray Eisenhower jacket which the young Enoch liked best.

The process of learning how to soldier began. Barry became proficient at polishing both shoes and brass so he could see himself clearly in their surfaces. When Springfield rifles were issued he learned to clean them too. Everything was done in ranks and the cadets marched everywhere. Barry learned to accomplish tasks as a team. Team spirit got the cadets through their demanding inspections and parade ground reviews. In addition they were taught how to act and to respect all levels of rank. The cadets ate at the colonel's table in the mess hall. They stood at attention until the colonel's wife was seated at one end, then waited until the

17

officer returned to his own seat at the other. When all the officers' ladies were properly seated the command "Seats" would be given. Then and only then could the cadets sit. No one dared move until the colonel had given thanks. Lessons on table manners were soundly adhered to.

Cadets were to be involved in sports and Barry chose football in the fall and spring. When the season ended he went out for swimming. As always, teamwork was the answer where success was concerned. Whatever the cadets did, if there was just one goof-off, the whole team suffered for his actions. The academy instilled in Barry an appreciation of what it was to be a teammate, which would stay with him throughout his military career. There were cadets from other countries at the academy as well and from these Enoch developed a respect for their backgrounds and personalities.

The only "mom" at the academy was the senior cadet in the dorm. Barry struggled with his grades, and the senior cadet—himself an excellent student—often spent time to help the younger man keep up. From this example he learned the proper relationship of the leader to his men, at one time helping kindly to see achievement and at another time becoming the strict overseer for whom no errors would be tolerated.

Upon going out for swimming Barry began to hear about the Navy. Tales about the Underwater Demolition Teams, or UDTs, were rampant. One cadet had a library book on frogmen and what they did to clear the beaches during WWII. Somehow Barry Enoch just knew he wanted nothing more from life than to become a frogman. A strong swimmer, he began working even harder to develop his swimming skills to achieve his goal.

He left the academy at the end of the school year and returned home. That single year saw deep roots put down which would nourish his life in the times to come. The academy molded the direction his life would take, and combined with the already strong roots of his formative years in Marion, they became a part of the bedrock foundation which would support the man to come.

That summer he attended a Kentucky Junior Conservation Camp for boys. Camp Currie was located on Big Bear

Creek at Kentucky Lake and was operated by the Kentucky Department of Fish and Wildlife Resources. Barry spent most of his time either on the rifle range or waterfront. He got his certificate in junior lifesaving skills as well as small bore rifle. It was during the Red Cross sponsored lifesaving class that he met Doug Travis, a Conservation officer who was the camp's Water Safety Director. Doug became a major influence in Barry Enoch's life over the next five years.

In September Barry started high school in Marion. He once again went out for football and was soon playing on the same team as the juniors and seniors. This wasn't surprising as it was a small school and everyone played on the same team regardless of grade. The older boys were tough, and it was hard for the younger players to receive their letter unless they truly excelled. Barry did, with the most enjoyable aspect of the effort being a part of a team.

Back in the swing of things in Marion he found himself taking up hunting again. Joining the Junior Conservation Club at school he once again came into contact with Doug Travis. Travis taught his students respect for the environment and its wildlife. He took them hunting and fishing, using the opportunity to "help make Kentucky a better place for the outdoorsman." That summer Enoch returned to Camp Currie where he passed the senior lifesaving course. He was allowed to stay on for a few weeks at the camp where he hung out with the lifeguards on the waterfront. Barry decided he'd like to come back the next year as an employee of the camp, working as a lifeguard.

Upon graduation from high school Barry attended the Aquatic School in Paducah, Kentucky. With Mr. Travis as one of their instructors the young men from the camp were motivated to be at the top of the class so they wouldn't let Doug down. They all became instructors, sewing on their new patches with pride.

Back at camp they approached Doug about making a long-distance swim on Kentucky Lake. It was ten miles from Aguness Ferry Bridge to the mouth of Big Bear Creek. Travis had made the swim before. Barry found a friend who could provide a safety boat and the details were laid out. Mr. Travis joined his instructors as they greased their bodies down to help insulate them from the cold waters. They entered the water at daylight and soon Barry learned not to look at the shore because to do so caused him to feel he wasn't making any progress. Everyone finished the swim as a team, and that night the tired but excited band dissected the event stroke by stroke. Enoch now wanted to become a Navy frogman more than ever but he kept his secret to himself.

Barry started college at the University of Missouri with a major in wildlife management. His grades once again became a problem and by spring he knew college and he would have to part ways. Coming home he called upon a little redhead he'd been dating throughout high school, and both agreed there were other things in their future besides a career in wildlife. Summer rolled around and Barry returned to his job at Camp Currie. He knew he needed a full-time job, but he wanted one last summer working with Doug and his fellow lifeguards on the lake. On June 24, 1955, Barry Enoch and his high school sweetheart were married. For Barry, it was the best move he ever made.

On August 17 of the same year he joined the United States Navy. He was nineteen years old and accustomed to being called "Bear" by his friends which was short for Barry. In time, the nickname would take on a different meaning as Enoch climbed the ranks as first a frogman and then a U.S. Navy SEAL.

G.A.W.

3

Combined Studies

The orders read: "You are directed to proceed on or about 1 March 1963 to Saigon, Vietnam, and upon arrival report to Commander U.S. Military Assistance Command V (COMUSMAC/V) temporary additional duty in connection with naval matters for a period of about six months. Passport and visa for Vietnam required. Commercial air authorized in the execution of these orders."

As I climbed the steep metal stairs to board the large Pan American jet, the skyline of San Diego seemed to bid me good-bye. This was the first time I had ever deployed courtesy of a civilian airliner, and the first time I'd had to carry a passport to do so. Our commanding officer, Lt. David Del Giudice, briefed the platoon although what information he'd passed along was sketchy, at best. We knew the mission was top secret, and that meant we'd only be told what we absolutely needed to know for right then. His last words before people were released to begin preparations were, "The information you will receive in Saigon could be detrimental to the security of the United States. Good luck."

Being wished luck was a first too.

Two SEAL Team One operators had been dispatched to

Vietnam in January 1962. The security around their trip was so heavy neither Chief Sullivan nor HM1 Charlie Raymond talked much when they returned stateside, and what operational information they'd gathered was locked down tight by the Command. When we deployed I believed our officers knew more about what was coming up on the horizon than ourselves but today I'm not sure that was the case. No one truly knew what to expect in Vietnam, or what our mission might encompass. We were left in the dark because that's the way some one above our level wanted it.

A new boat appeared just before our departure—also top secret—left tied up at our private pier on the Naval Amphibious Base in Coronado, California. An armed guard was posted at the head of the pier to keep the curious away and even we SEALs were required to present a special pass from the team office to step onto the pier.

The craft was called a Swift boat and I was told it was supposed to be very, very fast in the water. It was packed with sophisticated electronics which allowed it to move nearly undetected through enemy waters. Oddly enough there were no guns mounted and as a gunners mate this did not sit quite right with me. Time would prove this early criticism valid. The pilothouse was beautiful with its mahogany and teak trim. We were told civilian versions were available and being used to transport personnel to and from offshore oil rigs. No one knew what exactly the Swift was to be used for in Vietnam but BM2 Roy Adams was ordered to stay with the boat as it was crated and loaded aboard a seabound freighter. On February 25, 1963, my platoon and I were responsible for taking the first Swift boat to Vietnam where these rugged little craft would make quite a name for themselves.

The flight stopped in Los Angeles, Honolulu, and Tokyo before delivering its anxious cargo of Navy SEALs to Saigon. We'd been advised to wear suits, and old ones at that, because the tropic humidity would ruin good material in a heartbeat. My mom had given me one of Dad's suits after he'd passed away, a double-breasted beauty with pinstripes. She and I had never seen eye to eye about my clothing but under the circumstances I'd accepted the gift without a fight. Turns out it was just the thing to wear overseas on a classified mission.

Stepping off the plane the intense heat of Vietnam hit me full in the face. Within minutes I was sweating like mad beneath the old suit's layers. My footlocker failed to arrive with me so I was stuck with only what was on my back and draped over my arm. There was no way of telling how hot it really was inside the suit but I know I looked a sight. Elliot Ness must have been spinning in his grave at how poorly I presented what was his trademark during the Roaring Twenties.

A waiting truck moved us to a secure military compound near the airport where we spent the night in relative comfort. The next morning the platoon was once again loaded into a truck which took us to MAC-V in Saigon. I recall being in wonder at the huge number of bicycles that flowed around us as we wove our way down strange and crowded streets filled with Vietnamese. MAC-V itself was a large multistory structure with white masonry walls that shimmered in the boiling sunlight. Security walls of the same construction fenced the compound and its dwellers in, barbed wire like steel frosting running along their tops. Guards were everywhere I looked.

Once through the gates we stiffly unloaded the vehicle and were taken upstairs to turn in our orders. Along the way I lost count of the security doors we encountered on our way to the Combined Studies Group. Everyone I met appeared to be a civilian and we soon learned the platoon would be working for the Central Intelligence Agency, or CIA. President John F. Kennedy had authorized the agency to train selected Vietnamese in the conduct of covert operations against their enemies in the north. Our mission would entail instructing these personnel in clandestine maritime operations, the project the forerunner of what would become known as OP-34 Alpha. It had been Kennedy who had blessed the birth of both the Army's Special Forces with their unique green headgear, and the Navy's SEAL teams. The president believed the Navy needed a commando force which could operate in the maritime environment, his own experiences as a PT boat commander ferrying special operations teams around in the Pacific during WWII a certain influence.

Beginning in 1947, the CIA had taken on the responsibility of conducting resistance movements and guerrilla warfare because the OSS had been dismantled at the end of WWII. In a debate between the Army and the CIA it was decided that the agency would be permitted to conduct what was called unconventional warfare during "periods of declared peace." The Army would step in during declared war. The CIA, given the green light by a National Security Council decision, stepped up to bat and took over the entire unconventional/resistance warfare pie, to include the requirement for special soldiers to train and lead partisans in occupied countries.

As the agency didn't have a paramilitary core of seasoned combat veterans from which to draw, it turned to the Army for such assets. By 1962 Special Forces were operating in both Laos and Vietnam for over five years. When President Kennedy made sure the SEAL teams were brought on-line, it was only natural we'd come into contact with the CIA in Vietnam.

Despite the atmosphere of our first visit my only question was "Where's my footlocker?" I was assured all of us were going to be outfitted with new khaki uniforms that very day. No rank or other badges of distinction would be worn by our team. The Vietnamese tailor we met with told the group it would take five days for him to finish the uniforms . . . which left me in Dad's old suit for another week! Everywhere we went from then on I stuck out like a sore thumb. Questions from the peanut gallery seemed to be always directed toward me because of my dress. Even at the U.S. Embassy I drew more than my fair share of attention. Much later I would learn my footlocker was making its way around the world finally ending up in Oklahoma City.

Thus began a daily process of being trucked into MAC-V headquarters for endless security briefings, then back to our tents at the secure compound for an evening's rest. Each man in the platoon was told to come up with an alias for a first name and never to use our true last name. This is very difficult for military men to get used to as we are essentially called by our last names from the first day in uniform until mustering out. We made our choices and began working on getting used to a new procedure of identifying each other as well as answering to our new names without hesitation. Corrected time and again I finally began to get the hang of it, as did my teammates.

Our passports were ordered turned in and each SEAL was given an embassy ID card with only our new first names on it. The platoon began eating in the local restaurants so we didn't appear so military. This early on in the war there were very few Americans in Saigon in comparison to what was to come with the buildup. Eating out gave me a chance to begin learning the language. You can't imagine some of the things I got served because of this.

After three very hot and uncomfortable days in my old suit I was beginning to smell more like a bear than a man. One of the CIA fellas took pity and brought me over to his villa and loaned me a pair of pants and a shirt. Dad's badly treated suit went into the trash but I felt like a new man, and even smelled better I'm sure. New clothes were picked up by all several days later and we were ready to begin our new assignment.

The CIA was well established in Vietnam. The agency had shifted their emphasis from the long-running covert war in Laos across the border because of a diplomatic pact which made Laos supposedly neutral. Agency resources even in 1963 were impressive and included Air America, the CIA's private airline. Ordered to Da Nang the platoon was taken to an isolated section of the airstrip where a silver DC-6 with no markings waited. The crew was Chinese and I later learned they had thousands of hours flying these old but reliable aircraft. Once onboard we settled in for the short flight, all the time getting closer and closer to the war.

On the ground in Da Nang I found myself and the platoon being whisked away to what was called the "White Elephant." An old French civic center, the Elephant was the agency's operation and supply center and the largest building in town. It was just across the street from the Han River, which carried waterborne traffic in and around the city.

Our boss turned out to be a former marine who'd lost his left leg during the Korean War. Tucker Gougleman was a professional in the world of clandestine and covert warfare and I grew to respect him immensely. After the war would end, Tucker—living safely in Thailand—would slip back into Vietnam in an attempt to locate his adopted Vietnamese children. Compromised in what used to be called Saigon, Tucker was arrested and sent to a prison camp to be "reeducated." I have since learned Tucker died from all the ailments common to those mistreated in such camps. He is today buried at Arlington, his grave beside that of Francis Gary Powers, the U-2 pilot shot down over Russia.

Combined Studies ran its operations out of a secure compound at My Khe, a tiny village across the Han which occupied a beautiful chunk of oceanfront property. Monkey Mountain towered above the village and I often admired the long stretch of white sand beach which ran from this mountain clear down to Marble Mountain. I never knew until much later that Marble Mountain housed an extensive Vietcong tunnel complex. When I recall all the times I took a jeep and drove to the mountain to buy marble souvenirs for family and friends, I'm amazed at never having run into a VC welcoming party either coming or going. Marble Mountain became a good example of nothing in Vietnam being considered one hundred percent secure from the enemy. In fact, perhaps the only haven between Monkey and Marble mountains was a Catholic orphanage we used to visit now and then.

Settling into what would be our home for the next six months I was introduced to "Big John," our advisor from SEAL Team Two. He must have been using an alias because I've never been able to locate him since the war. Big John became a good friend and outstanding teammate whose personality drew people to him regardless of race or rank. We got on well together once he discovered I was a gunners mate and soon John was telling me about his "special" junks.

Big John's project involved outfitting junks which could travel up along the coast into North Vietnamese waters without drawing attention. They appeared to be simple fishing boats, with their crews playing the part to a *"t."* Always on the lookout for infiltrators and intelligence gathering efforts, the North Vietnamese navy used Chinese supplied SWATOW patrol boats to prowl the waters considered theirs. These PT-style boats were armed with 37mm guns and were near impossible for a simple sailing ship to take on without serious redesign. That was John's department.

The morning after our arrival at My Khe the platoon toured the small South Vietnamese naval base on our side of the river. I took off on my own to find Big John and soon did. He was aboard one of his junks, anchored just off the naval base. I was told to take one of the basket boats and paddle out to where John stood on the junk's deck waiting for me. A basket boat is just that. It is about four feet in diameter and made from bamboo. I discovered it was impossible to paddle the boat in a straight line unless I sculled my paddle in the direction I wanted to go. What a tub!

John and his Vietnamese crew got quite a laugh out of my efforts, the boat going in circles until I figured out how to navigate. A great show at my expense. It took about twenty minutes for me to reach John's junk, and my red face wasn't just from breathing hard. It was from this point on I began learning about junks.

Any boat that a full-grown water buffalo can stand sideways in amidships without touching the gunnel is a junk, pure and simple. Any boat smaller than this is a sampan. The trick is finding a buffalo who will let you take him for a boat ride in order to prove your point. Junks from the north flew red sails, which John was careful to point out to me. All of our junks used such sails as a means of deception. Each was also outfitted with a diesel engine giving them the ability to evade detection or to outrun, if necessary or possible, anyone looking to search or board them.

Belowdecks there was space enough to hide twelve men, or a team. Atop the deckhouse John had employed a row of V-shaped wooden troughs with open-end gutters. The troughs served as a launch platform for a brace of 3.5-inch rockets. These were wired to be fired electrically and covered with grass mats to conceal them from view. If a SWATOW challenged one of our junks at sea, the patrol boat would be allowed to come in close as if the junk's captain were going to allow boarding. At the right moment the junk would fire the rockets into the patrol boat's exposed flank. The rockets were aimed so they would actually skip off the water's surface and impact the patrol boat at its waterline or above. It was a very slick trick.

I began working with John to further improve the junks' ability to defend themselves. Wanting to put a .50 caliber machine gun up high, and a .30 caliber gun forward by the mast, we needed to build gun mounts which couldn't be detected. By fashioning 55-gallon oil drums with their tops and bottoms cut out the problem was solved. Now, how to mount the guns?

Our first efforts used two-inch pipe welded to a large steel plate. This plate was itself a half-inch thick and bolted into the junk's wooden deck. Still, when the .50 was fired, its intense recoil simply jerked the plate up from the deck causing the gun to come crashing down. John discovered if we used a second plate bolted underneath the deck, and a hard rubber pad as a buffer, the foundation with the rubber bumper absorbed the shock and held the gun firm. We tried it and were pleased to discover the arrangement worked.

With mounting and firing figured out to our satisfaction the task of training the crew came into focus. Split second timing was necessary as the Chinese patrol boats would be too close for comfort if someone missed his cue. The junks had high gunnels, high enough for men to hide behind and not be seen from another boat alongside. We concluded after some discussion with our Vietnamese counterparts that once the rockets were fired the crew—armed with submachine guns and hiding—would hose down the SWATOWs' decks until the oil drum covers could be pulled free by their gunners. Our target was the 37mm gun each patrol boat carried, and either the .50 or .30 possessed the firepower to knock this weapon out. Even as such a sea-borne ambush was taking place the junk's engineer would be firing up the diesel engine and backing up toward South Vietnamese waters at full speed astern.

Full speed wasn't that fast . . . but it was faster than full sail.

We trained at night to ensure the security of our operation. Normally I wanted to train after midnight when most everyone was asleep or inside. One night, while waiting for the clock to strike twelve, we beached our junk on a small island. The Vietnamese went right to sleep but I remained awake, staring out at the blackness of the jungle. After a while the tide went out and we were left high and dry . . . and one heck of a target. I stayed on alert at the gunnels in the bow until I noticed the junk's captain had begun waking the crew. He'd looked up at the sky for some time before doing so and I asked John why this was.

"If the Southern Cross has two stars under the horizon we're at low tide," John replied. "If the cross is above the horizon it's high tide." I don't know if this formula works at different times of the year or if it only applies to junks operating in Vietnam but from that night onward I held a great respect for that old junk skipper.

Our training went well for several months, as did operations against the North. When some of the junks failed to return from their missions we became worried. I later learned one junk sailor had showed up in Da Nang after evading being captured by the North Vietnamese after they sunk his boat. He'd reported the North had become angered at losing a SWATOW now and then to our sneaky little red gun-junks. As a response they'd begun sending two patrol boats out in tandem, with one boat standing off in overwatch as the other prepared to board stopped craft. The sailor's crewmates had successfully engaged and sunk the first SWATOW but the second got the upper hand. It sunk our junk with all aboard but for the lone survivor. He'd hid in part of the stern which stayed afloat, swimming ashore and making his way back moving only at night.

Warfare is a game of ever-changing tactics. We realized our project needed something more effective than a junk to continue, especially with the North's revised rules of the game. After submitting our reports to Combined Studies about the new manner of combating our junk navy we were told to expect some help. It would turn out to be the "Nasty," a Norwegian PT boat that became so effective in the Gulf of Tonkin that the North's aggressive response to this new threat would trigger the incident formalizing our war against North Vietnam.

My assignment changed at this point and I became responsible for training Vietnamese commandos. Our troops began arriving from Saigon where they'd been subjected to background checks and little else. Half were sick with TB or the plague. These we loaded right back on the Air America bird and shipped right back to the capital. It took several such personnel inspections before a class large—and healthy—enough to train was formed. The platoon housed them at a small compound at the base of Monkey Mountain.

As I would be responsible for weapons training I asked for some time to visit the armory at our compound at My Khe. The agency assigned two Chinese Nung mercenaries to me as bodyguards. There wasn't anything they didn't know about weapons. The Nungs were a proud race of people whose profession was the profession of arms. They traveled with their families at their sides and were staunch allies of the Americans in Vietnam. Having two of these fierce and loyal warriors with me was as good as having a platoon of anyone else's army, except if it were a platoon of SEALs. The Vietnamese troops didn't like the Nungs, nor did the Nungs cotton to the Viets although they never let on it mattered one way or the other. My Nungs just went about their business which was looking out for me.

When we finally got down to training I used the Nungs as assistant instructors. They taught field stripping and care of the weapons we'd located for our troops. On the rifle range I elected myself range master and we got down to brass tacks. Anyone who has tried teaching Third World country armed forces knows how difficult it can be. Poor nutrition leads to physical weakness and eye problems, both which will detract from accurate shooting. My commando hopefuls were as respectful of firearms and their safe handling as any U.S. troop I ever worked with. However, when it came to hitting the target they were more bad than good. In fact, they were real bad.

We demonstrated marksmanship basics until we couldn't demonstrate anymore. I drew sight pictures in the sand and explained the proper grip and trigger squeeze over and over. Still, they were lucky to even hit the paper once bullets went down range. After two days I was becoming discouraged. Noting my frustration one of my Nungs approached me and said, "Vietnamese no wink." It was only then I realized the commando candidates were trying to shoot with both eyes open. When I tried to get them to close one eye, both would close. Winking was something Americans learned to do at an early age but not these guys.

I divided the commandos into teams of two and had one lie in the sand in the classic rifleman's position. The other sat on his back and held his jungle hat over the shooter's left eye. As we began firing, the teams got used to this procedure and suddenly rounds started striking home! The men continued to practice and sure as shooting, that one eye began closing on its own accord. With time and many, many more trips to the range our commandos became fair shots.

Grenades came next and after the rifle range I was again having my doubts. Grenades, if handled improperly, go off near you and cause all kinds of grief. You don't mess around with them and you can't screw up, even once. The first day I placed a grenade inside a 55-gallon drum and detonated it using an electric blasting cap. I wanted to show the Vietnamese just what one of these explosive little eggs could do. My demonstration went off so well that to a man the recruits didn't want anything to do with grenades. I began all over, this time throwing the grenade. Time and time again I threw grenades to show if done right you couldn't get hurt. No way. The commandos weren't going to even pick one up.

By accident I asked one of my Nungs to throw a grenade as I explained the procedure from the sidelines. That did the trick because by relying on the Nung I put the Viets in a position of losing face. No one enjoys looking the lesser to anyone else, especially if there's an ethnic or culture barrier involved. The Vietnamese displayed an immediate change of heart and grenade training went very well thereafter. I'd learned my lesson too. From that point on I had a Nung demonstrate for any class I gave and few problems ever arose again under these circumstances.

As soon as the commandos were trained for the agency they were taken away and I never saw them again, or heard what it was they were supposed to do . . . or ever did. I'd made some good friends and hoped they fared well in their new assignment.

At the tail end of this program someone had begun

building safe houses on the beach between My Khe and Marble Mountain. Every house was alike: metal siding and roofs, barbed wire around each for security. No one house was positioned close to another, offering a degree of privacy and isolation. When the commandos pulled out I was handed a team of Vietnamese, most of whom had come from the north. These guys were operationally ready, meaning they were well trained to begin with. Quite a welcome surprise when compared to the crew I'd just graduated. The team chief was solely responsible for his men and he ran the unit with an iron hand. When I needed something I always went through the team chief, who was the single point in the chain of command for the unit. I never asked or was told where they'd got their training and experience. But whoever was responsible had done a fine job. These guys were good!

After introductions and administrative matters were addressed I sat down and talked with the chief. My recommendation was that we run some daylight patrols, just to gradually work into a routine. He told me we would begin working at night, right away. By doing so the VC wouldn't see us or become too curious about our activities. So be it. The very next night I found myself on Monkey Mountain, playing the role of the student.

And that became the routine. During the day I was the unchallenged weapons instructor for my team of North Vietnamese hard-core veterans. At night I took my place in the patrol file and kept my mouth shut. The chief acted as his own pointman, breaking trail and searching for any sign of the enemy. What I learned from this old team chief stayed with me throughout the 1960s when I was training my own SEAL platoons as their chief. It became the norm for me to dress in a black uniform much like the VC wore. We all wore black and learned to move silently, like wraiths in the night. The chief never used a compass during our patrols yet everyone knew exactly where we were and where we were headed. Some very bad men to run into if you weren't on their side of the fence.

After a time I was called in for a mission briefing involving my platoon. The brief included excellent aerial photos of the area showing its well-traveled roads and pathways. The target itself was described as a small but very modern North Vietnamese navy base. Roughly twenty buildings made up the compound which was located on a concave-shaped beach. A hill was present on the base's left flank, its elevation just over three hundred meters high. It offered a broad overwatch position of the compound. Combined Studies wanted to know if I believed it possible to hit the base with a 60mm mortar attack, avoiding going out to sea to be recovered by either surface vessel or submarine. My first question was why go after such a target in the first place?

The base, as I was informed, was being used by the North Vietnamese to train frogmen. As such skills were way out of the enemy's league to provide for themselves, a cadre of Russian military experts—probably SPETSNAZ (Russian special forces)—had been brought in. North Vietnamese frogmen were not an asset in the best interest of the South Vietnamese or their U.S. advisors, given what havoc they could wreak and intelligence they could gather if deployed. The agency wanted the base taken down, Russians or no Russians. I could understand that.

The mortar attack plan didn't sit well with me and I told the briefer so. "Let me talk with the platoon and see what we come up with," I offered. With permission given, along with a warning to maintain security during our discussions, I returned to the hootch with not a little bit of excitement running through me.

After much debate and brainstorming we came up with a plan. It seemed feasible to borrow a concept from our junks and apply it to the Russian frogman caper. Using 3.5-inch rockets with chemical firing devices and a launch platform we might be able to fire the rockets directly into the compound from the nearby hilltop . . . and not even be there when the attack actually occurred. I contacted our supply source at the White Elephant and asked for a dozen old PRC-10 radio packboards. These were located right away and we went to work.

The wooden V-shaped troughs used on the junks to hold the rockets were awkward and heavy. It took some time and a great deal of sweat to discover we couldn't mount them on the packboards with any reliability. I did learn the rockets could be fired from inside their hard cardboard shipping tubes, however. Each packboard could hold four rockets in series and these could be fired by a robotic device like we thought. The rockets proved capable of being fired over and over during training without damage to the packboards, which was a big plus during the train-up. As the tubes were black they were invisible at night.

My team of raiders was selected to accomplish the mission. I briefed the agency handler about the new plan, which went something like this.

The team would insert onto North Vietnamese soil using an IBS. This was the standard black rubber raiding boat used by UDT for just such infiltrations. It could hold up to seven raiders and their equipment, which worked out fine given the size of my indig team. The chief would send in scout swimmers to check out the lay of the land as well as to select a landing site. Once ashore, the team would patrol its way to the top of the hill where the chief would position his men, one at a time, ten meters apart until reaching the last man.

Each team member would carry a packboard with four rockets onboard. The base had been sectioned off using the intelligence photos we'd been provided, and each man had an assigned sector at which to aim his rockets. The cardboard caps would be pulled off the front and back of each tube, then stuck into the ground with the packboard/launch platform then rested atop it for elevation. A chemical timer consisting of a glass vial with an acid liquid inside would then be crushed, the acid eating its way toward the actual firing mechanism connected to the rockets. Once the acid did its job the rockets would fire, and the team would be long gone.

The chief would activate his timer first. Then, moving from man to man, he would tap them on the shoulder and they would crush their own vials. As each vial was crushed the firer would fall in behind the chief until the entire team was on its feet and moving back downhill to the landing site. From here, they would paddle quietly back out to sea and await extraction. The way I figured it they would be back home on the beach drinking tea when the rockets went off. We'd loaded each packboard with two high-explosive rounds and two white phosphorus. Such a mix would both

34

blast and burn anything in the surrounding area of impact, the devastation unbelievable.

Our handler liked the plan and gave it the go-ahead. The team chief liked it too and from then on he was working for me.

Before training began in earnest the Swift boat showed up. It had been a long trip for Roy and he was as happy to see us as we were him. Upon arriving at Combined Studies he'd been briefed, given a map and a .25 caliber pistol, and told where to find us. So outfitted, our teammate set sail from Da Nang, his crew less than happy about the whole state of affairs. Along the way the Swift was fired upon twice by the South Vietnamese navy who'd never seen such a boat in their lives. Adams fired back . . . with his .25 auto. He then opened up the big engines and headed out to sea, outrunning anything our allies had in pursuit. I was excited about using the Swift for our upcoming operation and told Roy so. It would give us a huge advantage over the junks and would be a great shakedown cruise for the new vessel. After hearing me out the platoon officer, Lt. (jg) Hawthorne agreed.

We spent the next day aboard the Swift looking for a suitable training site. The bay side of Monkey Mountain was perfect for our needs with a small beach and hill which fit the general description of the target. The chief and I went ashore and conducted a quick recon of the area. The terrain was about right but we still had a lot to do. The two best swimmers on the team became our scouts. Their specific training began right away. Surf training drills needed to be conducted for the others in the raiding party, as well as loading and securing drills with the IBS.

Simple codes using a red lens flashlight were worked out so the swimmer scouts could guide the team onto the beach. Dummy codes were used in training so we wouldn't compromise any portion of the mission due to someone being up late watching. The real code would be given to the team only when they received their mission order.

Rockets were only fired at night. A "hell box" was used so we could control when the munitions actually went off. The chief and his team worked with the glass timers at their safe house on the beach. In a short time everything was ready and the team was more than proficient. The agency received their final briefing and declared the mission a "go." To my knowledge the frogman training program hosted by the North Vietnamese and taught by the Russians came to an abrupt halt shortly thereafter.

All of us were working day and night and I began feeling lousy for no apparent reason. First it was the chills and then I would be burning up with fever. Then I'd be fine again. Without warning the symptoms would start all over and my sleep was plagued with dreams. I'd dream I was falling, wrapped up in my parachute. When I'd awake the bed was drenched with sweat and my sheet would be coiled around me like a sodden cocoon. I was finally taken to the nearby Marine base and their blood tests proved I'd come down with malaria. By the time I was on my feet again the team had carried out their mission against the enemy navy base.

The platoon started making parachute jumps on the weekends and we mostly jumped from C7-A Caribous. These were graceful cargo planes with rear-loading ramps just made for that perfect airborne exit. A Caribou blast was one of the best and Roy Adams served as our jumpmaster. The area on the far side of My Khe around the river was our drop zone and the jumps kept everyone current on jump status and pay. After a while someone got the bright idea we deserved Vietnamese jump wings and the paperwork came down. I really didn't feel much like jumping but it was something to do with my teammates so I did. With time I began feeling better but ever so often the chills and fever returned to haunt me.

After the chief and his team departed I was given another team to replace them. All these teams were very much alike in terms of their level of training and expertise. Like I said, someone had done their job well. I liked the new team chief right away, his ability to speak a little English making my day. Between my poor Vietnamese and his broken English we communicated pretty well. Rocket training was our first class as the method had proved its worth.

Two weeks later I got the word to report to the White Elephant. It sounded as if another mission were in the works. BMC Lloyd Cobb and I left the compound at My Khe and headed for Da Nang by truck. To get to Da Nang proper we'd have to leave the truck on our side of the Han River. A small boat would pick us up and deliver us to our destination in town. The agency employed an old Vietnamese man whom we called "Pop." Pop was always on the river waiting to transport us, day or night. The old man didn't speak any English but he understood his name. We tried to speak Vietnamese around him so he wouldn't feel too uncomfortable. Pop smiled a lot when we were onboard and I almost believe it was because our Vietnamese was so bad.

At the White Elephant Cobb and I were given intelligence pictures to study. This was how most missions began, a handful of photos introduced us to the proposed target area. This time it was a large fuel farm they wanted us to hit. Part of the farm was underground which made things somewhat more difficult. Huge round tanks managed most of the fuel, a moat dug around each tank for security. In addition, the tops of the tanks actually floated on the fuel and went up or down depending on the level of the tank's contents.

Cobb and I believed a high-explosive round would only punch a hole in the side of such a tank. This would damage the tank, but its fuel supply would simply run out and fill up the moat. We wanted to destroy the tank along with the fuel, and if enough tanks went up the entire farm would be put out of business. The trick was in how to pull it off.

I reasoned if we had an HE round with a magnesium head riding piggyback, the HE would puncture the tank with the magnesium head falling to the ground upon impact. When the piggybacked warhead ignited it would in turn ignite the fuel now rushing out of the tank and we'd have one fine fire on our hands. White phosphorus was considered but we discovered it would actually burn out, or be put out, by the sudden onslaught of fuel which would overpower its tiny flame.

It was also learned we'd need a primer on the magnesium warhead to prevent it from exploding too soon. There had to be some fuel on the ground to get things going so a premature burn wasn't in our best interests. "No problem," we were told. The agency would have them made up over on Okinawa at the secret spook laboratory they ran in support of our war effort.

The Army Counterinsurgency Support Office (CISO) was

formed to take over the agency's logistic support needs by sharing the Army's ability to handle such things with the 1st Special Forces Group, whose operators had been in-country since 1956. Under Project Parasol-Switchback, the program was given the highest priority possible. Anything we needed CISO could get or make. The founder of CISO was a young SF captain by the name of David E. Watts. He would retire a major general and to him goes a great deal of credit for CISO's effectiveness.

Heading back to our compound Cobb and I went over the training problems we could see right off the bat. Chief Cobb was concerned about the weight of the new magnesium warheads and how this might affect a rocket's range. Cobb was one of the finest chiefs I ever had and he was a great influence on me in the most positive sense. The chief had served with UDT 12 and was one of the legendary "Scouts and Raiders" in China during WWII. I've never respected a man more than Chief Cobb. We signaled for Pop and headed across the Han to where our truck was. Training would begin right away.

By now our six-month tour was nearly up. As the new warheads were being worked up at CISO we put the team on the rockets, knowing we'd need only a bit of adjustment once the agency delivered the goods. This team was even better than my first at their jobs. Once again it looked like I'd miss out on the fun of taking the boys in and seeing them do their stuff. All I could do was my best, knowing their lives and the success of the mission lay in our platoon's hands.

Everyone had teams of their own with different missions to train for. The North Vietnamese were getting zapped fairly frequently thanks to us, perhaps payback for all the trouble they were causing the South Vietnamese from their illegal bases in Laos and Cambodia. All is fair in love and war, they say.

Roy Adams now became responsible for training Vietnamese skippers and crews on the Swift boat. He was pulling his hair out trying to keep up with everyone's demands for boat training and support. Some of my teammates were working with support teams needed up north, others were training harassment teams like our own. Infiltration by sea was the most secure and easiest to conduct so Roy was constantly at the helm of the Swift. These missions and teams would continue as a project throughout the 1960s, their effect on the war effort merely a shadow in the classified files maintained somewhere very far away. By the time President Johnson sent in the Marines, I and my platoon had become pioneers at fighting the North Vietnamese as clandestine warriors.

Our time was up and I was headed back to the States to see my family. The fuel farm mission would be completed by our replacement platoon, all good men. I was ready to go home. But in doing so I was returning a far better SEAL than when I'd arrived. So much had been learned about the kind of war I knew we SEALs would be asked to conduct against a very tough and determined enemy. When SEAL Team One was first commissioned we plank owners wondered what it was SEALs would do . . .

I now knew. And I was determined to become the best operator I could possibly be so as to accomplish the mission entrusted to us. More importantly, I knew deep inside only the best would be acceptable to my teammates.

4

SEATO Operation

Our platoon returned home from Vietnam to SEAL Team One in Coronado, California. It was good to be with my family again and my wife was due to have our third child in October. In the teams I was assigned to the armory for the rest of the year. My wife had a baby boy on October 13, and we were thankful I'd been able to be home for that blessed event.

In early 1964 orders came down sending me to Foreign Weapons and Special Demolition school at Fort Bragg, North Carolina. It was an excellent school with many of the weapons systems I'd worked with in Vietnam present. There is always more to learn, but it was the teaching techniques of the Army's "Green Berets" which really benefited me for years to come as a SEAL.

While at Bragg I met new and old friends both from the Army and Vietnam. One night in the NCO club I enjoyed a dinner with M. Sgt. Antonio Duarte who'd been the senior NCO instructor for the parachute course on Okinawa. We talked quite a bit about our experiences in Vietnam, and I reminded him he'd been the one to tap me out the door of a C-130 in 1961 during my attendance at jump school. It was a pleasant evening which passed all too quickly.

Upon my return to Coronado we began training as a combat action platoon, or CAP. After two intensive months in California the platoon received orders to participate in a SEATO training exercise in the Philippines. The orders read "On or about 19 March 1964, you will proceed and report to Director, Exercise AUMEE III for further assignment." We were further authorized to make parachute jumps from both military and FOREIGN/FLAG aircraft.

Subic Bay was the home of the West Coast UDT teams and we were looking forward to visiting with our teammates there. During one of the several briefings which occurred after our arrival I learned we'd be making a parachute jump from a French aircraft called a NORD. We linked up with its crew and began preparing the plane for the operation, which would also include a Filipino UDT platoon as well as its jumpmaster. So now we were jumping from a French plane with its French crew, with a Filipino jumpmaster putting us and his own platoon out the door for a combined exercise. And I thought I'd had language problems in Vietnam! It was a short flight to the drop zone and everyone got out the door without a problem. The Filipinos had their personnel on the ground ready to receive us, including providing medical care . . . which thankfully wasn't necessary.

Soon afterward the platoon was briefed concerning a second jump, or parachute infiltration. The command wanted to jump us into the mountains on Mindoro Island, and from there we'd be tasked to conduct a reconnaissance mission against a large aggressor force without being detected. Our Marines were tasked to act as the enemy, a chore I'm sure they appreciated. The platoon was assigned a Filipino UDT senior NCO as our interpreter thereby sorting out the language problem. It is standard operating procedure today for platoons to receive at least fundamental language training before they conduct a mission in foreign territory, with attachments such as qualified interpreters likewise SOP if they are available. This is an evolution of the challenges we faced working in Southeast Asia with numerous different ethnic groups and nationalities both in wartime and peace.

As it was the Year of the Tiger the platoon was given a

number of formal certificates with a tiger depicted on its face. The certificate thanked whomever we might run into for cooperating with us during the exercise while explaining we were the "good guys" and that we needed their support. People are funny in this way. If you can give them a patch, or an emblem, or a fancy looking piece of paper they can hang on the wall it goes a long way in enlisting their help and empathy for your cause. We would present such certificates as the need arose, sometimes in a formal ceremony and other times upon immediate contact with the locals.

Every SEAL in the platoon checked his gear and weapons prior to being briefed on the patrol order. I and the others then grabbed some sleep before the jump, wanting as much rest as possible prior to what I knew would be a tough infiltration and patrol. Awakened some time later we were transported to the NORD again, but this time we found a different crew waiting for us. I recall the crew chief was a woman, and no one onboard spoke English. As none of us spoke French the best we could do was point out Julie Drop Zone on the Mindoro Island map, which the crew indicated they had been briefed on by pointing to a circle drawn around it on their own chart. The crew chief made sure we were strapped in before taking off and I could only assume the crew knew what it was doing despite not one word of real communication between us. Soon afterward, we were airborne and enroute to the DZ.

When I heard the sharp sound of the warning buzzer come on I stood up with the rest of the platoon and began preparing for the night's jump. We hooked up to the steel cable meant to stablize our static lines so the 'chutes would open once we left the aircraft, and conducted our equipment checks as trained to do by Special Forces. We were fully loaded down to include personal weapons, and maintaining our balance as the NORD lined itself up for the final run over the drop zone was difficult. Each SEAL was packed tight up against his teammate's parachute pack tray so we could all get out the door on the first pass. Once the line started moving there would be no stopping us until the last man in the platoon was airborne and under canopy.

Our jumpmaster was leaning out the open door searching,

I knew, for the island. Once spotted, he would then begin trying to line up the aircraft on the DZ which would be marked in some fashion so as to be seen from the air. The wind was whipping past him and the roar coming from both the plane's engines and the turbulence outside was deafening. Apparently the pilots had already spotted the drop zone as the red light on the door frame went from red to green, which meant we had to go and go right then. Even as I exited the aircraft in as tight a body position as possible I knew the NORD was flying at a higher speed than we normally jumped at. The force of the slipstream jerked me near parallel to the ground far below despite the combined weight of myself and my equipment. The opening shock transmitted from the blossoming parachute canopy down through the shroud lines and parachute harness was the worst I'd ever experienced. It was brutal. I absorbed the bone snapping force of the canopy exploding overhead up through the leg straps and around my shoulders with what I'm sure was an audible grunt even at altitude. The force of the opening shock took me by surprise . . . and it hurt too. Each of us was carrying a .45 caliber submachine gun which was secured to the "D" rings underneath our reserve parachutes with an eighty-pound test line. When my chute ripped itself open the force was so great that it snapped the test line, sending my subgun flying into the darkness of Mindoro Island. As it left me the weapon smashed off the tops of my boots, adding more pain to what I'd already endured.

The platoon landed safely despite the terrible drop speed but now I was a gunners mate on an exercise with no gun. After figure-eight rolling my 'chute and stuffing it into its kit bag I checked in with the drop zone medical crew to let them know I was all right. To my great relief (and surprise) one of the medics handed me my grease gun! As I had jumped in the center of the stick, the weapon had fallen onto the drop zone instead of into the surrounding jungle, nearly hitting one of the safety crew waiting for us on the ground. Beside the wire telescoping stock being bent into the pistol grip the weapon was fine. I pulled and tugged the stock back to true, and was once again a gunners mate fully armed and ready to continue the mission. I don't know that an M16 would have fared as well under the same circumstances as that old but finely built "grease gun."

Our Filipino NCO took off for a short time, returning with a man who owned a water buffalo. We gave him a certificate and he was tickled to death to help us. The buffalo was loaded with our heavier equipment and supplies and we headed down a trail off the mountain for a cave near the beach. The local had informed our interpreter about the cave's existence so we decided to use it as a command post for the exercise. It was an easy hike and soon we were once again on the ocean. The equipment was cached near the cave, with security put out just in case the Marines got lucky and stumbled across us.

The next morning small patrols were sent out to check the area for enemy activity and to get a lay of the land. We moved our equipment to a different cache point, one farther from the cave and more hidden. If compromised, we didn't want to lose the gear for having it too close to home. Our radio operator made contact with the base and we checked in every day at different times using different codes. Early in the evening the patrol order was given for the night's first recon operation. Per SOP every SEAL checked his equipment and weapons, then got what sleep he could before going out. This procedure was important to me as I knew firsthand how critical such preparations were prior to going into combat. Every little thing counted, from how your magazines were loaded to the fit of your patrol harness. Plus, every man had to be ready and alert, as well as aware of what was expected of him during the mission. I learned early on not to tolerate any chance of preventable error and worked hard with my platoons to ensure only the best performance from myself and those whose lives I was entrusted with.

We moved out in the darkness and throughout the night patrolled with no contact being made with the enemy force. At daylight the platoon located a small farmhouse in a tiny cleared area of the jungle. A watch was put on the house for some time and after we felt it safe the interpreter was sent in. He returned a short time later, informing us that the farmer living there had invited us to share a meal with him and his family. Not wanting to offend the man we accepted despite the risk of being spotted should the Marines have a patrol of their own out. Naturally, security was put in place for just such an event.

The house was built of wood planks with a tin roof providing cover from the sun and elements. Two very unhappy dogs raced out to greet us but at a word from their owner they slinked under the flooring to ruminate about our invasion of their turf. A long table was the centerpiece of what furniture was available, and it was covered with a beautiful tablecloth. The farmer introduced us to his wife and two daughters, both whom he proudly announced had attended college in the United States. We sat down to a meal of rice and meat, washed down with cold coconut milk. The family told us they had not seen any military activity at our end of the island, and once the meal was over we presented the farmer with a Tiger certificate which he proudly hung on his wall. Saying good-bye we patrolled back to the cave, electing to conduct a nighttime patrol of the beach later on in case the Marines landed looking for some action.

While on patrol that night we ran into heavy jungle which forced us to swim out into the ocean and around the obstacle before we could continue searching the beach. Soon after the refreshing dip and once again back on dry land, the patrol spotted a tiny flickering light coming from a house built high over the water. Investigating, we discovered an old fisherman who gladly invited us to stay and eat some of his catch of the day. During the meal he told us of "a big Navy boat" which had dropped men and trucks off on a small island about a mile from Mindoro. We also learned of a small village on a river some distance from our present location. I was beginning to appreciate the immense importance of information which could be gathered from the local population by our patrols. By treating them, their property, and customs with respect and announcing our intentions as honorable, much was learned which saved hours of often fruitless patrolling. We were always cautious and never accepted anything at face value, but intelligence gathered in this manner often led to successful combat ops later on down the road.

With the information about a possible enemy base off-shore we decided to move our area of operations farther down the island. The cache of equipment was dug up and a new place was found to live in relative security. Once the move was completed two of the men were selected to act as swimmer scouts. Their mission was to swim from Mindoro to the tiny island the fisherman had described, and to locate and identify what enemy might be present. Poncho rafts were constructed by stuffing green foliage and bush in between the ponchos much like those rafts I'd learned to make while attending Army Ranger School in 1962. The scouts would fasten their recon gear and weapons atop the tiny rafts and would infiltrate the island by sea. They waited until it was very dark before entering the surf zone, and soon I lost sight of them as the night and sea swallowed them whole.

Watch was set up on the beach that night and continued all the next day. Waiting for the scouts to come back with their report was hard and required great patience. We didn't know what they might have run into just making the swim, or what may have happened once they actually got ashore in "enemy" territory. It wasn't until nearly 2200 hours the next night when we saw their signal on the beach, indicating they'd returned from a successful swim and recon. Gathering the scouts up we congratulated them and then went into a hurried huddle. The Marines, the scouts reported, had set up their camp just below the military crest of the seaward side of the island. They appeared to be at company strength with light weapons, two trucks, and one jeep. It was our firsthard information of the exercise and we'd gathered it without being detected.

The next night we requested that the old fisherman guide us to the village he'd described by the river. It took most of the night to make this movement, primarily because we took all of our equipment with us. After setting in a secure cache point we observed the village itself until daylight. Early in the morning we sent a small team in to make contact with the people, a certificate changing hands with the fisherman who was then allowed to return to his home.

Our interpreter interviewed the village's inhabitants and explained what we were doing in their backyard. We asked for their help and they were eager to give it. The school-house became our forward operating base as the people told us there were no Marines on Mindoro Island at all! In the evening we set up our security around the schoolhouse and went to sleep. All of us were beat and needing of a good night's rest.

It was around midnight when I woke up to the loudest, most blood-curdling scream I'd ever heard. Lt. (jg) Fox had been bitten on the neck by the largest centipede most of us had seen. Its poison was being injected into the young officer through fangs deeply embedded in the meat of his neck and we literally had to pull the creature out of him to remove it. The centipede was just over six-inches long and a half-inch thick! Our Filipino UDT convinced everyone (except for maybe Lt. Fox) that he would be all right by morning. However, he did have us put salt around where each of us was sleeping to keep other centipedes away. I used more salt that night in putting up my anticentipede perimeter than I'd used on my food for the whole year prior. Sure enough, the next morning Mr. Fox was fit as a fiddle except for a sore neck and very little sleep.

We borrowed four sampans from the village, loaded our equipment, and moved down the small river to our pickup point on the sea. By now our platoon had established the lay of the land, located the enemy, made friends with the local population, and acquired our own little navy of sorts. It was shaping up to be a fine operation and I was learning more each day about operating both as a participant and a leader. Upon reaching the sea the call went out for pickup and soon a Navy PBM aircraft was circling overhead. We'd moved to the leeward side of the island and far enough out in the water to where the plane could spot us easily.

Once it had landed on its pontoons the crew began frantically waving for us to get aboard. Our sampan docking techniques were not yet perfected and we had a time of it trying to get the small boats positioned in such a way as to actually load the plane. Finally, the procedure was completed and as soon as the last SEAL was onboard the big plane began moving. We figured out what all the hubbub was about once inside. The PBM was in some need of repair as the water flooding in from the sea through numerous leaks in the flooring told us. I watched in horror as the crew began pulling up deck plates to check the water level! As the plane picked up speed the water began to run out of it, continuing to shower down on the ocean even after we'd become airborne. It was all in a day's work for Naval Air, but for this Navy SEAL it was something very new.

The platoon was exhausted but feeling elated after the operation. Command voiced its accolades on how we'd performed and I was to discover later the most important thing we'd done was to gather timely and accurate information. We'd performed as a Combat Action Platoon in such a way that it would become the format for conduct of operations in Vietnam in the years to come. This was where training and realistic training exercises paid off. We'd operated in a foreign environment successfully using our military skills and assigned assets to see the mission accomplished. I would review every little thing I could remember, and ask questions of my teammates about what they had observed, for some time afterward. Being a SEAL is a learning process that never stops. In Vietnam, intelligence and proper action would save lives and win battles. I wanted to learn all I could to accomplish those two goals.

Mr. Fox reported to sick bay and was declared to be in good health. We cleaned up and sat down to a good meal. For the first time since arriving we had the time to relax and enjoy the sights and sounds of Subic Bay. But we hadn't heard the last of AUMEE III.

Several mornings later the word came down for the platoon to report at quarters for submarine operations. Chief Cobb took charge and work began. He directed that two seven-man IBS rubber boats with four extra boat bottoms be checked out. In addition, the chief wanted two silent-running, seven-and-one-half-horsepower outboard engines from the UDT compound. We would use two of the spare bottoms to reinforce each of the IBS bottoms. From the other two we cut a foot of the bow end off. These then became large rubber bags with an air pump connection. Inside of each was placed an engine, its gas tank, and a handheld infrared sender/receiver unit. The open end of the improvised "sandwich Baggies" were then accordion folded and held shut with a diver's dry suit clamp.

To remove the air trapped inside we reversed the hand pump hose and sucked the air out, creating a vacuum around the stored equipment. A test was run on each bag with its contents to ensure everything stayed watertight. Towing bridles were attached to the "D" rings on the bow of the IBSs and outboard transom to the stern, and the boats were now ready. CO_2 bottles and lanyards were secured in place to inflate the IBSs when necessary. Platoon members not so engaged with the rubber boats were preparing lines and rigging for the submarine operation. Finally, we declared ourselves ready.

Quarters was held on the bow of the USS *Perch* (APSS313). Chief Cobb gave us a lecture on how our conduct was to be aboard the vessel. We were guests, he reminded us, and we were to remember that the sub was home for its crew. All respect and protocol was to be in effect as if on any other Navy ship. Of course, being the good chief he was Cobb made sure his speech was made within earshot of members of the ship's company. That way word would travel that we were here to work with them in their environment. The war bags were stowed, containing each SEAL's personal effects, weapons, fins/mask, and any other thing he might feel necessary to have along. Dive gear was stowed in the forward room with the war bags, which became our base of operations. The sub's captain passed the word that as soon as the SEALs were below decks the submarine would be underway. We secured the IBS and rubber storage bags in the sail, or the super structure above the main deck of the submarine, and went below.

Once at sea the platoon was told the submarine would be undergoing its annual test dive. It would go to its maximum depth and, among other things, check for leaks. Upon hearing this I couldn't help but remember the leaky PBM we'd flown off Mindoro in just days before. Leaks on a sub at max depth would be far different than on an old seagoing PBM. For one thing, the water would be rushing in and not out regardless of our position! SEALs were to stay in their bunks and out of the crew's way during the test. They went to general quarters and the next hour was very busy indeed. The boat dove at an angle which gave no doubt as to the seriousness of the exercise. The depth was called out as she dove, with each station reporting what was happening at intervals. I found it exciting to witness the test from an observer's point of view. These submariners certainly knew what they were doing.

Later in the afternoon we surfaced and began to rig the boat for SEAL underwater ops. It took an hour and every man was busy. We secured the two IBSs to the aft deck behind the sail, putting the equipment bags in them. These were checked once more for vacuum. The towing bridles were hooked to a towing line secured to a collar around the sub's periscope. The lines that secured the IBSs to the deck were tied with a quick release bowline so that one SEAL could hold the CO2 lanyard and release an IBS at the same time. The IBS would inflate as it was pulled to the surface by the towline. Another line was run from the collar forward to the ladder leading to the submarine escape trunk. This trunk was meant to be used in aiding surface ships in rescuing a submarine's crew. Two diving tanks were secured under the deck beside the trunk. Chief Cobb supervised the rigging and checked every knot used. We were finally declared to be ready and went below. The sub dove, its course set for Mindoro Island.

A platoon briefing was held with all of us dressed in our camouflage fatigues, with weapons and ammo. Fins and masks were also present. Once the concept of the operation was laid out and understood in fine detail we prepared the rest of our equipment and made ready. With the sub on station the platoon moved to the trunk, which was entered from an overhead hatch in the forward troop quarters. Once in the trunk, the bottom hatch was shut and dogged secure leaving two SEALs in very tight quarters at a time. To move, you would voice each command so the other man would be able to accommodate you as best he could. For many, working in the trunk was not a very pleasant experience.

To flood the trunk a command was given to un-dog, or unlatch the side door. Each command from this one onward would be repeated so there could be no misunderstanding what was taking place. Then the VENT valve was opened, followed by the FLOOD valve to let seawater in. The water was always cold. And it got colder the higher it rose on your legs. As the water came up to the top lip of the side door you closed the VENT valve, watching as more water continued to flow in for about two more inches. Then the FLOOD valve was closed and you would just crack the valve marked BLOW. This would increase the pressure to crack the seal on the side door so you and your teammate could exit the sub. Once the door was opened the divers would report "Divers Out," and the trunk operator would drain the trunk and stand by for the next two divers to enter.

Draining the trunk was accomplished by the trunk operator. He would first shut the door and then secure it. Then both the DRAIN and BLOW valves would be opened. This would force the water down and out of the trunk. It also caused the trunk to fog up, for some reason. When all the water was clear of the trunk the operator would close the DRAIN and close the BLOW valves, next opening the VENT valve. Air would now vent into the boat and the operator would have to remember to exhale as the pressure decreased around him. Then the operator would report being clear of the bottom hatch which would then be opened from inside the forward room. The next pair of SEALs would be standing by waiting their turn in the trunk. Should the trunk operator ever make a mistake in this procedure a member of the ship's company could override the process by operating the trunk from the forward room.

As our first two SEALs left the trunk they set about turning on the air in the two sets of dive tanks prestaged by Chief Cobb for their use. Breathing from the mouthpiece, even as they were putting the tanks on, the men geared up at sea for what was to follow. Moving along and up the ladder the divers pulled themselves along the deck toward the stern where the IBSs were. When in place they signaled each other, releasing the tie-down lines while pulling the CO_2 lanyards at the same time. The current quickly snatched the IBSs from the deck, pulling them away from the sub even as they were inflating underwater. Moving back forward to the trunk the SEALs secured their dive tanks and began ascending the towline up toward the surface. By now, two more SEALs were out of the trunk and following right behind their teammates. Once on the surface the two pair of divers would right the IBSs and begin rigging the outboard engines on the transoms, getting these started.

Soon, all the platoon had left the sub and were secured in

their assigned IBSs. The infrared signal lights were pulled from the bags even as the sub was towing us to our prearranged dropoff point near the island. The submarine's captain would use an infrared light through his periscope to signal when he was about to release us, which we would answer with a signal of our own. Then the towing bridals would be released from the towing line and a platoon of SEALs were inbound, armed and ready.

Using a compass to guide us the two small rubber boats headed toward the infiltration point. Roughly two hundred meters off the beach the scout swimmers went over the side to pull a quick recon. The rest of us lay as low as possible in the bobbing boats while they did their work. When the proper infrared signal was received we headed in. The scouts brought us in at a point where the boats bottomed out on the rocks about fifty meters from the shoreline. Stepping out of the IBSs our feet found a solid but rocky bottom which was covered with sea urchins. Everyone was wearing coral booties which are very much like tennis shoes in construction and design. It made for difficult walking as we dragged the IBSs in with all our gear, each step a possible puncture wound as the sea urchins' spines could easily penetrate our footgear.

Finally on the sand we rapidly pulled the boats into the dark safety of the treeline. An odd noise came from one of the men and we found Dale McCleskey out like a light underneath a large palm tree. A big, burly coconut lay beside his head where it had landed after striking him soundly as he sought cover under the tree. When we brought Dale around he couldn't remember what had happened, or believe what had hit him. There was a large knot on his head, though, and he must have suffered some kind of headache afterward. I learned not to trust coconut trees after this incident.

Our mission was to pick up two downed pilots and take them out to sea for pickup by the submarine. Assisting Naval Air in the off-shore continuation of escape and evasion networks was even then a SEAL task, and it remains so today. We found the two "pilots" and learned they were in fact SERE instructors from the school at North Island Naval Air Station in Coronado, California. As

SEALs we'd attended this school on survival, evasion, resistance, and escape, doing time in the mock POW compound they'd set up for "realistic training." I and the others began telling our two charges about how we planned to lock into the submarine, wondering aloud if they'd be able to hold their breaths underwater for sixty-some feet and then get back into the trunk. It was payback time for all the crap they and their fellow SERE instructors had subjected us to at North Island, and believe me, they were beginning to get scared.

The submarine came straight up out of the sea once we'd established our bona fides using infrared. We boarded, secured our equipment to the deck, and went below with our two new friends. I've never seen two guys happier at the turn of events than these two when they realized we'd only been joshing with them about the trunk. Back at Subic Bay everyone began working on his feet, which had been punctured or pricked by sea urchin spines during and after the infil. Some were festering while other wounds were easily treated. One variety of sea urchin found in those waters is poisonous but we had no way of knowing which variety we'd stepped on. Since no one died it was assumed we'd hit the nonlethal type. Dale was pronounced good as new except for the sizable knot where the enemy coconut had dinged him. Again, the platoon had pulled off a great training mission with many lessons learned which we would apply later in Vietnam.

For four months we'd been training together under realistic conditions. Concepts and skills learned from attending Army and Marine schools were tried, tested, adapted, and incorporated into our SOPs. We were heading back to the States having moved yet one more step forward in our evolution as a CAP. I was proud of myself and proud of the men. We were a team in every respect of the term with no one individual standing off by himself when work needed to be accomplished.

It was good to be a SEAL.

5

"HOOYAHH!"

*Speak softly and carry a big stick; you will go far. If the
American nation will speak softly and yet build and
keep at a pitch of the highest training a thoroughly
efficient Navy, the Monroe Doctrine will go far.*

—Theodore Roosevelt, September 1901

At the beginning of the new year in 1965 I was facing yet
another crossroad in my life. I was a plankowner in SEAL
Team One, meaning I was one of the original handful of
SEALs to activate the team when it was commissioned. I'd
made two overseas tours with One and spent most of my
time when in the States attending various Army and Marine
schools which I'd never even heard of before becoming a
SEAL. Still, there was something lacking in my professional
life. I finally determined what it was. I wanted to be an
instructor in UDT Training, or "BUDS" as it is now called.
There were no other men in my book who were as tall or
drew as much respect as a UDT instructor. So, I reenlisted
for UDT Training at the Naval Amphibious Training Command (NAVPHIBSCOL) in Coronado, California.

When I reported aboard I felt the heady satisfaction of
being a frogman once again. Some of the men had been my
instructors in 1960. There was Dick Allen, the "Fighting
Frogman," All-Navy boxer whom I had trained with while
we were on the Navy Amphibious Boxing Team when I was
assigned to UDT 12. Bud Jurick was still there, and it would
be he more than anyone who would teach me how to be the
proper instructor. Kevin Murphy, who knew more about

being underwater than most of us knew about being on land, was now a peer. And last but not least was Chief Price, the leading CPO who was the best coordinator I've ever served with. Would I ever be as good as these men, I asked myself? At the time I certainly thought not.

As a gunners mate I drew classes on weapons and demolition. Lesson plans were required and I soon realized I needed to know more about the subject and how to present it than I'd ever imagined. The library became a regular place to find me as I worked at rewriting these in order to accomplish the training objective. Everything had to be done within strict time constraints. My classes had to start on time and end on time. I was studying the manuals more than ever before so I could answer the students questions . . . on time. Just knowing about military explosives wasn't enough anymore. I needed to know their exact composition and understand how each worked down to the final second. Weapons were my strong point and didn't require the amount of study that demolitions did. One very important phase of instructor training occurred when we were allowed to sit in on an instructor's class before being required to teach it ourselves. Bud Jurick taught the classes I was soon to be responsible for, and I made it a point to also sit in on his land warfare classes so we could overlap as coinstructors. Often times Bud would sit in the back of the class with me after a session was over, taking extra time and being extra patient. His critiques were classes in themselves and I owe him a debt for such attention.

Still a young man, I wanted to be the tough guy and do all the things to the students, or "tadpoles" as they're called to this day, that I could remember being done to me when I went through training. When we received our first class I was ready for them. If it was to my liking I would drop a man for fifty push-ups in the blink of an eye. All instructors were involved with the class and its various training evolutions outside of the classroom and I enjoyed every minute of it. One of the older instructors was always present to keep us younger pups from getting out of line or going too far, so I didn't make life too unbearable for my charges.

The first month was devoted to physical conditioning, UDT style. Each morning the class would fall out and double-time to the ball field. They would be yelling "HOOYAHH!" at the tops of their lungs, the battle cry and byword of the frogman and SEAL. We would have them form a circle around Dick Allen and after each exercise they would be given a "right face, left face, on your stomach, on your back, on your feet, right face, double-time march, halt, left face, next exercise" and so on. This type of PT went on for nearly an hour. While Dick was making the men stronger we would be prowling the outside of the circle watching for anyone who was corking off.

When a tadpole gave up on an exercise he would be told to begin doing push-ups or SCUBA flutter kicks until the next exercise began. If giving up became a habit we would send the man into the San Diego Bay at a run where he would complete the exercises dripping wet. There were some instructors who demanded more from the men than others and whenever the tadpoles would be double-timed around in a circle they hated being stopped in front of such an instructor. We would do the exercises with the students, but we never took our eyes off them while doing so. It reinforced the team concept and told the tadpoles we wouldn't ask them to do anything we couldn't . . . or wouldn't . . . or hadn't ourselves. With PT over we'd run them back to the barracks where they'd prepare for the next evolution in training.

Back at the ranch they were allowed no more than five minutes to change into dry uniforms. Then the students had to fall out with their assigned IBS, boat paddles, helmets, and life jackets. They were given sheets with song lyrics on them to learn, and they would fall into ranks singing until an instructor came out to take them to the mess hall for breakfast. It was not at all uncommon for an instructor not yet finished with his morning coffee to yell out the office window that he couldn't hear the class singing, even though they'd be doing so at the tops of their voices mere feet away. Down they would go in the front leaning rest—or push-up—position until said instructor came out to retrieve them. When ordered to recover, or come to their feet, the class would do so with an earsplitting HOOYAHH! It was as much a morale builder as an act of unified, acceptable defiance in the face of our intentional harassment. Boat paddles would be secured in the IBSs and the boats would be carried to the mess hall. For four long weeks the tadpoles carried their IBSs wherever they went, and always at a double time.

After a satisfying Navy meal the students would follow— at a run—their instructor to the beach and the obstacle course. The Silver Strand hosts a most remarkable "O" course which was built by the training unit. It features rope climbs, parallel bars, monkey bars, barbed wire, sand crawls, tower climbs, and more. The goal is to run the obstacle course successfully in better and better times. Many a meal has ended up in the sand trying to do so. Afterward, the class would pick up its IBSs and move to the log PT area at a horizontal ledge partway up the slope of the beach called the Ocean Berm.

Log PT is done by seven-man boat crews. The logs are old power poles which have been soaked in saltwater from the efforts of many a tadpole in years gone by. At the command of "stand by your logs" we would hear the ever-present HOOYAHH! as the tadpoles broke ranks to rush to their assigned power pole. The commands for the exercise were "right ankle log, right hip log, right shoulder log, and overhead log." These were repeated for the left side. If and always, when a log hit the sand, Instructor Vince Olivera would have that log's crew hit the surf with their log to wash it off. Naturally the crew would get some unexpected relief from the sand that was driving them crazy from where they'd picked it up at the obstacle course . . . but not for long. After rejoining the class the command "right hip log" would be given. The crew in question would receive an additional command of "on your cans." In the sitting position with the now clean log in their laps they would do sit-ups in cadence, rolling the log up onto their chests each time they went back down. In this position they would be ordered to press the log as a team. So much for getting over on the instructors.

All wet and sandy the class was now ready for IBS surf drill.

The morning's lead instructor would have the boat crews stand by their IBSs on the berm, all the while giving them the instructions for what was to come next. His eyes would rove the surf as he spoke, patience rewarded as the highest possible series of waves would be coming in when he released the tadpoles. "Hit the surf!" the instructor would yell, the students sounding off with the SEAL battle cry as they grabbed and tugged at their IBSs, paddles in hand.

Running through the hard sand, coxswains began ordering the men into their assigned boats by number. He would be at the stern pushing the boat into the surf passage even as his crew was digging their paddles into the water, furiously trying to help bring the IBS to bear. The coxswain would then jump in, and if the passage was timed right and everyone was working as a team, the IBS would bust through the foaming waters and be outside the surf zone's control. Success is short-lived as the order comes to "dump boat!"

All paddles are now passed to the coxswain and with these in hand he slips into the sea, holding on to the stern line. Two men rig the bowline along one side of the IBS to a "D" ring on the stern. This is where the rest of the team will reenter the boat. Now, two tadpoles stand on the opposite main tube of the inflatable boat and pull hard on the rigged bowline. The IBS gracefully flips up and over, landing upside down in the water. Two more students already in the water hang onto the spray tube and kick hard so they roll up onto the boat's bottom as it is turning over. Now the roll is repeated so the boat is put right side up with the first two men coming back into the IBS. Frantically they pull their teammates in, only to repeat the drill over and over as the boats are ordered in, then back out into the pounding surf. For over an hour the exercise continues, with paddling the boats around given as a brief but welcome respite from the capsizing drills.

Surf drills completed it would be time for the morning run. . . .

Tired, wet, chilled, and numb students secure their life jackets, helmets, and uniform shirts to their IBSs and fall into ranks behind an instructor who most often was an officer. Upon command he would begin jogging on the hard sand, warming up for the long run down the beach. Other instructors like myself would run alongside the formation giving encouragement to the class. As it began to spread out, the leader would circle around to pick up the slower runners and stragglers, which only stretched the formation out that much more. Now the stronger runners, having to run twice as far as their slower brethren, would begin giving their own version of "encouragement." Our runs would begin at two miles, growing to four in the weeks to come. Sometimes I would form up the slower runners and take them into the soft sand dunes south of the Del Coronado Hotel. I would run them up the dunes and then down, and then back up again. Some would feel I was harassing them but after a few sessions in the soft sand they found their legs getting stronger and their wind capacity becoming greater. Soon "Enoch's Mountain" became a challenge rather than a penalty. The men would push themselves to see how fast they could climb to its top and how much faster they could run down to the base. It was a motivator and I often saw my "class" of runners dwindle as they rejoined the formation in perfect step.

The run completed it was time to return to the UDT Training Unit. With IBSs on their heads the class would double-time back to wash their equipment out in plenty of fresh water. They'd leave them hanging on the dry racks, changing into clean uniforms and falling in for noon chow. We'd head for the mess hall at a double time, of course! After the meal the tadpoles reported to the classroom for an hour of related training and then it was into swim trunks. The base swimming pool was our next stop, its fifty-meter length perfect for continued specialized water instruction.

They would begin with stretching exercises to warm up before entering the pool. Quarter-mile swims progressed to half-mile distances before they earned their fins. With fins, the swims increased by another quarter mile with the class transferring to the open ocean for swims up to four miles when we felt they were ready. Now, it was said, the tadpoles had legs.

After the pool swims we went back for more surf drills, runs, and classroom projects. The evening was reserved for night operations involving the ocean, the IBS, and rock surf drills where the students had to paddle in tune in order to perfect their teamwork as a crew. Even as we were teaching the individual how much more he could expect of himself mentally, physically, and emotionally we were also teaching men to work together as a single unit. It has been said that teams survive and individuals die, and certainly this is true for SEALs. Anyone who ever promotes himself as being a solitary SEAL has missed the whole point of the teams. What we accomplished we accomplished as Team One. That is why our combat record and heritage is so greatly respected today.

During the first four weeks each day was much the same as the other with only one objective in mind: to get the students into exceptional physical shape for what lay ahead. Students could quit any time they wanted to. All one had to do was tell an instructor he wanted out and poof, he was *gone!* Men quit for many reasons, some suffered physical injury and had to. SEALs like Harlen Funkhouser broke bones in training. In Harlen's case, he is the only SEAL to have broken a leg after Hell Week, recovered, and then gone back through Hell Week a second time with the class he was reassigned to. You don't get much tougher than that in the teams.

HOOYAHH! became an ever-present part of the tadpoles' vocabulary. I never learned where this yell, this password into our fraternity, came from but I understand it. When a bear is hurting he growls. When a bear is threatened he growls. When a bear is angry he most certainly growls and when that bear is happy about something he growls too! Well, this Bear's growl is *HOOYAHH!!!* and so it goes with all tadpoles, Frogs, SEALs, and even Snakes.

At five weeks the tadpoles had names and faces. They also had strengths and weaknesses. The quitters were mere numbers which had been crossed off the manning roster. We'd have a class of men to work with after the fifth week, and they would face the hardest challenge yet to come.

Hell Week. HOOYAHH!

Every SEAL has gone through Hell Week, meaning every instructor has been there, done that, and got the T-shirt. I had endured the mental and physical stress of this period.

Each instructor was concerned about "his" students and we wanted all of them to successfully complete—or survive—what was to come. However, we knew from past experience this would not be the case. The men were all physically strong enough to last but did they have that unexplainable need way down deep in their guts to really want to be frogmen? Did they truly want this distinction regardless of how much the pain and misery to be laid upon their shoulders would be? For those who would make it the formula for success would be mind over body, with everything coming from the heart. As a Navy boxer who'd done all right by his teammates in the ring in countless smokers I'd learned men with heart can, and will, beat excellent technical fighters who lack heart. Heart was what would get a tadpole through Hell Week, because heart would be all that was left him.

It began Sunday at midnight. It would not end until the next Saturday at noon. The days were essentially the same as they'd been for the first five weeks. But at night there was no sleep, no rest, no breaks. Unexpected exercises were created to put the mind under additional stress. Simple problems became nightmares once the rest factor was taken away. The students would sing proudly in the ranks when Hell Week began. Soon after they'd be told to hit the racks for some sleep. In two minutes the lights would be out. Three minutes later they would come back on with an instructor entering the barracks from both ends of the building, orders barked to fall out into the street in swim trunks. Life jackets, helmets, and paddles in hand the men would scramble for the doors. Any man late would hit the bay at a run while his boat crew went into the front leaning rest until he returned. "Stand by your IBS and double-time to the beach!" Night surf passage. Afterward, it was head north to the "Rocks" behind the Del Coronado Hotel and come back in from the ocean on the red light.

Hell Week was underway.

At three in the morning the students would be found double-timing back to the training unit with their IBSs on their heads. Freshwater wash the IBS and fall in to return to the beach. Run south this time. Would the goal be the state park fence? That was only six miles away. . . . After a blistering pace at one mile we turn them around and return to the start point.

"Class! Fall in one column on the berm facing the surf. Do you want to see the sun rise? Then *sing!*"

My fellow instructors and I would move up and down the ranks dropping first one and then another student for push-ups. Daylight would arrive at last. Our tadpoles would be shivering in the early morning's light, wet from water and sweat, chilled to the bone from the cold night's air. The wind would come slipping up over the white sand, striking the class's formation and making the physical discomfort even worse. Time to get back to the training unit. We'd wake everyone up with our singing, running by at a double time—cold, hungry, and wetter than while at the berm. Five minutes to change into a dry uniform and fall in for chow. It is only Monday morning and the spirit is still strong.

Bud Jurick and I are in the armory. It will soon be "So Solly Day" and we are preparing the half-pound explosive charges for this evolution. "So Solly" is a holdover from the first UDT men who fought the Japanese in the South Pacific during the Second World War. Bud and I remove the metal ends from TNT charges to prevent injury to the tadpoles when these go off. Moving to the south beach where the demo pit is we begin laying the charges. The pit, dug out by a bulldozer, was below sea level and so the ocean's water formed a pond in its belly. Some charges are placed at the bottom of the pond, others in the sand on the sides of the pit. Around the outside of the pit is a barbed wire obstacle course, with two poles at either end of the pit supporting a crawl cable over the water. Charges are set all around the barbed wire course, with one set dead center of the course itself. The students are finishing a four-mile run and we sit back to wait for their arrival.

They come. Today they are dressed in green utility uniforms, helmets, and boots. The demolition course has been explained to them and you can see apprehension in varying degrees surface in each man's face as he looks us over. The class is formed up in four ranks, all on line facing the course. When the order is given they hit the deck and begin crawling under the barbed wire, their heads buried in the sand at all times. They are used to this as the "O" course features a similar obstacle which they've run a hundred times by now. When they reach the end of the barbed wire course they're told they must monkey crawl across the wire cable over the water-filled pit. At first, this seems to be no problem.

I fire off the first charge which is the one set dead center of the course the tadpoles are now crawling on. They hear and see where the TNT has exploded and realize it's in a direct line with them. Their heads are up, looking around as they wonder if there are more charges on the course and if so, where? We order them to stop gawking and to get their heads back down! Now begins the careful and slow detonation of charge after charge as they make their way under the wire and across the sand. The tadpoles are being blasted by sand and pummeled with shock waves. The noise is deafening and many are hearing the sound of explosives for the very first time in their young lives.

No one is singing.

Coming out at the other end of the course each student is told to report to the instructor at the top of the pit. Everyone else remains where he is in the sand. They cannot see the pit from where they lie. Ordered to monkey crawl across the cable the student is warned about the dire consequences of falling off the cable and into the pond below. As he moves out into open space an explosion greets him, sand peppering his exposed skin. Then another as water erupts upward, shaking the cable and nearly throwing the student off. One by one they cross until the entire class is safely on the other side.

There are many lessons here. Teamwork is one. Learning about what you will do under such conditions is another. Plus, each man sees the man next to him going forward despite the fear and dread of the unknown. You can trust him, he'll be there when you need him, no matter what is going on around you both. Teamwork and teammates. It's the SEAL way of doing business.

As the day is passing I can pick out the ones who are going to pack it in and quit before the week is out. Students who have what it takes will dedicate themselves to each other even outside of their own assigned boat crew. I'd spot the men who stood out because they were helping others, sometimes even carrying their teammate's load as well as their own. I once saw two students drop out of a run, circle back to another student who had fallen and been left, grabbing him up under the armpits and pulling him along while all the time talking him past his pain so he could finish with the class. I have seen boat crews hoist a crew member atop their IBS although his feet were so badly blistered he couldn't stumble, much less walk or run. They carried him. Most every student who finished Hell Week did so without a voice—having spent it by giving encouragement throughout the week to each other and all those around.

This, then, is what makes a SEAL.

Early Tuesday morning the class is told they may get some sleep. It is a mind game, a calculated scenario meant to draw them down, to cause them to drop their guard, to make them believe it is safe and okay to relax for a few precious minutes. Five minutes later, with many of the students already in a dead sleep, instructors turn on the lights and begin running through the barracks firing M1 rifles with blank adapters on their barrels. The noise is deafening and the shock it brings on is self-evident. Students are ordered to fall out in swim trunks and life jackets, boat paddles in hand. Once this is done they are educated about "Enoch's Fishing Line."

My fishing line saw each student snapped onto a role of cod line by the chest snap of their life jackets. They were then ordered to back down the boat launch ramp into San Diego Bay and to keep the line straight—at all costs—by using their boat paddles. I always timed the exercise to occur with the tide running either in or out because this made it near impossible to keep the line straight under any conditions. After an hour of fruitless labor I'd drag my fishing line back in and we'd put the class to bed, this time for only three minutes. When they snapped back onto the line they were in wet trunks and life jackets. It was miserable. Some of the men became so cold they would begin shaking without control, but they went back down the ramp. Others would unsnap themselves from the line as fast as they'd been snapped onto it. They would quit.

Officer or enlisted, all tadpoles were treated the same. No one had special demands placed upon him unless it was for his physical well-being. Likewise, no one was cut any slack due to his rank or personality. Sometimes, however, there were students that it was impossible not to have your attention drawn to. One such student was Lt. Theodore Roosevelt IV, relative to President Roosevelt of "Rough Rider" fame. One instructor upon learning this fact dug up an impressive piece of driftwood timber roughly the size of a fence post. Mr. Roosevelt was ordered to "speak softly and carry a big stick" which he did without complaint. The lieutenant kept his magnum-sized stick with him until we felt it was becoming a little too much to ask of anyone. Lieutenant Roosevelt proved himself to be a good sport and went on to become a fine UDT officer and teammate.

I found great favor in the "Mud Flats" which became another traditional exercise during Hell Week. The south end of San Diego Bay was very shallow which gave us four-to-five feet of blue-green tidal mud in which to have our students play. It was sticky mud, very soft and mushy and the smell could bring vomit to your throat on a good day. The boat crews were ordered to paddle from NAVPHIBSCHOL at Coronado to the southwest end of the bay. Once there they would report to instructors they would find on the beach.

The trip was a race between IBS crews. Six-or-seven man crews had been working together as a team since Sunday night. Each team was receiving points for each evolution conducted during the course of the week. The mud flats were a place where one could either build up points, or lose them. The crews who were trailing behind would be given a chance to close the gap at the mud flats. Total point count was important at the end of the week for one reason alone. Crews were released from Hell Week on Saturday based upon their standing in the polls. Simply put, the higher the point count the faster the pain ended and the sooner uninterrupted sleep began.

The last crew to arrive was the first to fall in at the mud

flats. They were instructed to move through the mud searching for any foreign matter such as glass or sticks . . . anything that might injure them later. This finished, the other crews followed the same instructions until the crew that arrived first was the last to make the search. This crew got the most rest, but they'd spent the most energy getting to the mud flats to begin with. Even better, by the time they went into the flats the mud had been churned to the point where it was thicker, deeper, and stinkier than ever before. This meant it took more energy to search through while everyone else was waiting. The crews which had completed the mud flat exercise were kept on their feet singing in order to keep them awake. We continued the exercise through most of the afternoon. Crews raced against each other for points and soon were covered from head to toe with oozing, foul-smelling mud. Some became so cold they started shaking, mud flipping off them in gooey little hunks.

When a halt was called in the exercise the students were allowed to take a good swim in the bay to clean up. Each student was inspected for any mud still present after the first swim, and if mud was found after our generous allowance of time for a bath we would send the offender back into the bay. When everyone in the crew was nice and clean, the IBS was paddled back to the base as fast as the students could move it.

Upon their arrival back at base the crews were checked in for points. They would clean their IBSs and life jackets, then hit the showers. From there they went to the corpsman to wash their ears out in order to prevent infection. We allowed no hot water for the showers as this would cause the men to go to sleep while standing up! Cleaned up and inspected by the medic the men could dress, fall back outside, and prepare for chow. Of course they sang until the last man joined the formation. Our greatest concern was injury or infection. We wanted them to succeed and that meant watching closely so that stupid accidents did not happen.

To push the men past their self-imposed physical and mental limits, we instructors always kept them under close observation during Hell Week. When a man goes without sleep for a week it is the instructor's job to step in between the man and the dumb things he will try to do as the days progress. Keeping their wounds clean and ensuring they were more than well-fed was foremost in our minds. They would scrape themselves, bust their knuckles, skin their knees, get cuts, blisters upon blisters, open sores, and everything else during Hell Week. These we could treat and did, all the while letting them know nothing was so bad it could keep them from making the grade. When they ate, they ate well. Calories were needed to keep the engine running and we never kept food from our students. If a man quit he did so only because internally he didn't have the heart to become a frogman.

One of my favorite night operations was "Treasure Hunt." After their evening meal the students would return to the classroom for a briefing. Information given included uniform for the exercise, air and water temps, IBS criteria, and anything else of importance. Instructors move among the students to make sure the dry, warm clothing and good food in their bellies didn't put them to sleep. Each boat crew officer was given an envelope with directions to a start point. With a room thundering HOOYAHH! the men were off for a night's fun and games.

At the starting point the crews would find an instructor in a jeep. He would take the envelope and give them their first clue in return. It might be "meet your instructor where the big birds land" or something like that. The students would have to discuss the clue, come to a decision, and then tell the instructor where it was they thought they were going next. If they were wrong the instructor whom they found would simply give them a note which read "try again." Where the big birds land was the North Island Naval Air Station fence, four miles up the beach to the north. If this was a crew's objective they would load their IBS on their heads and head down the dark beach at a double time. When they arrived at the right location the next instructor would hand them a note which might offer they needed to "try the other one." This would be the fence ten miles to the south at the state park. Once again the IBS is loaded and off the crew goes.

The treasure hunt went on through the night with each clue getting harder than the last. It was meant to force the men to fight through their physical exhaustion and growing mental fatigue in order to solve the problem at hand. In combat, decisions which render battles won or lost must often be made under the worst of conditions and in a fraction of a second. We were teaching the men this fact of SEAL life and seeing who could pull together as a team to solve the riddles as they came. It became an effort for the men to agree even on a direction of travel. A clue stating "A magazine you can't read tonight" could be the base library or the ammunition dump. Crews who got into loud argument over this or that lost points. The boat crew in the lead would be pulled out of the treasure hunt at four in the morning. They would secure from Hell Week and be ordered to hit the rack. The last boat crew would normally see their reprieve sometime after daylight on Saturday.

It was the responsibility of the duty instructor to keep an eye on the sleeping tadpoles. We didn't want any of them trying to drive home until they had a minimum of six hours sleep. I watched men shower, dress, and fall back asleep in the front seats of their cars after Hell Week. Once I woke a student up who I found in his car and told him to go back to bed. The only way I convinced him he couldn't drive yet was to point out he'd only put on his shirt and shoes after waking up. That seemed to do it.

Hell Week might have been over but training was not. It would continue for many weeks to come. By early 1966, I could feel a coming change in the instructors at BUDS. Reports coming back about our brothers fighting in Vietnam were real, and when men returned they shared their hard-won experiences with the cadre. We, in turn, adjusted training to meet the threat. The others and I felt a greater responsibility than ever before to better prepare our men for battle. We had to create new ways to make the difference between life and death. We asked questions of every man who returned to Coronado. Our staff meetings were always open to new ideas and methods of accomplishing the mission. Some were good, some were not. The fact remained that we were flexible and willing to improve ourselves so that the teams would benefit.

Hell Week created teammates of our students. After it

was over there was nothing we could throw at them that they couldn't work through either individually or as a cohesive unit. It was tough, sometimes brutal, and as often as not comical in one way or another. It made warriors out of young men.

HOOYAHH!!!

6

The First to Fall

RD2 Billy W. Machen
KIA 19 August 1966
Rung Sat, RVN

It was August 20, 1966, and I was at the armory, UDT Training Base, Coronado, California. We'd just returned from a particularly challenging phase at San Clemente Island and I was field stripping the weapons our students had turned in before their graduation. A good job had been done cleaning them, especially given what the students had just gone through. But I wanted to assure myself they would be ready for the next class and if you want something done right . . .

BM2 Vince Olivera burst through the doors disturbing my work with the weapons. "Hey, Bear! Did you hear about Billy Machen yet? He was killed in Vietnam!" Vince had just come from SEAL Team One where he'd heard the word about my friend Bill Machen.

"No," I answered quietly, "I hadn't heard." My watch said it was just 10:00 in the morning. After asking Olivera how he'd heard, I watched him as he disappeared into his office down the hall. For a short time I continued to work with the weapons, not knowing anything else to do. Bill and I were the best of friends. Before he'd left for Vietnam he'd come over to our house to wish us good-bye, asking me to walk with him to his car.

"Bear," he said quietly, "I don't believe I'm going to make it back."

"You're nuts," I responded. But I could tell he was sincere and that unsettled me somewhat. Carol, his wife, was pregnant with their child.

"Promise me you'll take care of Carol and the baby if something happens to me," Bill asked.

"I will," I said. "But, Bill, ain't nothing gonna happen to you over there." It would be the last time I spoke to my friend while he was alive.

Turning to the phone I placed a call to SEAL Team One to confirm what Vince had told me. It was. Casualty Assistance Officers were already with Carol. I then called my wife and told her Bill was dead and that I was coming home. Fifteen minutes later I was in our living room, the shock starting to set in. Eatsie, my wife, said we needed to go see Carol. Bill's house was right behind ours so we left. It was the hardest walk I have ever made in my life both before and since. We spoke with Carol for a while and decided I would go with her and the kids to Texas. Her sister, Karen, would come along and her husband, Martin Mapes, who was also a SEAL, was picked to escort Bill's body home. There was an airline strike taking place at the time and it took some doing to arrange for tickets. But we did and soon enough we were on our way.

As the plane gained altitude I could see the lights of San Diego below us. Then darkness took the city away from my view. I walked back to the stewardess station and, for some reason, told them why we were going to Texas. A short while later one of the stews moved us to First Class as it was nearly empty. It was a kind gesture. The children were asleep but sleep would not come for the rest of us for some time.

After a while I found myself studying a drop of water on the outside of the window. It formed, then broke into tiny beads which shot off in different directions as the pressure of the wind broke it up. Strange how people will stare out a window even when there is nothing to see. Even more surprising to me is remembering this fragment in time after so many years: twenty-eight to be exact.

My thoughts drifted back to when I first met Bill. It was

the third week of UDT Training and we were working our way through a one-mile pool swim. Another student had brought me in to the base that morning and as I watched, he left the pool and began talking to one of the instructors. Then, he left. At lunch I learned he'd quit and when a student quit you never saw or heard from him again. I told Bill the man had been my ride home. Machen offered to drop me off and from that point on our friendship grew. Bill and I helped each other get through each day's training. We pushed each other, encouraged each other, and looked out for each other as only teammates can.

Upon graduation we found ourselves assigned to UDT Team 12, 1st Platoon. Not only were we the new guys but we were the youngest too. The men of the 1st Platoon were all Korean war veterans and we looked up to them from day one. In turn, they accepted us right away and began showing us the ropes of being a frogman. Even after getting to UDT there was a bit of a letdown between Bill and me. Things were slow and we wanted some action. As the new guys we were driven even closer together and began plotting a means of testing ourselves.

My wife and children took to Bill from the beginning. They loved him and my wife must have seen how close we had become since meeting. If I had ever had a brother it would have been Bill Machen. I didn't know of anyone else who could stay out half the night then come into our home and sleep on the couch without a word from Eatsie. He was so at home with us it wasn't unusual to have him give a quick knock at the door then come in, raiding the 'fridge as if it were his own. A smile crosses my face as I realize even now that indeed he was at home!

In our quest for action we ended up volunteering for Project IceSkate. It seemed the U.S. Naval Ordnance Laboratory wanted divers for some Arctic based underwater demolitions tests. We decided that was for us so we beat feet to Lieutenant Freeman, our platoon officer. Freeman was a fine officer and we learned later how he would go to the wall for one of his men. Bill and I must have done a great job selling the program because the lieutenant wanted to go with us! Our request was approved and after drawing new dive suits we were on our way to Alaska.

Upon landing in Fairbanks, Bill and I couldn't resist going "steaming." Apparently we had a bit too much fun as we fell asleep under a tree outdoors. No one had warned us about the mosquitoes and when we awoke neither of us could hardly recognize the other! It could have been worse, a moose or something could have stepped on us during the night. With liberty over we hopped on a plane to Point Barrow, Alaska. There we reported aboard the USS *Staten Island* (AGB-5).

Our team was briefed by Naval Ordnance personnel on a new type of military explosive which we were to test under the ice. Not just any ice, but Arctic ice. Such ice is found only far up north. It is a hard, gray-looking form of ice and to get to it we had to travel some eight hundred miles past Point Barrow. The ship ventured in excess of seventy-five degrees latitude and Lieutenant Freeman, Bill, and myself became part of the first Navy ship to make the farthest penetration of Alaska's winter frontier for that time. The explosive boys wanted us to place different-sized shots under no less than eighteen feet of Arctic ice. Our mission was to discover the precise amount necessary to blow a hole large enough to allow a submarine's sail to fit through if it had to surface under an emergency.

The commanding officer of the ship put Lieutenant Freeman on watch in the crow's nest. His "job" was to look for this specific ice flow. The assignment upset us and it was dumb. When the ship found the ice it did so by hitting it . . . which stopped the *Staten Island* dead in its tracks!

Machen and I were swim buddies and we made the first dive together. We were supposed to take the shot one hundred and eighty feet back under the ice at a point determined to be "just right." On the surface the ice was flat but below the sea it was rugged, sometimes twenty to sixty feet deep. The explosives had to be pulled behind us along with the firing cable. It was hard, back-breaking work and at one point Bill pulled so hard on the line that he jerked upward and hit his mouthpiece on the ice above us. The impact knocked the mouthpiece from his mouth and out of the dive suit's hood. As the cold water hood was part of the suit itself it had a hole cut in it especially for the mouthpiece. This hole was no larger than a dime making it a very snug fit when everything was in place. To reinsert the life-giving mouthpiece we'd have to stretch the hole around it while wearing thick gloves and stranded one hundred and fifty feet under the ice and away from help.

It was quite the struggle but together we got Bill's hood stretched back over the mouthpiece and he was breathing on his own again. I remember him having a mask full of very white eyeballs for a while, however. We made two dives under the ice. There were six of us in the team and two divers had to be suited up as safety divers while two others were actually working underwater. It was fairly comfortable when you were submerged but on the surface the wind and snow made it some kind of cold. When we would come to the surface the safety divers would pull us out of the water quickly, wrapping us in blankets because the wind would freeze the dive suits in seconds! We learned to keep our masks on too, because to take them off in the twenty-eight degree water could cause our faces to freeze before making it back to the ship.

It was a great trip and both Bill and I had a good time. We'd handled ourselves well during Arctic diving and learned a lot. And there were great stories to tell the rest of the frogs back on the Coronado Silver Strand.

I came back to reality when the pilot announced it was time for us to fasten our seatbelts and to quit smoking. The stew told me we were preparing to land in Denver, the strike rerouting us. I asked if we should move back to the coach section, but the stew told me to wait as First Class didn't fill up often late at night. A few new passengers joined our flight. I took note as the stewardess talked quietly with one of them, an older man. He shook his head up and down and moved to the rear of the plane where he took a seat. As he'd passed us he'd looked at Carol. Once we were airborne again I went to the stewardess and thanked her for keeping us up front. The passenger I'd seen had given up his seat for us and when I heard this I went to thank him. As we spoke he told me he'd served in the South Pacific during WWII and he appreciated what we were trying to do in Vietnam. Thinking back today I do not recall any other civilian I met during that time period ever thanking us for supporting our country by answering its call. But then, he knew more than most civilians.

By the time I got back to my seat everyone was asleep again except for Carol. Thinking she might want this time for herself I returned to my lonely window to watch the water drops fall away.

Again, my thoughts were swept back to better times. When we'd returned to the Strand our team was standing down for deployment to WESPAC, or West Pacific Command, to relieve UDT 11. All hands turned to for the next two weeks as we loaded the ship taking us to Hawaii. Our good-byes said, we got underway, next stop Pearl Harbor.

Our first task upon arriving at WESPAC was to requalify on the fifty and one hundred foot free ascent in the Submarine Training Tank. It would be the first time I had ever qualified at one hundred feet. When a diver does a free ascent he breathes air under pressure, exhaling all of his air as he rises to the surface. A training tank instructor would punch you hard in the gut to make sure you were out of air before letting you go, a safety diver shadowing you as you made for the surface and a fresh breath of air. Any one having trouble would be pulled into a safety lock by the safety diver. The point of the exercise was to practice an emergency ascent as if escaping from a stranded submarine on the bottom. It was very exciting for both Bill and me, to say the least.

After a week's training the ship left for Japan. Before arriving, though, half of us were dropped off in Okinawa with orders assigning us to the Army's 1st Special Forces Group. We were about to become paratroopers! Machen and I were once again paired up and would support each other in training. I needed support because I just didn't think jumping was for me. Bill gave me a good talking to, reminding me about how tough we were and how we couldn't let our teammates down by quitting, especially quitting an Army school. I wasn't really convinced when he finished but it did help me feel better.

The first instructor we met was M. Sgt. Antonio Duarte. He had a special aura about him which demanded respect from all of us frogmen. In fact, all of our Special Forces instructors enjoyed our mutual respect but we tried hard not to let them know this. They had been in Southeast Asia for a long time and were the most professional soldiers I'd ever met.

We were in great physical condition and the training was a lot of fun. Not easy, but fun. The last day was jump day and it was the hardest of all. Our first actual jump was from a C-130 and it was a morning "blast." Everything happened so fast it was over before I knew it. We went to chow and Bill was beside himself with excitement. The jump was all we talked about and I had a lot to say about that drop zone! It was hard, real hard. They'd named it Yomitan DZ and my body became very well acquainted with it before the day was over.

After lunch we once again loaded aboard the C-130 but this time Master Sergeant Duarte stood me in the door. I was to be Number One Jumper. It was an honor but one I would have gladly given to Bill. Duarte pointed out how the ocean looked and all sorts of other things as we climbed to altitude. I could have done without the tour, believe me. Finally Yomitan DZ loomed into view below my boots and Duarte hit me hard on the leg, sending me out the door with a single bound. Again, I hit hard but in one piece. After rolling up the 'chutes we dropped them off at a 6X6, grabbed another parachute, and reported to a H-21 helicopter for yet another jump. We did this three more times until the required five jumps were tallied and we'd qualified for our jump wings.

That night we partied with our instructors and were pinned with the silver wings of a paratrooper. Bill somehow learned that C Company was making a jump the next morning and he got us manifested. It would be our cherry jump, meaning the sixth jump which made us more than just qualified military parachutists. There is no way of describing how bad my body felt already but Bill got me up and to the plane that morning. Once again I was floating high above Yomitan DZ, thanks to my teammate Bill Machen.

A day later we climbed aboard a C-130 headed for Japan and the rest of the team. When I arrived I found a set of orders sending me to something called "SEAL Team." No one knew what a SEAL or a SEAL Team was and I was not happy. I was a frogman and that's all I ever wanted to be. But orders are orders. Bill stayed with UDT 12 and I returned to Coronado to start up SEAL Team One, whatever that was.

My return to the States was met with orders for all sorts of Army and Marine schools. From there I went to Vietnam and when I returned Bill was out of the Navy. My new orders took me to UDT Training at Coronado as an instructor. It was one year later and I had my students in the front leaning rest when a nearby car blew its horn at me. It was my old friend Bill Machen. He had reenlisted and had orders to SEAL Team One. Bill brought me over to the car and introduced Carol, his wife, and his little daughter. I was overjoyed at seeing him again, especially with a family in tow.

A year later Bill was gone, this time forever. And I was keeping my promise.

The plane landed in Dallas and one of Bill's brothers met us at the airport. He drove the family to Gilmer, Texas, to the home of Bill's father. East Texas was green and hot in August. Their home reminded me of my parents' home in Kentucky. The family was introduced and they thanked me for bringing Carol and the children back to them. I felt right at home in Bill's house.

It was a three-day wait before Bill's body arrived. It was in the morning and I was setting quietly on the front porch when a car pulled into the driveway. It was Bob Henry, a SEAL who was helping escort Bill from Vietnam back to the States. Bob and I were both plankowners in SEAL Team One and had known each other since 1962. It would be Henry who would tell me exactly how my friend had died.

"Bear," he began, "we were working about fifteen miles southeast of Nha Be on the Dinh Ba River. The day before, the eighteenth of August, our patrol had found two large hootches filled with rice. It was a big cache and too much for us to carry out.

"There was so much rice we couldn't get it to burn so we called in air strikes on the cache. When it was finally destroyed we continued our patrol. The next day we got a report from a helicopter about two camouflaged sampans upriver. Naturally, we went to check it out.

"Bill was on point and he was doing a fine job of it. First he found fresh tracks which led us to a series of bunkers and fighting positions along the river. I'd never seen bunkers like these, they were like huge beehives. We checked them out and moved on.

"We finally came to a clearing where Bill halted the patrol. We waited for a while, then Bill moved into the clearing alone. But before he got across it he suddenly dropped down and opened fire on a bunch of VC. He'd seen them lying in ambush for us but he knew we were already moving into the clearing. So he opened up from inside the kill zone to both warn and cover us."

Bob went on to say it was just like live fire training on the Salton Sea in southern California. He'd never heard so much firepower going downrange. The SEALs returned fire and Bill was able to make his way back to the team before dying. According to Bob, Bill Machen had saved his teammates' lives at the cost of his own.

The next day Martin Mapes came with Bill's body. Bob and I went down to the funeral home to make sure everything was in order. The funeral director let us see Bill. I asked him if he would pin my silver jump wings on Bill's uniform, which he was being buried in. It was a simple request to grant. The funeral was held at the First Baptist Church in Gilmer with all military honors. The pastor elaborated on how special Bill was. He said his selflessness, his courage, his devotion to duty, and his personality live on in our memories.

Carol returned to San Diego and began trying to put her life back together. Bob returned to his platoon in Vietnam and was wounded aboard a Medium Landing Craft (LCM) when it was ambushed by an entire Vietcong battalion. His wounds were so serious he was medically discharged from the Navy. I went back to Coronado and my students. But I was different inside. A new outlook on my responsibilities to my men had been birthed by Bill's death. There was a new emphasis on what I was teaching, and a new awareness of how important the lives of my teammates were to me. For the first time in my life I felt a deep rage coming forth. Like an angered bear I was reacting to the death of my closest friend, and what I was feeling would result in the deaths of many of the enemy while also ensuring the survival of those who were my fellow SEALs.

It was a grizzly bear's rage which was now consuming me. In Vietnam, I would turn it loose with what many later told me was deadly effect. In late 1995, the Navy would formally commission Camp Machen, named after my friend Bill. I am proud to say I was there to see this monument to his heroism and sacrifice dedicated.

7

The
Long Rehearsal

After I'd returned to Coronado with the training group I found my teammates were filled with the same mixed emotions that were eating at my own guts. Loss and anger were challenging us, the question on everyone's minds being how we could improve our training so our students would be better prepared for war in Vietnam. Already an additional class had been added to build up the number of men in the teams. Talk was going around that we'd next be making the UDT course eighteen, and maybe even twenty-one weeks long instead of its now sixteen-week cycle. SEAL Team One would lose five more teammates to enemy fire in 1967. However, their actions against the enemy in the Rung Sat Special Zone were not unnoticed. Because of their operational success the Navy demanded more SEAL combat action platoons for the Mekong Delta. Each instructor, to include myself, became motivated from deep within to turn out frogmen and SEALs who were better than ever given what was coming. We would not drop the quality of training, however, just for the sake of adding to the command's numbers.

To qualify as a SEAL the enlisted men first needed to graduate from UDT Training, then made one successful deployment to the Western Pacific (WESPAC) as a member of a UDT Team. Rankwise they needed to be at least a third class petty officer as this meant they'd spent some time in the Navy and knew the ropes. Vietnam changed these requirements as the war intensified. By 1967 a graduate from UDT Training could be assigned to SEAL Team One right off the Silver Strand. From here he'd go straight to jump school at Fort Benning, Georgia, and then back to the team where he'd be trained by a SEAL cadre. Probation at the team was six months and if the man made muster he'd be assigned to a combat action platoon. This meant that in a little more than a year our tadpoles could find themselves in Vietnam. Everything in training needed to be reevaluated as the students were younger and going to war sooner. In a sense, we more experienced SEALs were feeling perhaps a bit older in lieu of the faster pace of things.

Our teammates were the Navy's elite. They'd been tested under fire in WWII and Korea, and in Vietnam since 1963. By 1966 SEALs were engaged in a major turf battle with the Vietcong in areas where "Charlie" had once been safe as a babe in its cradle. SEALs were undertaking intelligence gathering missions which took them far from standard amphibious activities they originally trained for. Combat action platoons were going out on search and destroy missions, and were many times outnumbered by the enemy they faced. No matter the odds, the SEALs inflicted heavy tolls on the VC but not without a price paid. Training was the only way to close the gap and to hone our edge that much sharper!

Training Command relied upon the old .30 caliber M1 Garand rifle. I say old because the M1 was the standard military rifle of the WWII era. Blank ammunition for training was available throughout the military and could be expended during training without a thought for resupply. They were big, heavy weapons and very good for making an impression upon a student as a training aid. The problem was the SEALs were not using the M1 in Vietnam. When our students graduated and went to the teams they went back to basic training weaponwise in order to learn about the new rifle we'd adopted. This caused unnecessary delays for everyone involved.

The new rifle, adopted in 1962, was the 5.56mm AR15. Developed by Eugene Stoner along with the Armalite Corporation, the AR15 was a new battle rifle and thought to be a vast improvement over the M1 and even M14 rifles. Colt Firearms obtained the rights to the new rifle and it became known among SEALs as the Colt Armalite AR15, with the Navy officially giving the weapon its beginning as a service arm thanks to its SEALs. Colt went on to develop an upgraded version which it called the M16, the Army adopting the rifle for standard issue to its troops. In the teams, we continued to update and modify the weapon in the armory during the 1960s and UDT Training soon had enough AR15s available to use them in training for the benefit of the students. SEAL Team One's requirement was met in this manner as we covered field stripping, basic rifle marksmanship, and battlefield employment of the new rifle in class. Still, the old Garand made its bark heard during field training exercises because we still had more than enough blank ammo for our tadpoles to fire.

The other instructors and I made every moment possible available to our students. We also met with as many SEALs coming back from Vietnam as we could. Just hanging out with them could key you into something new which could be integrated into training. At UDT Training we couldn't create SEALs nor did we want to. That was the job of the SEAL cadre at the teams. Our responsibility was to turn out UDT operators who were capable of charting ocean beaches for potential amphibious landings and demolitions. Frogmen cleared the beach of manmade or natural obstacles using swimmer delivered charges. At training we could create the core fiber of the Navy SEAL but frogmen were what we were about primarily. Still, it was clear frogmen were becoming SEALs and that was where we as instructors found ourselves challenged.

An officer returning from Vietnam told me about being caught up in a clever river ambush laid by the Vietcong. "The support boat was hit by rocket fire and many of the boat's gunners—as well as SEALs—were killed or wounded by the initial attack," he explained. "Even with our teammates bleeding they pulled themselves up and manned the fifty caliber machine guns, suppressing the VC fire so everyone could escape." How could they do that, I wondered to myself. "Bear," the officer added as if reading my mind, "the only way they could have done that was because of their physical training. Whatever you guys do in training, don't ever let up on them!" Our training program was geared to build a strong foundation for both the UDT and SEAL teams. After hearing his story I vowed in my own mind we wouldn't let up, instead we'd make the foundation that much stronger.

When students completed Hell Week their physical training slowed to a point where they could recoup what Hell Week took away. Then it gradually increased in intensity again so we could begin building the men up to an even greater degree of physical prowess. Morning PT and the beach runs were ongoing but the students were in the classroom more. Combat beach recons and swimmer recovery drills kept them in the sun and physically active, as well. I usually enjoyed my students' presence in the afternoons during classroom sessions. It was right after noon chow and many times they had trouble staying as awake as I liked them to be. A short trip to the bay, only fifty feet from our classroom, brought them around although they were always a bit wet around the gills afterward.

We changed very little from our old training program, adding more new ideas and evolutions from our discussions with returning SEALs and UDT men. For example, conventional explosives training was enhanced by adding a class on the kinds of booby traps which would be found in Vietnam. These were simple but effective man-killers. Grenades with trip wires, punji stake pits, and all manner of other creative disasters were proving dangerous to our teammates. The SEALs were running into booby-trapped ammo boxes, weapons, and even bodies. To help the students recognize the wide range of traps awaiting them we developed a unique exercise where they made their own booby traps.

The students were provided with MK2 firecrackers and an array of items with which they could devise a booby trap. The firecrackers provided the realism of an explosion if the trap was set off, an experience no one but the instructors and those other students watching enjoyed. Those traps which weren't found were disarmed by the students who emplaced them. It was a fun exercise, however, our objective was to firmly install in the students' brain housing groups that booby traps were killing and injuring our people.

Other explosive training continued. We trained our new teammates about how the explosive haversack normally used for clearing underwater beach obstacles worked in a satisfactory manner in Vietnam. The twenty-pound sack had an oral flotation bladder which could be used when inserting or patrolling rivers, canals, or other water-related areas. The haversack could be broken down into two-pound charges for smaller shots, or divided among patrol members during long-distance movements.

One item of explosive ordnance which became a favorite subject of mine was the claymore antipersonnel mine. Night ambushes on rivers were a common and much favored tactic of SEALs working the Rung Sat Special Zone. With the killing place, or kill zone facing the river itself the ambushing unit would use claymores to protect its flanks and rear area. Once the VC were wiped out or the operation terminated for whatever reason, the mines could be detonated to cover the SEALs' extraction from the target site. Claymore mines were light, easy to carry, and effective. We taught the students how to place them, wire them up and fire them, and how to use them to create overlapping fields of fire. The mine was used by Army Special Forces, Marine Force Recon, and the Australian Special Air Service (SAS) in Vietnam. Its internal C4 explosive charge would direct over seven hundred .30 caliber steel balls in an aimed arc once detonated. Not much lived through a claymore explosion.

Training after Hell Week now varied, with demolitions joined by small arms, land warfare, beach reconnaissance, cartography, and underwater diving.

On a beach reconnaissance the students would be dropped off by swim pairs at sea in a line parallel to the beach. The swimmers would start toward the beach, taking soundings using a lead line along the way. This measured depth. They would also free dive to check for obstacles unseen from the surface. All this information would be recorded on a Plexiglas swimmer slate carried by the swim team. The men would shift twenty meters to the right or left and then swim back out, creating an overlap procedure which was repeated until the ocean's bottom as it applied to the entire beach was charted. When finished, the teams would be recovered by a high-speed boat using a method taught them beforehand. Today's beaches around the world are subject to SEAL curiosity, and no one does it better than we do.

Back in the classroom the students studied cartography. This was a graphic exercise in chart making where the swim teams turned their information into a map. Some men would be assigned to record the information on paper while others prepared a large piece of chart paper for the map itself. Still other students were responsible for cutting out smaller sections of chart paper to log beach gradient and other marginal information critical to a good chart. Students would mark the positions of obstacles, such as large rocks or sandbars. When the chart was completed they would have to check it for accuracy. Once graded, the swimmers would either come away pleased with their work or start all over again. Always, they improved.

Until the Korean war the Navy's UDT teams carried out demolition efforts underwater, primarily to clear beaches. The North Koreans provided us with targets on land near their coastline where demolition attacks were feasible. These were primarily troop and supply routes from the north to the south, to include bridges and tunnels. The Navy noted it always had UDT men aboard a ship offshore somewhere and that they could be used to interdict North Korean traffic.

In the beginning the targets were very deep inside enemy territory. Demolition teams soon found themselves engaged in heavy fighting and the frogmen learned they were "fish out of water" under such conditions. Solutions had to be arrived at if such raids were to be successful. More effective light arms had to be carried, along with ammunition to feed them, but this meant less explosives could be man-packed to the target sites. The distance to a target from the water was looked at more closely, along with using other combat units trained in land warfare to provide support during a mission. The Navy was of the firm belief this category of inland raid could be successfully carried out by its frogmen. At one point, British SAS commandos were used to provide a perimeter defense around American frogmen as they laid their charges. The first example of what today is called a "joint operation" worked well in North Korea! UDT teams began to rely upon this procedure and they learned from the SAS. Soon hit-and-run missions involving UDT men were able to be conducted using only American personnel and the frogmen perfected this type of working defense. It became standard operating procedure in Korea and I still remember us teaching it as part of UDT Training in the 1960s.

The SEALs and UDT frogmen soon discovered their missions and the terrain in Vietnam to be quite different from what they'd been during Korea. SEALs were operating in heavy jungle such as that poised by ops in the Rung Sat Special Zone. They were hunting guerrillas and this kind of work did not compare to the hit-and-run raids and demo attacks of Korea. Basic UDT training, however, had not caught up with the evolution faced by our men in Vietnam. Until 1967 new SEALs relied upon Marine Force Recon, Army Special Forces/Rangers, and the SEAL cadres to learn the new tricks of the trade. After 1967 the demand for SEALs to immediately move into a wartime theater caused us at UDT Training to begin teaching land warfare at Coronado and its surrounding training sites.

After beach and dive training came the next phase of training. It was where the students would be asked to pull together everything they'd been taught. We moved them to San Clemente Island off the coast of southern California. At the time Chief Price would swing into action coordinating this movement of troops long before it actually took place. Concert obstacles needed to be loaded aboard landing craft such as the LCU. These were then transported out to San Clemente where they were placed in the Northwest Harbor under Price's direction. The LCU would then move surplus tanks and steel for the demolition ranges. Explosives and ammunition needed to be taken out, as well. The students staged their IBS rubber boats, personnel equipment, and "war bags" for the trip at the training unit. But Jurick and I would fly with the advance party to the island to set things up properly. Everything was arranged, from food to classroom supplies. The support team knew its job well and made the camp ready for the students' arrival. Bud and I checked the demo range and built targets for day and night training, to include raids along the northwestern end of the island.

Navy aircraft flew the students from the North Island Naval Air Station to San Clemente Island. Upon their arrival the duty instructor moved their equipment onto a truck, with the students running to the camp in formation. The run took them around the runway and back up the other side to Northwest Harbor. This would be their home for the next two weeks. At the camp they were assigned to a hootch, or small set of stark quarters, by the boat crew. There was enough time to put equipment away before the evening's meal. After chow a crew would be asked to clean the mess hall, turning it into a classroom. Rules and regulations for the camp and island followed.

The camp was located in Northwest Harbor and high ground watched over it except for a concave beach to the west. To the south on high ground was a large wooden water reservoir which rose over three hundred feet above the camp due to its placement. Students were advised to conserve fresh water and would learn all about the water tower in the days to come. The first morning's reveille found them formed in their PT circle outside of camp. We kept a large pile of wooden pallets nearby which always drew the students' attention. The pallets were important to the "Flight of the Wooden Butterflies," a motivational exercise we'd developed to help our students learn better and faster.

If a student encountered a problem completing an exercise he would be pulled out of the PT circle and instructed to draw a set of "wings" from the pallet pile. From this point he would be sent to check in with an instructor staged at the water tower. The student's only task was to ask the instructor what the water level in the tower was and to bring this figure back down so he could inform the instructor at the PT circle. To do this, the student would balance the pallet on his back and shoulders, becoming a wooden butterfly . . . of sorts. At the double time—and always at the double time—he would run up the hill to the tower to visit with the instructor who had the answer to his question. Sometimes the hill would be filled with wooden butterflies—so many the tower instructor would have to put them in landing patterns to keep things straight. Around and around they would run in circles until each individual answer could be given. I understand the wooden butterfly, a rare breed, is only known to inhabit San Clemente Island.

The student officers and sometimes senior enlisted personnel would be briefed on each morning's activities. From here they became responsible for preparing and issuing a warning order on the operation or patrol to the men. Operations were normally a beach recon complete with graded chart. In the afternoon we'd visit the demo range for hands-on explosive training. The students learned how to cut steel with plastic explosives, how to create and use shape charges, or how to blow tank traps with ammonium nitrate. They were graded on their ability to create the proper charges and to use the right formulas to solve the explosive problems we gave them.

One of the first nighttime problems the students faced was that of being a swimmer scout.

Swimmer scout teams would be briefed and then dropped off in swim pairs at sea. Each drop time and place was staggered so the teams wouldn't get in each other's way. The objective was to slip into camp without being detected; few teams were successful. Many of those "captured" by the waiting cadre would spend long hours in the front leaning rest position waiting for their buddies to arrive. One objective was to crawl to the center of Bird Island where they would bring back a sample of bird dung. This was to be analyzed within the scenario to see if the enemy could make a form of gunpowder from it. We might not see or hear them during this exercise, but you could sure smell them afterward.

The next morning a student officer would be called in and given a chart from the beach recon conducted the prior day. He would also be assigned an objective to clear off underwater obstacles using swimmer placed demolitions. At morning chow the officer called for a warning order in thirty minutes. During this period the men would be given their assignments, going on to build firing devices and charges. They would also waterproof their gear and draw additional equipment such as extra line and wire. Once the explosives were prepared and deemed ready, the students would get the operational order which described how the mission would actually be executed. There are a hundred little things which must be done to ensure an operations order is given properly and within set time constraints. By now the students were not being ordered to do this or that by their command structure. They knew what was required and were asking how they could further help. We were creating teammates, or men who didn't need to be run down and cornered to get a task done.

After the operations order was given to the cadre's satisfaction the men would move their equipment to the beach where it would be loaded aboard a beach landing craft. The LCPR was painted with a shark whose open red mouth exposed its razor sharp white teeth from the bow. A large eye was painted above the mouth on either side of the craft. When the boat was at high speed it looked like "JAWS" on the warpath to a swimmer waiting to be picked up. An IBS with a towing bridle securing it to the LCPR was present to allow for swimmer cast and recovery.

The deploying team was taken to sea. As the LCPR began its run an instructor in the forward end of the boat would raise his hand signaling the first pair of swimmers to slip over the gunnel. From here they moved to the outboard main tube of the IBS. The next pair followed them into the IBS, with everyone moving forward a position in preparation for their own drop. Watching the shoreline the instructor would drop his hand, sending the first pair of swimmers into the water at high speed. At the same moment another crew member would throw the demolitions bag over the stern so the swim team could recover it and begin their task. Needless to say, all eyes were glued to the instructor and his signal hand.

By this point in their training the students were very good at this procedure. They found themselves placed in a line parallel to the beach, each swim team roughly five meters apart. They would begin swimming in toward the beach while towing their explosives behind them, looking for their underwater targets along the way as identified by the charts they'd made.

When a target was found the hard work began. Coming over an obstacle the swim team would review their plan of attack within seconds. They would deflate the flotation device on the demolition haversacks with their knife, which was normally a Navy issue combat/fighting knife. The divers would then hyperventilate and conduct a foot first surface dive together. Reaching the obstacle they would hang their haversacks to it by the sack's carrying straps. The obstacles were most often concrete and steel structures with plenty of protrusions from which to attach the sacks. Returning to the surface they would begin diving one at a time to work on the obstacle. This pace allowed each man to rest for a while, plus it provided an on-site safety swimmer as each could observe the other during the combined effort. A sash cord was pulled from the haversack and then tied behind the obstacle. Extra line was pulled around and tied, with final efforts made to secure the explosive charge to the obstacle.

While swim teams were working on the obstacles other divers would be preparing the trunk line. This line was tied onto a horn, or protrusion, of an obstacle at one flank of the entire obstacle field with the team then swimming a role of wire-bound detonating cord to the opposite flank, securing it to a horn on the final obstacle in the field. They would then secure what were called branch lines between the trunk lines thereby completing the firing field. This procedure would be repeated until all the obstacles were tied in and could be blown at one time. One last administrative branch line would be run from the inboard trunk line to the beach. If the sea surge caused the detonation to cut off, or in case of a misfire, the field could be blown from the beach by an assigned instructor.

The individual swim teams would pull two lines of detonating cord from each haversack, tying these into the trunk line. Instructors would always be swimming the field to check the swim teams' work as they finished. If something wasn't done right it would have to be corrected by the students and then rechecked by an instructor. Once the entire obstacle field was wired and checked, the swimmers would head out to sea and form a recovery line. One swim team would stay at the field to act as fuse pullers. The LCPR would make its run to recover our swimmers with a second boat following. Its job was to snatch anyone who missed the first pick-up run out of the water. This was fairly common as swimmers by this point were very tired. When the boats finally had all swimmers onboard they would head out to sea. A red smoke was pulled to signal the fuse pullers to attach their firing boards to the seaward trunk line. Now they were cleared to ignite the fuses. Once done, they would swim like crazy out to sea where they would be picked up.

The fuses were timed to go off in twenty minutes. After the massive explosion took place the boats would wait an additional thirty minutes for an instructor to check the field. It was important that the entire obstacle field be destroyed with one shot. Once this was done the students went back to the classroom for a critique. They would receive their next mission with beach clearing tasks the work at hand for the next several days until all the placed obstacles brought in by Chief Price were destroyed.

Training continued. The days were filled with demolition work using explosives the students had only been exposed to in the classroom. They would clear underwater channels using an Mk-8 explosive hose. Other challenges might include a demolition ambush on land. Physical training increased to include a four-mile ocean swim and twenty-two-mile forced march conducted at night. Night training placed the students in an outdoor classroom which provided them with the opportunity to scout and patrol using all the techniques and classes we'd taught up until then. San Clemente Island put everything together in one tightly wrapped, well-oiled package. Most frogmen and SEALs when they talk about training only recall the misery and pain of the event. What they forget, because it was in the course of their normal day, are the skills that were inbred into them, skills meant to keep them and their teammates alive in combat.

I remember one of the night ops with my last class on San Clemente. The target for that evening was a radio transmitting station built by Bud Jurick and I a week before. At night it did not look like the intended target, a lesson everyone learned when working by day or by night against selected target sites. The student officer had briefed his men well and they, in turn, had likewise properly prepared for the mission. The IBS was loaded and put to sea. Bud and I took the ambulance and drove to the target site, moving to a vantage point above the beach so we could watch the students arrive to do their thing.

This was late in 1967 and I was rotating back to SEAL Team One after this class. My mind was filled with questions. Were the men I'd helped train ready to go to a team? Had we done all we could to prepare them for war? Would I have the privilege of taking some of my former students into combat with me? Were we now as ready as we could be? I was a first class petty officer and there was a good chance, given all I'd seen and done to date in the teams, that I'd become a combat action platoon's leading petty officer. Did I have what it took to keep my men alive? This last question burned me inside with its implications.

I started sharing my thoughts and concerns with Bud as we waited high above the darkened beach. The sound of the surf smacking the hard-packed sand at the water's edge kept us both company as we searched the sea for our waterborne raiders. After listening to me for a while Bud offered his thoughts. "Bear, I've known since Machen was killed what you've been carrying around inside you. I've watched your attitude about the students and their training change. The men we've sent over have done well and these men, here tonight, will do well too.

"You've always looked on them as teammates even though they're still just students. I know it's been a long rehearsal for you as well as for them. Don't worry about it. You're going to be all right."

Bud stopped, pointing at two black apparitions which had just appeared at the surf line. It was our swimmer scouts looking for the best, most secure place to bring their teammates in on the beach. I appreciated Jurick's professional as well as personal reinforcement. He was right and I could only agree. It had indeed been a long rehearsal.

8

Tools of War

*He trains my hands for battle, so that my arms can
bend a bow of bronze.*

—Samuel 22:35

On December 27, 1967, I received new orders taking me
back to SEAL Team One in Coronado, California. The team
was located across the street from the amphibious base in
Coronado, a beehive of activity which included and supported not only SEALs but UDT frogmen, as well. SEAL
Team One had been built a new headquarters building in
1966 which was connected to the UDT complex sharing the
same compound. In short, SEALs and frogmen were once
again together as a community.

The team had changed in many ways since my leaving in
1964. SEAL One had grown from ten officers and fifty
enlisted men in 1962 to over two hundred officers and
enlisted by 1968. Many old and trusted faces were there to
greet me upon my return, with not a few war stories shared
between us due to so many of the men having seen action in
Vietnam. There were quite a few men I knew from past
UDT training classes and seventeen graduates from Class
42 had just come from across the street to join our ranks.
They were preparing to leave for Fort Benning in Georgia to
attend parachute training. In six years the team had come a
long way.

After checking in I was assigned to the armory. There was

a great deal of work to be done and the team had an armory like no one else's. A primary requirement for any SEAL was to have maximum firepower available to him in combat. This meant specialized weapons and ordnance. The development of such materials had begun in earnest in 1967 due to our unique operational environment. We had an exceptionally high priority when it came to all manner of firepower and explosives, much of what could not be found in the normal Navy supply system. Taking a tour of the armory I found over a hundred pieces of ordnance equipment then being either tested or fielded, with other items still in the developmental stage.

Competition for what the armory held was intense. Our time and space were spread out over three different training elements which made coordination a number one concern of mine. Those SEALs first in line belonged to the platoons soon to deploy to Vietnam. Their needs revolved around weapons for the ranges, training operations, preparing their weapons for deployment, securing spare parts, and staging their weapons and other equipment for shipment overseas. Next came the students who were participating in the six-week cadre course, or SBI. These fellas showed up at all times of the day and night, moving equipment to their training camp near Niland, California. Whenever they returned from training the armory had to be opened and the weapons cleaned, inspected, and then checked in. Since the students were all eager to be released we worked hard and fast, with instructors and all armory personnel pitching in together. Finally there were the students attending the four-week special operations program which provided SEAL advisors to the PHOENIX program. Their camp was located in the mountains east of San Diego and weapon support was critical.

Naturally all three elements believed their needs should be our highest priority at the armory. To their way of thinking we needed to be open twenty-four hours a day, or at least whenever they were in town . . . even if elements were back on base at the same time! Security was my number one priority and it was strictly enforced. Not just anyone was given a key to what many considered a giant firearms toy box. Coordination was a big headache for myself and the other armory personnel, but we made the best of it.

The combat action platoons were just beginning to use shotguns on patrol in Vietnam, these carried by our point-men. The first choice for such a weapon was a modified pump action shotgun with a choke. The choke would expand the shot as it left the muzzle and the one we decided upon was called a "duckbill." Other shotguns were being developed and tested too. Some were semiautomatic or full automatic, others used extended magazine tubes. We used primarily OO buck in Vietnam, each round containing nine buckshot pellets. Some SEALs preferred #4 buck with its twenty-seven pellets per shell. This round wasn't as effective as OO buck in terms of being lethal, but it offered the operator a more generous shot pattern when fired.

We used the standard M60 military machine gun, but this weapon also was highly modified for SEAL operations. We cut the barrel off just forward of the gas port, then re-threaded it in order to reattach the flash suppressor. The rather heavy and awkward bipod was removed for two reasons. First, it always got hung up in thick jungle terrain and second, we hardly used it for its intended purpose. Individual SEALs often removed the issue butt stock and replaced it with the aircraft butt stock seen on Army and Navy helicopters. All of these modifications made the M60 lighter, shorter, and more easy to wield during a firefight. Our experience in Vietnam proved we needed the heavy punch of the 7.62 NATO bullet the weapon fired, and the SEAL version of the M60 made it an excellent close quarters fighting weapon in the jungle.

Every individual SEAL was assigned a team number and then issued an M16 rifle and .38 caliber S&W revolver or 9mm pistol. These weapons were all marked with the team number so we had strict control over where the guns went and to whom. The operator cleaned his own weapons, and if he didn't, they didn't get cleaned for him. Very few of these items actually saw use in Vietnam but the men kept them spotless and well oiled. One thing about SEALs is their appreciation for a fine gun.

The M79 grenade launcher came our way, this handy item firing a 40mm grenade much like a handheld mortar although it resembles an oversized single barrel, sawed-off shotgun. I believe the M79 was very effective in support of SEAL infiltrations when used on the boats which took us in, but on patrol they had their drawbacks. The worst of these was the fact it was an individual weapon, meaning someone ended up carrying both a rifle or machine gun and the M79 on patrol. We soon saw this problem solved when the XM148 grenade launcher was introduced. This was a compact launcher which mounted underneath the barrel of the M16. The package was lightweight, offered enormous firepower options, and was usually carried by the radioman.

SEALs trained with 60mm and 81mm mortars, the 57mm recoilless rifle, and the .50 caliber heavy machine gun. All of these could be found at a SEAL firebase and were used in either the offense, defense, or support mode. There were special use weapons too. The MK22 pistol—known as a "hush puppy"—was a SEAL trademark of sorts. The pistol was a modified S&W Model 39 in 9mm. An MK3 suppressor was threaded to the specially made barrel and subsonic ammunition was used to make the weapon effectively quiet when used. The pistol got its name because we used them against dogs which the VC often put out as their first line of warning against our patrols. If a dog started barking it could cause us to lose the element of surprise which is so important to a successful operation. The enemy's own AK47 assault rifle was also a favorite tool of the trade and we used these for special operations or as a matter of individual preference.

But there was one weapon which captured my imagination and attention immediately. It was the Stoner 63, a 5.56mm weapon system configured as a light machine gun.

To say we SEALs were excited about the Stoner 63 is an understatement. The weapon had already seen combat in Vietnam when I arrived in 1967 and good reports were flowing back to Coronado about its performance. Predeployment platoons were training with the Stoner at Niland and were constantly devising ways to stage an extra one to take with them to Vietnam.

To my knowledge we were the only troops to employ the Stoner as a light machine gun during the war. I have seen pictures of Marines firing Stoner rifle and carbine versions in Vietnam, but these were experimental deployments of the weapon in a variant form. Also, I am aware of unconfirmed reports the Army's Special Forces have claimed their operators used the Stoner system too.

I wanted to learn all I could about the system. It had been designed by a former Marine, Mr. Eugene Stoner. He'd likewise designed the original version of what was now the M16 rifle. Cadillac Gage in Warren, Michigan was selected to manufacture roughly 2,400 prototype Stoner systems which were then tested by the Army and Marine Corps. The Corps conducted extensive testing in 1963-64 and designated the system as the XM207. They were looking for a rifle and light machine gun which used the same ammunition, making logistics and the grunt in the field's equipment load easier. The Stoner 63 was designed to fit this Marine Corps requirement and they were in favor of adopting it. General Wallace Greene, then the USMC Commandant put this in writing but in the meantime the Army had just adopted the M16 and elected to retain the M60 light machine gun. The secretary of the army lobbied the secretary of defense to block the sale of the Stoner system to the Marine Corps, offering the Corps needed to adopt the M16 so as to simplify overall service logistics.

The Army won.

But as a result of the Marines' testing of the system a number of modifications and improvements were made by the manufacturer. These included a stainless steel gas cylinder, an increased barrel life from 8,000 to 30,000 rounds and a longer retracting handle. Cadillac Gage expected other changes were in the works and redesignated the new and improved weapon as the 63A. The SEAL community was not under the same restraints as the Corps and the Navy adopted the 63A light machine gun (LMG) and typeclassed it as the MK23 Mod O for our exclusive use. Feedback from those using the system in Vietnam continued to find its way to Cadillac Gage until 1973. The 63A remained such where the manufacturer was concerned, with SEALs calling it the MK23 Mod O regardless of modifications or evolutions in the weapon.

With my manual in hand I began intensely studying the Stoner. I discovered the first Stoners we'd received were not only LMGs but the complete weapon system! Searching around behind the security cage of the armory I found a large wooden box filled with component assemblies. These allowed me to configure the rifle, carbine, light machine gun belt-fed, tripod machine gun belt-fed, and light machine gun magazine fed Stoner. I decided the best way to learn was to put them all together and go to the range. Building one of each weapon I headed for Niland and ran the guns through their paces. The results proved my teammates were right. The best configuration for the 63A was the 150-round drum magazine fed light machine gun. It gave us maximum firepower and reliability in the field and that was our goal.

Still, I was fascinated by the Stoner carbine. I liked the way it fit my hands due to the weapon's eight-pound weight and perfect balance. It was only thirty-five inches long and if I relied on the folding stock this could be dropped to twenty-seven inches. We'd gotten the new 30-round M16 magazines by now, an item which was then very hard to come by. The carbine was magazine fed and the new 30-rounders gave it some serious firepower for so compact a weapon. I learned the Marines had tested the carbine version and designated it as the Stoner Carbine XM23. It had performed well for them on the range which was my experience too. Its weight and balance allowed me to engage a target at one hundred yards and hold a very tight shot group. By pushing the selector switch from "SEMI" to "AUTO," I could cut the same target in half with a few short bursts.

The carbine version of the Stoner would become my weapon of choice in Vietnam, and according to my teammates it became my trademark in the teams. Returning to the light machine gun version I had to ask myself why our patrol and assistant patrol leaders hadn't taken advantage of the carbine more often in the field? I filed the question away for later thought and spent many satisfying hours putting rounds downrange with Eugene Stoner's LMG.

In Vietnam the SEALs operated in what were unfavorable conditions at best. Our environment produced mud, sand, saltwater, and heavy, unforgiving rains which took their toll on both SEALs and SEAL equipment. Like the men, the Stoner stood up and took anything Mother Nature could dish out. The 63A became our favorite weapon of choice, with its many variations and modifications adapting to the combat environment of Vietnam nicely.

The MK23 we fielded in 1968 was a left-hand fed weapon with a cyclic rate of fire of between 700 to 1,000 rounds per minute. This rate was set using the LMG's gas regulator. We appreciated the 150-round drum magazine and used it from 1966 until 1972. There were also plastic bandoleers (boxes) which could be hung from the left side of the weapon where the feed tray was located. These held 100 rounds of 5.56mm ammo. Most of the operators I know rejected these as they placed the weapon off-balance contrary to the drum which hung directly below the gun's receiver and actually added to its stability during firing. A 250-round drum was developed at China Lake, California, but it proved to be too bulky and heavy for our use. Some enterprising SEALs jury-rigged the Russian or Chinese RPD drum magazines so they could be fitted to work with the Stoner 63A and these worked fairly well.

In war not all things go the way you want them to regardless of the tool or quality of preparation. Word came back to us at headquarters that teammate BM1 Walter Pope was killed by nonhostile fire somewhere in the Kien Hoa Province, RVN, on April 29, 1968. As it turned out Pope's platoon was aboard an armored landing craft with him and his fire team forward inside the bow compartment. His Stoner LMG had begun firing on its own, the rounds ricocheting inside the small space and devastating everything they struck. When a cat goes crazy and you try to control it, sometimes the thought process is to hug that wild cat in close and smother it against you. That's what Pope did according to his teammates that day. He stood up and pulled the muzzle of the weapon into his body to protect his fire team and took forty rounds in the stomach. Still, other men were wounded but none died.

The investigation of the accident showed they were just arriving at their infiltration point when the Stoner went off. The weapon offers a feedcover and receiver group that locks to the trigger group using two pins (a pivot pin and a take down pin). The bolt is held to the rear in the receiver group by the sear located in the trigger group. If the rear take down pin comes out for any reason the receiver pivots upward, disengaging the sear from the bolt. The result is a runaway gun if rounds are present.

It was determined the vibrations coming through the boat hull jimmied the take down pin free as Pope was resting the weapon's butt stock against the boat's deck, muzzle up. The pin itself has a tiny wire detent spring holding it in place. It was never discovered if this spring had been worn or if the pin wasn't fully engaged. What was determined was we needed Cadillac Gage to correct this deadly fault and they did so immediately after we went to work on the problem at the armory.

Our armory personnel found the take down pin for the carbine and LMG feed tray cover were manufactured differently than the pin for the LMG receiver group. The carbine/LMG pins were made of two parts which threaded together. The first part of the pin fit the holes in the receiver and trigger group. This pin was hollow and had female threads on the inside. The second part of the pin was smaller and had a male thread pattern. Both were to be threaded together, one from the left side of the receiver and the other from the right side. This would secure both groups together as a single unit. We passed this along to Cadillac Gage and within days the new pins for the LMGs were on their way. Once installed, this tragic malfunction never repeated itself.

One of the USMC tests put the 7.62mm M60 up against the 5.56 Stoner LMG. The two weapons were fired at multiple targets on a one hundred-yard range. The larger dispersion pattern of the M60 LMG resulted in more than one target being hit with each burst of fire. The Stoner, on the other hand, demonstrated such a tight pattern when fired that its burst did not cover more than one target at a time. For this reason the Stoner came in second for hits on multiple targets due to its greater accuracy.

Depending on the reason for the test, did the Stoner "fail"? The 63A is the only light machine gun I have ever fired that delivered automatic fire with a high degree of accuracy from the shoulder. Placing two Stoners with one M60 in a SEAL fire team delivered a firepower and capability to engage various categories of targets which was unequaled. In our case, the line of march looked much like this; Pointman/Stoner, Patrol Leader/CAR 15, Radioman/M16-XM148, Stoner, M60, Stoner, and Rear Security/CAR 15. Each platoon changed the order around depending upon the weapons available and what the team felt comfortable with. Maximum automatic firepower delivered with accuracy was the right way to go.

Ammunition for the 63A came in standard 5.56mm ball and tracer. The Stoner used a method of feeding which required a belt using a disintegrating metallic link similar to the standard M13 push through link as seen with the M60. The ball ammo left the muzzle at 3,250 feet per second with approximately 1,300 foot pounds of energy. When the round hit a human target it often began to tumble due to the high velocity and the bullet's light weight. I have witnessed a single such round enter the rib cage on one side of a body and take the arm off at the shoulder on the opposite side. Regardless of its size, or what ammunition/gun writers might say, the 5.56mm is a killing round without question.

Still, the Stoner carbine (now known as the XM23) intrigued me. I liked the weapon. The cocking handle was located on the top of the receiver and the carbine was fitted with a folding stock which made it handy in tight quarters. The XM23 also fired from the closed bolt position whereas the LMG fired from the open. I appreciated this feature. In my hands the carbine performed better than the M16 or CAR15 and I knew I would most likely be placed in the position of either rear security or assistant patrol leader, or even patrol leader once back in Vietnam. To me, the Stoner carbine was the best weapon I could have under these circumstances. The gunnery officer in charge of the armory as well as the new platoon officer didn't have any objections to my training with the carbine. I took issue magazine pouches for the twenty-round magazines and modified them to hold Stoner thirty-round mags. This weapon served me well on two tours to Vietnam without once ever failing under combat conditions. No, not even once.

Stoner 63 historian Ralph Stafford shared information taken from three letters written by Army Captain Mack W. Gwinn, Jr., to Cadillac Gage dated from January to February 1969. Captain Gwinn reports that on January 17, 1969, his troops captured a Stoner LMG found in a VC weapons cache stored underwater for some time. The weapon was badly pitted but was otherwise functional. Along with the LMG there was a drum magazine with more than seventy rounds in it. Captain Gwinn wrote that less than ten minutes after hauling out the Stoner the drum and its contents were fired without malfunction! Gwinn later learned from an enemy POW the VC had captured the weapon over a year previously and much of the time it was in the underwater cache.

Scrounging some necessary parts for the weapon from some SEALs in the area the captain rebuilt the gun. He changed the barrel and the butt stock and began taking the LMG with him on operations. In one of his letters he describes taking down two Vietcong at over six hundred yards, the Stoner supported on a rice paddy dike. Gwinn was so impressed by the 63A he wrote his superiors and encouraged them to obtain and issue Stoners to specific Special Forces units. His letter dated February 6 reveals he had fired twelve thousand rounds up until then and only suffered a broken feed pawl. My favorite comment from the captain was "Most people who see the weapon can't believe it still works much less that I use it in combat." Captain Gwinn's letters are a Stoner 63A testimony by themselves.

SEAL teammates during the 1960s were often fond of saying the only thing that never changes in the Navy is that there will always be more changes. Not only changes in the way we operated took place, but changes in the number of SEALs sent to Vietnam and their equipment occurred as well. The Stoner 63A was no exception, as I've mentioned earlier. In 1969 the teams deployed the 63A with a new quick change 16-inch fluted barrel. This item was designated the MK23 Commando barrel. It made the weapon easier to handle and became the barrel of choice for our pointmen. However, the gas port was now almost at the end of the muzzle which caused port pressure to drop immediately as soon as the bullet left the end of the barrel. This resulted in faster piston acceleration and this sometimes caused problems with reliability.

Some Commando barrels were used on left-hand feed 63A weapons already in service and relying on 150-round drum magazines. The new 63A gave the operator a right-hand feed cover as well as 100-round plastic ammo boxes which centered under the receiver like the drums did. This new evolution made the Stoner lighter (14 pounds 12 ounces as compared to 16 pounds with the older model) and balanced the ammunition weight center of the weapon.

The feed cocking lever was relocated from the right side to below the forestock. The new right-hand feed prevented spin back of empty (and hot) brass into the receiver itself. This most often resulted in a temporary jam which took the gun out of action for precious moments as it had to be cleared by the gunner. Now such a malfunction was a thing of the past. We machined a four-inch cocking handle to replace the new one-inch handle under the forestock. One inch was too small and easy to miss under the stress of a firefight, or to slip off if your hands were slippery or wet. New butt stocks of a stronger material were realized, with the sling swivel moved to the top of these stocks. This made carrying the LMG in the combat ready position easier and more secure. All of these and other changes initiated by my teammates were dutifully passed along to Cadillac Gage during the course of our war in Vietnam.

Throughout the 1960s the Stoner 63A or MK23 Mod 0 in all variations and configurations played a major role in SEAL Teams One and Two. The Stoners and the teammates who carried them are part of Naval Special Warfare history, and I am both humbled and proud to include myself.

Because of Eugene Stoner the SEALs were truly armed with our "bows of bronze."

9

Chubbie's Raiders

Since my youngest years I've always had a problem with my weight. It was a struggle to maintain myself at 175 pounds even while with the teams and I have to admit I was a bit sensitive about the subject. Until, that is, I became a member of ALFA platoon. ALFA and HOTEL platoons were running operations from the USS *Weiss* APD 135, just off the coast of Vietnam. Our platoon had a combat action platoon for about four months and I'd reached a trim 160 pounds during this period. I was one proud SEAL! However, I was about to find out that my teammates still thought of me as "chubby."

In every frogman's war bag you would find a reversible blue and gold (Navy colors) T-shirt. These were worn when doing PT, to keep the chill off after a long ocean swim, and so on. My guys wanted to remind HOTEL platoon who they were and how proud they were of it. Turning the gold side of the T-shirt out each man carefully printed "Chubbie's Raiders" with a dark marking pen on his shirt, complete with a cartoonlike drawing of me. Then they put them on and showed up on deck, much to my surprise and HOTEL platoon's delight.

Not to be outdone, a SEAL I'll call Ski did the same. But

his crude message read "Chubbies' Raiders Are Faggots" and when he showed up in it on the fantail, all creation hit the ceiling. ALFA responded by throwing Ski over the side . . . at night . . . while the ship was underway! If we notified the captain that a man was overboard I knew we'd be in *big* trouble, no doubt about it.

Now a SEAL going into the ocean is no big deal. The sea is our environment and we're as comfortable in the water as most folks are on dry land. However, it was dark and the ship was underway and we were in potentially hostile waters as there was a war on. Someone said we ought to throw Ski a line but it took us some time to find one, with our teammate all the while swimming for his life. Finally finding a line which would do, it ended up taking three throws before Ski could be hauled back aboard ship.

I knew I should chew my guys out for their reaction to Ski's T-shirt, but I just couldn't do so. HOTEL's soaked SEAL took his dunking in good humor and all of us needed the comic relief. For me personally it was great to feel the pride of belonging to a bunch of guys who were more than just a platoon, but the best teammates I could ask for. To understand why I would feel this way we have to go back ten months when ALFA, or "Chubbie's Raiders," were formed.

It was while I was working administratively at the armory that I was assigned to ALFA platoon. Seven of its members were from Class 42 and had been sent off to jump school. In addition, the platoon was short its full compliment of fourteen operators so I became a body meant to bring the platoon to strength when we all got back together. One of my armory duties was an explosives driver. Many of the trips I made hauling explosives for training were to the SEAL Basic Indoctrination (SBI) facility at Niland.

I enjoyed the trip over the Cuyamaca Mountains which were quite pretty. However, when I hit the desert below I also hit the desert heat which was brutal. I remember the truck's firewall becoming so hot against the bottoms of my boots that I would pull the fuel hand throttle out and open the windshield, poking my feet out the window just to cool them down. In retrospect, I'm sure it made for an odd sight to other drivers on the road. Here's a military truck carrying explosives roaring across the desert with its driver hanging both feet out over the hood, a contented look on his face and one hand on the wheel.

The Niland SBI training site wasn't much more than a collection of old Navy trailers parked together on a piece of property. The Chocolate Mountain bombing range was just three miles from Niland and we could shoot or explode just about any kind of weapon or ordnance we could get our hands on. When I went to instructor duty at UDT Training, the SEALs were having a tough time acquiring a range for things like this. Except for the Marine base at Camp Pendleton there wasn't a proper open range for SEALs to practice their trade. Even then, the Marines rightfully enjoyed first priority and even if we scheduled training nine months out it could—and sometimes was—canceled in favor of the Corps. Niland was a "must have" for the SEALs. Two small rivers ran into the Salton Sea, both studded with heavy undergrowth along their banks. Niland was a great training area for night operations. It offered us a range we could use for weapons and explosives training and was located in southern California.

As it would turn out Niland and I would once again come together although many years later and under far different circumstances.

ALFA's new paratroopers soon returned from Fort Benning and were granted leave so they could enjoy some free time. The platoon began training together with weapons, medical, and land navigation our first priorities. Word came down we'd been selected to attend the six-week SBI course in preparation for deployment to Vietnam. SEAL Team One was commissioned in January 1962, and its plank-owners went through a four-week course in Marine basic infantry tactics and antiguerrilla warfare with the Marines at Pendleton in March of the same year. I was sent to the Army's ranger school and was pleased to be the first Navy SEAL to graduate from this impressive light infantry leadership school in May 1962. They taught me a lot there, much of which I would later use with success in Vietnam. In June of '62, Jungle Warfare School in Panama followed, with my knowledge base growing by leaps and bounds as a result of what this fine program had to offer. But this was 1962 and times had changed by 1968. SEALs returning from Vietnam were sharing valuable experiences with their teammates and SBI had been developed to prepare us in the specifics which we would face in Southeast Asia. I knew I had much to learn and was eager for the opportunity. To be attending SBI with my new platoon made everything that much better.

Our new platoon officer was Lt. (jg) Rip Bliss. Although new—like most of us in the platoon—Bliss would go on to become a fine Navy officer. I learned to respect him more and more as the platoon developed into a fighting force to be reckoned with. Second in command was WO Scott Lyon. Mr. Lyon had already seen action in Vietnam as an enlisted SEAL with SEAL Team Two. He was a warrant gunner and that captured my respect from the beginning. Scott Lyon had been there and he knew what we needed when it came to relevant training. He joined the platoon at SBI although he didn't have to, which demonstrated his commitment to us. My level of respect for Mr. Lyon was so great I'm sure it overshadowed Lt. Bliss, which could not have made things easy for him. I guess that's a part of human nature, sir, and I apologize if it caused you grief.

ALFA packed its war bags, checked its weapons out, and loaded the truck up for the trip to the desert. I recall it was a long ride in that 6X6, especially when we hit the heat on the desert flats. We finally arrived at the compound, stowed our gear, and were assigned to our trailers. That first night the cadre took us to the range for a night firing exercise, which was just fine by me.

It began with a demonstration which included two M60s and four Stoner LMGs. The tracer rounds lit the desert up and all of us were duly impressed with the level of firepower now available to us. We'd loaded our M16 magazines with a tracer every fourth round for the night's activities and it was soon our turn to show our stuff. Needless to say our effort wasn't nearly as impressive as the cadre's and on the way back to the trailers we discussed who would get to carry the M60s and the Stoners over our assigned M16s.

The next morning began with our introduction to Chief Guy Stone. Stone was the senior enlisted man in charge of SBI training and I liked him from the start. He'd been in the Army during the Korean war and had the field experience which complimented stateside training. His briefing was carried out in a Southern accent he'd managed to maintain throughout his years in the military. No doubt existed in any of our minds that Stone was serious about SBI. Chief Stone was a committed frogman who, while attached to UDT 12 in 1970, would earn the Navy Cross for his actions against the Vietcong.

We loaded up a truck and headed back to the range after the chief's briefing. Once there the platoon went on-line and began moving through the desert, firing our weapons every time the left foot hit the ground. The objective of the exercise was to train us to keep contact with the man on the left and right of us while firing live ammunition. We did this over and over, and then over again. As we improved the exercises progressed in difficulty. Soon we were firing while leapfrogging from individual position to position. Then we began training to attack targets from the flank in squad-sized elements, all the while firing live ammo. ALFA did this so much we nicknamed Guy "Left Foot Stonie" and the name stuck for as long as I knew him.

Tired, dirty, and often a bit scuffed up from rolling around in the desert the platoon looked forward to cleaning weapons at day's end. Standing around the cleaning table we could relax and let off steam. The men joked about the day's activities and mishaps, and I enjoyed getting to know them better under these spartan conditions. Any platoon I've ever been associated with always has a self-appointed morale booster. Ours was no exception.

John Ware became the caretaker of ALFA's spirit. He demonstrated a quality of character that at times made him the most important member of the platoon. John always sensed when it was time to turn it on and I never knew him to get out of line with his unique brand of humor. Ware was an excellent pointman and worked for the second squad. He was slim and alert and could always be counted on. To this day John Ware is there for his teammates. You just have to call and ask and he's on a plane to be by your side. I don't think of John as just a friend and teammate from the past, but as a friend and teammate whose friendship just keeps on growing with time. I'm not sure, but I'd bet John was the ringleader in the "Chubbie's Raiders" incident aboard the *Weiss.*

Usually around four o'clock in the afternoon we'd get a warning order to prepare for an operation that night. Weapons and equipment were checked and double-checked. Magazines were stripped out and then reloaded with blank ammunition, blank adapters attached to our weapons so they'd fire the blanks just like the real thing. Before darkness fell around us the instructors would drag an old blackboard out and one of our officers would give the patrol order. It takes a while for dark to settle in the summer and we used this period of time to our advantage in preparing for the exercise right up until the last possible minute.

The SBI training missions were as realistic as they could possibly be made. Most of the men didn't realize how much so because they hadn't worked in Vietnam's Delta region yet. Some of the exercises were river ambushes where we actually attacked captured Vietnamese sampans! Other times we'd snatch a prisoner from a hootch exactly like the ones we'd find in Vietnam. There were times the platoon was ambushed on purpose to test our ability to react and survive. I remember we came out on top during a couple of these. Even to this day I believe this was the best training for war I have ever received, given the kind of combat SEALs conduct.

It was halfway through SBI when ALFA realized who would be our M60 gunners. Don Crawford and Paul Bourne were naturals with the weapon and had developed personal attachments to the guns which all of us could see. Bourne was tall, quiet, and very strong. He handled the '60 as if it were a part of him and could make it talk like no one else in the platoon. Crawford was smaller than Paul but just as strong. This attribute was important as the M60, even after being modified by ourselves, was a heavy weapon whose ammunition load required a small mule to tote. Crawford's skill with the LMG matched Bourne's and between the two of them we knew we could count on accurate and constant supporting fires when the chips were down. Don became a gunners mate and left the Navy after completing one tour of Vietnam. The next time I saw him was in 1986 at our

SEAL/UDT reunion in Coronado. He was reporting aboard SEAL Team One as their new operations officer. Proud of him? You bet I am!

Training continued and we began spending more time with special weapons. The 57 recoilless rifle became a platoon favorite. You needed to fire the weapon with your body at a forty-five degree angle to the tube because it belched flame from both ends. I never used the 57 in Vietnam but in 1970 we did come to rely on a 90mm recoilless, so our training was not wasted.

ALFA trained with the 60mm and 81mm mortar, as well. Both were easy to load and fire but learning about how to get one's rounds on target took lots of classroom work and even more range time. I don't recall if we ever got beyond the trial and error point at Niland but the introduction to mortar gunnery paid off when we used these extensively in Vietnam for indirect fire support.

By the time the platoon finished SBI we knew who would be our radioman. Communications in a small unit environment are critical to the unit's survival. Radio work is a hard-earned skill and quality communicators are valued like fine wine. Larry Hubbard and Steve Frisk fit the bill perfectly. Being a radioman under fire is a job only for those who can keep a cool head and make good decisions. Larry was our corpsman and was already looked up to by all in the platoon. Naturally, we hoped never to have to use him for his primary talents. Hubbard went on to become a master chief and stayed with the teams until he retired. Steve Frisk is still in the Navy but now he is Commander Frisk with his own unit in the San Francisco area. Yes, I am wonderfully proud of both my teammates.

Back from the desert we spent a week around base and then left again. This time it was for PRU Advisor Training in preparation for supporting the PHOENIX program in Vietnam. Training would take place in the Cuyamaca Mountains in southern California. Our first night would be as aggressors for the students already in training. We were able to attend some classes on who and what the PRU were during daylight hours and I found this quite interesting. The night problems were fun but the training during the day was about the PHOENIX mission, which was to target the Vietcong infrastructure.

Easily the most important thing I learned during the training program was this: You can't get intelligence out of a dead man. Real world accounts told us a captured Vietcong cadre would talk his head off if given the motivation to do so. "Your next operation may depend upon what this man has to tell you" we were instructed in class. It made good sense to me. The cadre also impressed upon us the importance of field "impact interrogation." This was information that paid off time and time again, meaning it had a positive impact on our operations when properly collected and interpreted. One of the cadre was Gary Gallager and he was especially helpful to the platoon. Good at most everything I ever saw him do, Gary was adept at hand-to-hand combatives. Every time that man got within arm's reach of me I got hurt . . . other than that, he was great!

With this evolution in our training completed ALFA returned to Coronado. Everyone was preparing for an upcoming change of command and there wasn't a spot on base that wasn't spit shined and polished. On July 5, 1968, Lt. Comdr. David Schaible relieved Lt. Comdr. Franklin Anderson, with the ComNavAirPac Band playing on. When you're in the Navy for a while you get used to seeing men go down the gangway for the last time. I always wondered what the new man would be like and this time was no exception. Captain Schaible had been an enlisted submarine sailor in the South Pacific until 1946. He'd reenlisted at the outbreak of the Korean war and volunteered for UDT Five, but was in UDT One from 1951 until 1956. He went on to be commissioned as a naval officer and became the captain of UDT Twenty-Two on the East Coast. We knew we now had a commanding officer who'd been around, but we were soon to learn just how far around he'd been.

A week passed by before Captain Schaible asked me to step into his office. ALFA was still one man short and we discussed who was available to fill the platoon out. He felt the man needed to be a senior petty officer and I agreed. I asked the commander for some time to do some personal research and he gave me the day. The first man I spoke to was MM1 Harlen Funkhouser. I told Harlen our platoon would be deploying to Vietnam on August 15 and asked if he'd want to join us, with me being the leading petty officer. "Yes," he responded immediately, "I'll go with you."

Pleased with his response I returned to the captain's office and told him of my choice and why. I'd watched Harlen go through UDT Training and during his first go-around he'd broken his leg after "Hell Week" was over with. Rather than quit, Harlen had returned with the very next class and gone through Hell Week a second time! Needless to say he graduated from the course. Also, I'd asked him to go with ALFA and he'd said yes. Captain Schaible told me my platoon was now complete and asked me to send Funkhouser to see him.

The next morning Harlen reported to ALFA platoon. He told everyone the story of his broken leg. "We were on a run down the beach when I went down," he recalled. "The Marines were also out training and Enoch grabbed me up from the sand so hard all the buttons came off my shirt!" Harlen went on to say I told him that he was never to let a Marine see a frogman hurt and that he finished the run before reporting to sick bay. It wasn't until then he was told his leg was broken.

ALFA began training as a full platoon under our platoon officers. Lieutenant Bliss asked me to make out a list of support items we'd need and to include their cost if they couldn't be found in normal Navy stores. We had roughly three weeks before deploying overseas and I went right to work on the list. Having helped other platoons stage their equipment for deployment I was fairly well advised as to what was needed and the next day I reported to Mr. Bliss with the list in hand.

A short time later the master-at-arms contacted me and said the captain wanted to see me. When I entered the office I could tell Captain Schaible was having a bad day and he let me know it. Handing me back my list he asked if it was indeed mine. "Yes, sir," I replied.

"Don't you know this is Lieutenant Bliss's job to prepare this list?" he yelled.

"No, sir," I responded.

"Didn't you go over this list with him?"

Again the best I could come up with was a negative.

"What's this about wanting olive drab T-shirts?" the captain roared. "I've been buying my own underwear since joining the Navy and why should I buy your platoon underwear now?"

I answered that the mens' clothing allowance only covered Navy uniforms and the olive drab T-shirts were not Navy issue. Plus, we were going into a combat zone where white T-shirts would not do in a tactical situation. Schaible stopped me in midsentence and asked me to close his door and have a seat. He signed the list without a second thought. Then he told me my job was to help all the men in the platoon and not just the enlisted. That meant taking care to educate and encourage Mr. Bliss as well as anyone else.

As I was excused the captain asked me to have Mr. Bliss step into his office. The young officer was standing in the hallway when I left and I imagine he'd been able to hear every word spoken. To this day I'm sorry not to have discussed the list with him before sending it forward for signature and I felt then like I'd really let my lieutenant down. At the same time I'd learned I had a commanding officer who was second to none and who respected his enlisted men and wanted them to succeed. Still, it was a bad day for me.

In a few more days our equipment was staged and all training had been completed. We were ready to go to Vietnam. I took a week off to spend time with my wife and children. My leaving was hard on all of us, especially my wife. When the time came my family accompanied me to the North Island Naval Air Station where our plane was waiting. As gear was being loaded the men joked with their families and made to be lighthearted about the whole thing. My wife remembers them calling me "the old man" even though I was only thirty-two then. She also remembers how young they all were.

But ALFA wasn't young to me. We were all exceptionally well trained and motivated and each one of my men was ageless . . . and they were my teammates . . . and we were going to war.

10

ALFA
In-Country

The flight to Saigon in the Navy C117 was long and tiring. Landing at Tan Son Nhut Airport we could sense Saigon just out of sight from where we now stood. The cargo door slowly ground its way open revealing our equipment, which had to be off-loaded and secured as soon as possible. The heat of Vietnam has often been described but there is no description for it. It bows over those who have never experienced its ferocity and humbles those who have suffered its fiery blast before. I remember hearing Scott Lyon mutter under his breath, "I cannot believe I'm back again. . . ." Since my first trip to Vietnam the airport had expanded greatly. Things were certainly different than they were in 1963.

A gray Navy deuce and a half truck backed its way up to the plane's cargo door as WO Jess Tollison greeted us. Jess was with MIKE platoon, or what was left of it. ALFA was in Vietnam to relieve Jess and his men; three who were killed and the rest who were wounded during their tour. It had been a bad time for them. Mr. Tollison was one of two new officers who'd relieved the platoon's original leadership. They had been wounded in May and the platoon had needed to try and heal itself under new command.

We unloaded the plane and were on our way. For the next two days ALFA spent time at the naval support facility in Nha Be. A SEAL Team Two platoon was operating out of Nha Be, their missions taking them into the infamous Rung Sat Special Zone (RSSZ). We bunked with them while checking in and getting our "welcome to Vietnam" briefing. Soon enough we were on a Mike boat heading down the Mekong River toward Vinh Long. The night was spent with JULIETT platoon and it was great seeing old teammates from Team One. The platoon chief was John Fietch and I bled him for all the information I could get in such a short time. A good man and trusted comrade, John gave me all the help he could.

Morning found us back onboard the Mike boat and on the river. As we sailed toward a point of land the PBR sailors called "Snoopy's Nose" the river nearly doubled in size. It not only became wider, it forked as well. The fork to the north became the My Tho River with the one to the south becoming the Ham Loung. The widest part of the river above this fork would be our home for the next three months. YRBM-18 was a yard craft with three decks above the waterline. It had large flat bottom barges on both the port and starboard sides, with three barges to the stern. One of the stern barges had a large sheet metal building which was used as a club. The other two were meant to tie up two PBRs (Patrol Boat, River) sections. These were Section 534 which covered operations downriver and Section 535, whose area of responsibility was upriver. There was a LCPL and LSSC also present from our Mobile Support Team, or MST.

Our Mike boat came alongside of the tiny floating city and we were escorted to a covered area topside aft to store our gear. Personal metal footlockers and weapons lockers saw quick attention, with equipment lockers taken care of as well. Our sleeping quarters were below decks and a bunk was assigned to each team member. Later we were given a small office where platoon records could be kept, and administrative actions could take place.

Up the north fork on the My Tho there was an Army base called Dong Tam. Flying out of this base was a naval air unit (HAL-3) which supported SEAL and riverine force operations in the region. Called Seawolves the Navy HU-1 helicopters were outfitted with miniguns which provided massive and accurate aerial fire support for us. All SEAL platoons in Vietnam would sooner or later have their bacon saved by the Seawolves. These pilots and their crews risked their lives for men they might have never met time and time again. A common and very special bond developed between the two units and it has never been broken.

Down on the Ham Loung rested the city of Ben Tra. It was the home of the Kien Hoa Provincial Reconnaissance Unit, or PRU. The unit's SEAL advisor was one Frank Bomar, a Team One veteran. ALFA platoon would be engaged in joint operations with Frank's PRU. Because of the working relationship between Bomar and ourselves a mutually beneficial exchange of intelligence and other operational considerations existed. Kien Hoa would be our target area for the next ninety days. The support was in place and the stage was set. It was show time!

The platoon settled in for the next forty-eight hours and prepared for our first operation. This would be critical as it would test us as no training exercise or course had. If it went well, our spirit and morale would be sky-high and we'd know we could work as a team from the get-go. If anything but the worst of luck affected us, then rebuilding would have to occur and that would take time.

We first received a briefing on the area of operations to include a detailed map study. It wasn't much of a problem to obtain an area to conduct a mission in as we simply requested clearance through the Navy Operations center (NOC) on the YRBM. This office cleared us through the Army tactical operations center, or TOC, at Dong Tam. TOCs in district villages were usually compromised due to ARVN counterparts in the intelligence area being penetrated by VC agents. However, U.S. TOCs were considered to be secure.

We began by working with RS 535. Our second night aboard the PBR we made contact at Snoopy's Nose running into a large enemy troop movement using sampans to cross the river, even though the SEALs were not involved in this unit's operations. The PBRs ran in pairs and the first of these moved upriver to distract the VC. As they kept their attention on the boat the sampans began crossing the river behind it, never suspecting a second boat was hanging back and watching them. When the sampans were in the middle of the river the PBRs went to work and had the upper hand from the first shot fired. A bunker on the north side of the river opened up in support of the VC and although its fire was ineffective the PBR gunners were forced to deal with it. The bunker, well constructed and hidden with great expertise, had caused this same problem before. It became an ALFA platoon target.

It was two days after this action that VC bodies began to surface on the river. Mr. Lyon took his squad upriver in our LCPL to recover the dead and to check them for weapons and documents. They only found combat webbing with ammo magazines still intact on the bodies, but the body count was a solid eighteen which was very satisfying.

ALFA executed its first break-in operation on August 18. We were going to conduct a hootch search on the Ham Luong River, looking for signs of enemy presence and/or supplies and weapons. The first squad was inserted by PBR using RS 534 at about 0300 hours in the morning. The terrain was open fields and rice paddies, making movement uncomfortable as there was little cover or concealment available. The patrol moved to within five hundred yards of the target area and then stopped to observe and listen. They'd spotted a light coming from a hootch and moving in closer it was confirmed. We set up around the hut, cutting off any avenue of escape if anyone was inside. Two SEALs entered and checked it out, scaring a VC who attempted to flee. It was a bad move and we added our first enemy soldier to our body count. Moving back to the river we called for extraction by LCPL prior to daylight.

The next night the second squad undertook their first operation. It was an area reconnaissance and they were inserted from the Ham Luong at about 0300 hours. The team moved inland and found six hootches filled with elderly Vietnamese. Nothing was found and the squad came out at daylight by PBR.

Our officers put together an operation centering on Snoopy's Nose. The warning order was given on August 21 and we prepared our gear. The weapons were test fired to assure their performance in the field and then got some rest. We were taking a nonelectric firing device along on this one and made sure it and the explosive got loaded aboard the LSSC. Just before dark Mr. Lyon gave us the operations order. He suggested we could leave our boots behind and go barefoot if we wanted to. Some elected to try it, others didn't. This frogman kept his boots on.

Final inspection was held just before midnight. Ammo was checked, weapons were checked, and everyone checked each other for anything that might be missing, not properly carried, or noisy. Anything that might give off a shine was taped or somehow covered up. We duct taped and spray painted any problem areas. Our face camouflage was heavily applied in whatever pattern or design the individual preferred. Hands and neck areas were likewise painted. By the time these preparations were completed we looked like anyone's worst nightmare. It was no wonder the VC and friendly Vietnamese considered SEALs to be demons. We certainly looked the part and our reputation in battle only added to the growing legend.

The platoon loaded as quietly as possible into the waiting LSSC and we were soon underway. RS 535 provided two PBRs which were tagging along to relieve their boats waiting on station. Our boat moved in between the two PBRs. Slipping away from the YRBM it became very quiet. No one was speaking and I suddenly noted how very dark it was on the water. The other boats were only blips on our radar even though they were not far off our port and starboard sides. Approaching within fifty meters of the insertion point the PBRs took up their overwatch position as ours headed for the shore. The team was down low in the boat, keeping still and quiet. As the LSSC's bottom touched the thick mud of the riverbank we slipped over the sides. Empty, our craft moved out and a PBR made its way in and dropped off the second squad. I checked my watch. It was exactly 0300 hours.

ALFA lay on-line for about twenty minutes. We didn't move. It was time to take stock and listen for anything out of the ordinary. Getting in and getting out were the most dangerous times for a SEAL operation and patience was our greatest weapon. The time wore by slowly. Tall grass surrounded us with overhanging trees masking the sky. Most of the Delta in Vietnam is covered with overgrown rice paddies and palm groves laced with tropical plants. There are impenetrable barriers of nipa palm and bamboo mixed with trees. These create a single massive canopy overhead, a living jungle roof. Small canals, as well as large waterways, snake throughout the Delta. Snakes that bite and ants that sting abound, not to mention mosquitoes wanting to suck one's blood and leeches willing to compete with their vampirelike flying brethren. In the quiet you begin to hear the noise made by the millions of insects surrounding you and your teammates. Some popped, some buzzed, but many others simply slithered by or over you.

The signal came to begin moving. We fell automatically into our order of march. I pulled rear security and from this position I could only see maybe three or four of the platoon in front of me. Each SEAL kept an interval of space between himself and the next man, covering their assigned fields of fire as we'd drilled so often in training. ALFA moved slowly, taking its time and remaining alert. I recall thinking I was wet, wet all over and wet through and through. It was warm, but all of this was probably a mixture of nerves and the humidity. The platoon eased into the tall grass leaving the cover of the trees behind us. Now I could see many more of my teammates, and then the unexpected happened.

Whoomp!

Two hundred meters to our front in the treeline the sound washed over us like a sharp slap with a wet towel. ALFA split to the right and left and then came on-line. Within three minutes the morning was once again broken by the sound of a mortar. I could see the quick flash reflecting off the underside of the leaves around the tube. A bright pop of light and then nothing as the round headed toward its unknown target. It was a big tube by the sound of it. Maybe an 82mm. I noted the sound was muffled and seemed farther away than it appeared. Mr. Tollison passed the word that the tube would have a security force around it. Maybe as many as twenty-five VC given their priority on such weapons. These men would be well armed with automatic weapons. Thirty minutes went by but nothing happened.

* * *

119

This SEAL's mind was racing. How far was it to Vinh Long? John Fietch told me they'd been taking mortar fire like this at the base located there. Could an 82mm hit the base from where we now were? Suddenly the tube fired again but this time it was about four hundred meters to our right. Were the VC moving the mortar or was there a second position? SEALs had often gotten into firefights with numbers greater than their own, I told myself. This could be one heck of a break-in patrol for ALFA platoon.

The patrol moved swiftly to the cover of the treeline and we headed in the direction of the last three shots. Just before reaching the area of the second firing position another three rounds were launched from yet another position! This time I clearly saw the reflection of the flash and it was likely the crew was firing from a hole dug in the earth, the living jungle providing a camouflage net for its security. We moved closer yet but no further rounds were sent downrange. They must have been content with their performance and shut down.

We patrolled to the area of the third firing position and found a deep canal. Its banks were steep and it was about twenty-five feet from the top down to the water. There was a small landing spot which I could see and it was clear a sampan had recently grounded itself there. All of us could still smell the burned powder from the mortar rounds. We followed the canal back in the direction we'd come and found another landing point. Then we found the first landing/firing point of the attack. The VC were moving the tube by sampan to prearranged firing points, taking their best shots, and then moving quickly to avoid being ambushed. The height of the canal bank explained why the mortar's sound was muffled at times.

ALFA quit looking for mortars and went back to our original operation. We moved about four hundred meters more and conducted a hootch search. Again, a single surprised VC bolted from the target hut and ALFA racked up another body count statistic.

We arrived at Snoopy's Nose before daybreak and put a defense perimeter in around the target. The platoon was in a dry canal bed which was laced with what looked like honeysuckle vines. Mr. Lyon told me to blow the target, which was our bothersome little bunker. Sneaking up to the fighting position I pulled up short when I spotted three trip wires across its dark opening. One was about head-high with another about three inches off the ground. The third wire was between the first two. I pulled my KA-BAR out and began probing. Digging under the bottom wire I placed my explosive in the bunker and slipped its fuse into place. Pulling the lighter I moved swiftly for cover.

Fire in the hole!

Linking up with Mr. Lyon I told him about the trip wires. When the explosive went off the bunker was ripped apart. The explosion was far more powerful than I expected from my charge and I figured there had to be some ammo or other ordnance in the bunker, as well. Suddenly three of our men yelled we had incoming and John Ware called for the corpsman. Bud Gardner was hit. When Hubbard went toward Bud to give him medical assistance he stepped on a punji stake which went through his bare foot. Others moved to help the wounded men, all of whom were barefoot. They'd stepped on small concrete blocks with barbed metal prongs sticking out of them. Each prong was about the size of a framing nail. I went to Bud and he'd been hit in the leg by a small log. Thankfully, he was all right. Mr. Lyon ordered everyone to freeze where they were. Funkhouser and I were wearing boots and we began moving men out of the canal bed. At 0810 hours Steve Frisk called for extraction "Blacksheep" and the LSSC came in. Two PBRs covered us as we loaded our wounded and made for the middle of the river. In the end, we all agreed it could have been much worse.

Back at the YRBM the injured were taken to sick bay and given tetanus shots. They all returned to duty. Hubbard had puncture wounds in his feet which would heal in three or four days. Bud's leg was bruised but okay. The platoon went through the debriefing and we figured we'd learned a lot for the first platoon patrol. We took a few days to heal and put our equipment in shape. Mr. Tollison wished us well and headed for the States, his job done.

ALFA ran some more operations without much intelligence information for a few nights. We were stationed aboard a million dollar barge in the middle of a river. We had no captured VC to use as an intelligence source or guide and had only been ashore to conduct combat operations. About all we could do was set up an ambush on a canal and wait. Most of the time we were coming up dry. The platoon needed help from someone in the intelligence business. That meant Frank Bomar and both Mr. Bliss and Mr. Lyon headed downriver to Ben Tre to visit. When they came back it was with an invitation to operate with the Kien Hoa PRUs. So, by operation #6 ALFA's luck began to change.

On August 30, thirteen SEALs from the platoon loaded up on an LCPL and went to join Frank Bomar's forces. Our teammate was on the pier at Ben Tre to greet us, a truck waiting to take us to our destination. Our mission was to hit a meeting of district level VC cadre. Frank told us, as we were getting our patrol order, the PRU chief was also giving his men theirs. ALFA would take up the defense for the flanks and rear. The PRU would make the assault and hit the hootch. It sounded like a good, simple plan so we took some time to rest after everyone was briefed and ready to go.

At 2400 we loaded in the truck and moved to the pier. Eighteen PRU were waiting for us with four PBRs from RS 534. Counting Frank, there were thirty-two of us. We loaded eight to a boat and headed downriver. At 0245 hours in the morning we inserted at coordinates XS752012, a mangrove swamp at low tide. Movement was ugly as the mud was knee-deep, with wall-to-wall roots making things even tougher. We got out of the swamp and into the rice paddies with their always present and hungry leeches. The hootch was at coordinates XS745008 and we brought the patrol to a halt fifty meters to the southwest of the target. Mr. Bliss took three SEALs and an M60 to the right flank. Mr. Lyon took three more and an M60 to cover the left flank. Four SEALs remained with me and we secured the rear approach. When the raid was in place Frank Bomar and his PRU chief moved toward the hootch.

The operation was going ahead just as planned. Then during the initial moments of the assault the rear security came under fire from a force of between four to six VC. We returned fire and began putting 40mm grenade rounds into the attacking VC force. During the action the PRU, having lost the element of surprise, hit the hootch with everything they had. There were no friendly casualties. Enemy dead numbered four with another probable but not recovered. Two VC were captured. The wounded were treated in the field and then taken in by the PRU.

ALFA patrolled back to the river and called for extraction. We were out by 0715 hours, stopping in Ben Tre to say good-bye to our new friends the PRU. Frank gave us a short debriefing which we appreciated. I was sorry about not being able to capture all the VCI chiefs, but we did get two who recovered from their wounds and went on to provide valuable intelligence from then on out. The mission cemented our newfound working relationship and from here on out we'd work closely with the Kien Hoa PRU and their SEAL advisor, Frank Bomar.

11

Phuang Hoang

The SEAL advisor for the Kien Hoa PRU was Frank Bomar. He reported to the officer in charge (OIC) of SEAL Detachment BRAVO which was under the operational control of Commander MAC-V in support of the PHOENIX program.

The PHOENIX program was developed to target the guerrilla leadership of the Vietcong Infrastructure and to collect high-level intelligence from the VCI. SEAL advisors preferred to snatch (capture) VCI as opposed to eliminating them. Bomar worked hard to convince his PRU to understand the priority for their operations was not to kill, if at all possible. To obtain intelligence from the VCI they must try and capture them alive.

The program received its name "Phuang Hoang" from the Vietnamese, after a mythical bird. The PRU became the primary action force against the VCI in 1968. The first to become PRU were those who were native to their assigned provinces. VC and NVA deserters also became members of PRU by going through the *chieu hoi* program. This program was specially designed to offer amnesty for enemy deserters and defectors.

PRU and SEAL platoons acting together nearly eliminated the Vietcong as a combat force in areas of the Mekong Delta by removing their leadership. Kien Hoa Province was one such area.

Frank Bomar's PRU was the most effective Vietnamese troop I had seen in the war. Frank was a big man with deep respect for his PRU. They returned that respect to him by proven loyalty and performance. The PRU were in their own backyard and could move deeply into the enemy's territory where the VC had been left alone to dominate the land and its people for far too long.

Frank always operated in the field with his PRU. If they were on a mission you would find Bomar leading the patrol. His PRU went on patrols based upon their own intelligence, and averaged ten to fifteen patrols a month. Their target would always be related to VCI except for the times they were with ALFA platoon. Frank was the only American operating in his assigned area of operations which earned my respect as this required great courage.

Sometimes the intelligence came in on more than one target at a time. It was necessary to act quickly before this information became cold, or unreliable. The first time we were aware of this happening it was in early September. Bomar briefed our officers on a mission to snatch a district level chief. He wanted the man taken prisoner and he provided us with three of his PRU to act as guides for the patrol. We left the YRBM around midnight by LSSC and moved down the Ham Luong River. The platoon inserted just before 0300 hours. The terrain was mostly rice paddies and palm groves and it was easy going for the patrol. The moon was full and the weather clear, and we elected to move through the palm groves as much as possible given the good light and their cover.

We set up at the hootch where the district chief was reported to be. The PRU, Scott Lyon, and John Ware assaulted the hootch and captured three suspected VC, but missed the VCI. When we found that he wasn't home, Ware handcuffed the three detainees and put a piece of tape across their mouths so they couldn't cry out. We put the VC in a bunker found inside the hootch and set up once again to wait for the chief. Still, he didn't show. Just before 0700 hours we broke our position and moved back to the river with the POWs. We were extracted by LSSC and returned to the YRBM, stopping at Ben Tre to drop off the PRU and the detainees.

On September 11, ALFA platoon inserted with the PRU by PBR from RS 534. The operation was down the Ham Luong River into the Kien Hoa Province. The mission was to capture a village chief and to sweep a VC village for whatever we could find or capture. We patrolled through rice paddies, coconut groves, and canals to the village, discovering it had fortified stone bunkers when we got there. The platoon captured four detainees from a nearby hootch without hostile fire and took five more detainees prisoner who were questioned and then released. Four of the captives were held for interrogation. No doubt the heavily fortified village was Vietcong, however, the civilians living there told us that forty VC using the village weren't there. An ARVN force had swept the same area the day before causing the VC to melt away for a while. We patrolled back to the river and were extracted by PBR.

That same night we inserted with the PRU by PBR from RS 533 to capture a VC hamlet chief. This time we got the chief but had to engage his guards in a brief firefight. The results were two VC dead, no friendly casualties, and one captured M3A1 .45 caliber submachine gun. We extracted by PBR at daybreak on September 12.

Two days later the platoon and PRU inserted by PBR from RS 534 on the Ham Luong. The mission was to capture a village/district chief. We patrolled to the suspected VC village and found it deserted. An old man whom we questioned told us the VC would be returning in the morning. ALFA put in an ambush and an hour later we executed it on a VC squad. This time we killed two VC and captured an M1 .30 caliber carbine. There were no friendly casualties.

ALFA platoon was beginning to change. They were getting good at what they were called on to do and were learning from the PRU each time we operated together. One teammate in particular was Gary "Abe" Abrahamson. Abe was in my squad and due to the order of march we were almost always together. I think we developed an unspoken bond that grew from our very first patrol. Not to say that

Abe always stayed out of trouble, quite the contrary. However, when he was in the field he was above all else an operator. You could always depend on Abe and his Stoner 63. Whenever I was called on to lead a patrol or to pick some men and join Frank and his PRU I always took Abe along.

Sometimes Frank would send us a crazy message like, "Show tonight and the monkey has no grinder. Send me six grinders for my circus. Show time 2230 hours." No problem for ALFA. Bomar wanted six SEALs with Stoners at the PRU headquarters at 2230 hours. Scott Lyon handed me a message just like this and told me to pick five other men with Stoners, to brief them as well as the LSSC crew waiting to transport us. Working for Frank Bomar was always a pleasure.

On one of Frank's calls we left Ben Tre on the PBRs which would be inserting us. Bomar informed us that we were to have a long night and a long walk. We were going after a district chief and after being inserted we would patrol back to Ben Tre when the operation was over. I released our LSSC and told them I would call them in the morning when we were ready to be picked up.

The first part of the operation was much like the others. When we got to the village he was not at home. We received some information from an old man that they would be back in the morning. We set up an ambush and waited on both ends of the village. It was past daylight when one of Frank's men came and got us. We formed up and off we went through a jungle of heavier than normal undergrowth. After about an hour we came upon a clearing that was about thirty meters wide with the trees hanging right down on the water on the other side. Our side was clear with a well-worn path along the bank that we were patrolling down. Abe and I were at rear security and the patrol was moving fast.

Suddenly there was a gunshot that hit the water behind us. Abe was already on the deck. The patrol kept going and we had no place to take cover on that muddy canal bank. We lay there for what seemed like a long time but it was really only a minute or two. I said, "Abe, lets go!" and he was up and running with me right behind him. We found the rest of the patrol moving on down the trail as if nothing had happened. When we returned to the PRU compound I told Frank about the shot and what occurred. He called his chief in and told him to debrief his men about the patrol. We called for the LSSC and were told to stand by for two hours. No problem, we had some green tea with the troops and suddenly a lot of yelling was heard out at the compound gate. Frank and his chief went to check on what was going on.

Frank called me in the back and said, "You've got to hear this."

It turned out we had walked through an ambush and the VC were afraid to shoot at us! The commotion at the gate was caused by a VC who was surrendering because he was mad at his officer. The officer was the one who refused to shoot at the "men with green faces," or us. I had heard that the locals called the SEALs this and were indeed afraid of us. They had hung this handle on us because of the amount of green camouflage we used on our faces during an operation. It all sounded like a good story until now. Apparently, it was true.

Frank continued telling us the story of the ambush. "The VC came and surrendered. He brought an SKS rifle with him, as well. He's the one who shot at you and Abe after we'd all walked through their kill zone." After hearing this we all went out back where the PRU was questioning the VC. He looked at me and said something which the PRU laughed at.

The PRU chief told me, "He said you are one of the devils," and everyone laughed again. I didn't think it was so funny; after all, we had just walked through an ambush. I was having trouble with my stomach and sure needed something to drink besides green tea.

On one of our joint operations we were to target a VCI but found he had been there the day before. However, he was supposed to return after dark that night. Also, intelligence told us the VC would return to the village after daybreak en masse. We set up an ambush on the only trail that entered the village. Our patrol had not used the trail so we had no sign for the enemy to find. Abe and I were placed on the right flank away from the village and had good cover. Abe was positioned to my right where his Stoner would have a field of fire giving him the best advantage, and we waited.

Just after first light we heard voices. Two VC came into view with a large gun over their shoulders. It took both of them to carry it and to me it appeared to be a .51 caliber machine gun. We held our fire to allow them to come into the ambush kill zone. First, the VC didn't allow a gun like this one to be moved without security, so we expected a squad or more to be in tow. Second, it was a PRU operation and they were to initiate the ambush. The terrain was heavy and the two VC were soon out of our sight. No one opened fire and we only saw the two VC. We waited. Why hadn't the PRU opened fire?

After we broke the ambush, I reported what we saw to Bomar and he sent two men down the trail to investigate. They found that the trail forked and the two VC had slipped out of sight by taking the trail leading away from the kill zone. To this day Abe and I wonder if holding our fire was the right thing to do. If we had opened fire it could have been an easy hit and we would have had their .51 caliber, but we could have been flanked by a security force and had our hands full too. We sure wanted to capture that gun. Sometimes when you think you have done all the right things it doesn't turn out the way you want.

It was September 20 and we had seven SEALs and thirty PRU that were inserted by PBRs from the Ham Luong River in the early hours of morning. The VCI target was moving again and we were coming up dry. It was easy terrain to move in and after daylight we went from hootch to hootch questioning the folks who lived there. We stopped for a break at the largest hootch I had ever seen. One of the PRU came out of the hootch laughing and motioned for me to come in. The family had five or six children and the mother was the only one who could see. The father and the kids had eyes that were about the size of a quarter and actually stuck out of their eye sockets. I didn't think it was funny at all. They looked like they came out of some kind of horror movie and I was sorry for them. The inside of the hootch explained why it was so big. There were large storage bins filled with rice around the outside area of the hootch next to the rice fields. The living area was no larger than what was normal for a family of that size. Most of the hootches I had been in were without furniture except for sleeping beds, however, this hootch had large tables that looked like some sort of picnic tables with benches that the old man and kids were sitting on.

Just as I came out of the hootch the PRU began to move on-line and were saying "VC! VC!" As we moved into position I saw some twenty VC moving about one hundred meters to our right in the open. They were about to enter some heavy jungle and the PRU opened fire on them. There was something different about them. They were all dressed alike wearing Smoky the Bear type hats, dark blue shirts, olive green pants, and backpacks.

We followed them into the jungle. We had blood trails to guide us. The jungle was so thick that you could only stay on the trails. To the side of the trails were small shelters with personal gear and olive green backpacks in them. NVA type ponchos were spread out under some of the shelters.

I was glad we were following the PRU because we were moving fast, too fast for me. A firefight broke out ahead and the patrol stopped. I moved forward with two other SEALs and came into a deep draw with a clearing to the right about thirty meters across. Frank was with his point element firing into the clearing. He told me that VC were in a spider hole in the clearing and to bring up the Stoners. We began to return fire. The firing stopped and the PRU went forward all the time talking to the VC. The VC came out of the hole with their hands in the air and were taken into custody by the PRU. One of the PRU jumped into the hole and handed two AK47 assault rifles out. Then they recovered a body from the hole.

The body was searched and laid on the trail by me. It was a young woman in uniform. The only way you could tell her from the other two was the long black hair and two jade earrings she wore. She looked as if she were asleep except for a five-inch hole in her head. There was nothing inside the head. It looked a little like the inside of a turtle shell after it has been cleaned. One of the PRU ran back to the spider hole and came back with something which he laid on the woman's stomach. It was her complete brain. The PRU looked at me then smiled. He must have read the question on my face. He said only one word, "Buddha." Later I asked Frank what this was all about and he said their religion required the body to be all in one piece to go to heaven. Anyway I got the idea. When they pulled her out of the hole the brain must have fallen from her skull. Another story for the Stoner 63 and its power in battle.

On the way out Bud Gardner and Leonard Horst were handling the two NVA prisoners. Bud's prisoner was moving slowly and Gardner kept pushing him along. Just before we reached the river the prisoner turned and kicked Bud. Bad mistake. The POW received a horizontal butt stroke from Bud's Stoner. I was upset not to mention how Bud felt about it. This guy must have been some kind of hard-core NVA. When I started to stand him up my hand was covered with blood. Checking him over I found that he had been shot just above the hipbone. A small hole in and small hole out. We put a battle dressing on him and let him go a little slower. Tough little soldier, he was.

At the same time we hadn't known how hard the VC had been hit during the 1968 Tet Offensive, and we sure hadn't given them any slack since. The VCI had just about been eliminated in most areas of the Delta and their army had been without leadership. However, they were being replaced with NVA cadre. Some of these new VCI were as high-ranking as a colonel in the North Vietnamese Army, especially at the province levels. With the NVA came new security and support. We had just hit an NVA medical team moving into our area. The recovery of the NVA medical packs and important enemy documents verified their identification.

On October 15, Mr. Lyon called for me and said, "Do you remember the PRU operation you went on last month where you reported uniformed troops?" I said yes and he said, "Are you sure?" I said yes again, and Scott wanted to know what they looked like. I asked what this was all about and he told me that COMNAVFOR V wanted a follow-up report on what the uniforms looked like because it was the first report of uniformed enemy troops in the Delta. We sent them back a message and told them what we'd gotten that day. It was a good score for ALFA platoon.

Between the YRBM and Ben Tre was a long island that

we called "Banana Island" because of its shape. The island was twelve hundred meters long and three hundred meters wide. The entire island was a free fire zone. That meant that anything that moved in it was free game. The boat crews used the island to test fire their weapons on a daily basis.

The PRU intelligence system found out the VCI were not at home in the Kien Hoa Province because they had moved across the river into the lower Vinh Long Province, possibly to avoid our operations. They also reported there was to be a large VCI cadre meeting behind Banana Island. We decided to go to their meeting.

We went by LSSC and met the PRU already aboard the PBRs just downriver from Ben Tre. We inserted two hundred meters below the island on a very dark night. As we patrolled toward a big treeline we could hear the VC talking on a megaphone. It sounded to me like they were making a speech of some kind.

We just knew that this was going to be a hot operation. Then the unexpected happened. The patrol stopped and I tried to communicate with the PRU in front of me but with no luck. Then we saw Bomar coming with a man over his shoulder. As he came by he said, "Snake bite," and went into a small nearby hootch and put the PRU in a hammock. He left two men with him and the patrol moved only a short distance and then stopped again. The chief had told Frank that his man would die unless they got him back right away.

Frank aborted the mission and we started back. I gave my weapon to the PRU in front of me and carried the PRU who had been snake bitten. He was unconscious and so hot that his body actually felt like a bad sunburn against my neck. When we got to the boats I wouldn't have given a plug nickel for his life. We offered to call for a medevac but the PRU chief said not to, in fact what he said was, "Gunshot wound U.S. doctor number one, snake bite number ten. We go to Chinese doctor, snake bite number one." That is just what they did and not only did the PRU live but he made the next operation with us!

Lt. (jg) Bliss was very good about letting his petty officers take out squad operations. By November, Harlen Funkhouser had been reassigned to Detachment BRAVO to assist

PRU advisor Frank Flynn in Can Tho. Bud Gardner was the next most senior petty officer and he took Harlen's place in the second squad. Bomar had asked for a squad of SEALs to go with them and Bud was to take the operation. Bud also asked me if I wanted to go with them. I agreed to.

On November 27, Bud's SEAL squad joined thirty PRU for what was to be our deepest penetration yet. We were inserted by PBRs from RS 534 down the Ham Luong River into the Vinh Long Province. We patrolled almost all night to get to our objective. PRU intelligence sources directed us to a small hamlet where a province level VCI meeting was to be held. We reached our objective just before daylight on the twenty-eighth. There were three hootches and we set up an ambush. No one was home.

The hootches were about fifty meters apart with a very wide, well-used trail between them. The PRU was in the middle hootch and the hootch on our left. We had one PRU with us and were set up in the last hootch. Across the trail from our hootch was a small hootch used for a barn and bunker. Right after daylight it began to rain and we could hear voices. Soon we could see people coming our way, some with weapons. One VC was coming up the path to our hootch when Bomar initiated the ambush. The PRU with us dropped the VC at our back door. We opened fire and men began to fall and run back toward Bomar when we heard them open fire and the VC came back toward us! We opened fire again and they ran back into Bomar's fire. We broke out of our hootch and advanced on the trail to our front to check bodies and here they came again. We fired and two VC ran around the small hootch in front of us. I managed to drop one but he got up and headed for the bunker. When I reached the bunker it was so muddy that I fell. I put a grenade in the bunker just in case the VC had fallen like me and hadn't been hit. I saw the second VC running in the rice paddy and *lai day*-ed him. He had on a white shirt and had a rice mat bedroll under his arm. I stood up and he turned to face me. The end of his bedroll turned red from the muzzle of the weapon hidden inside it and rounds hit all around me. I went down on one knee and my Stoner jumped and his face turned red as he fell backward. I never forgot that few seconds and it painted a picture in my mind that was to repeat itself again another time. I pulled the first body out of the bunker and searched it.

It was still raining hard, very hard. There was some scattered gunfire. Our people were talking and yelling in two languages, exciting to say the least. I turned and found myself face-to-face with the largest water buffalo I'd ever seen. He was tied from his nose by a small piece of string which was tied to a small section of bamboo in the three-sided hootch. He had four bullet holes in his side and he wasn't happy at all. For the first time that morning I was out of my element and scared, really scared of that buffalo. I couldn't shoot him because our guys were on the trail behind the hootch he was in. I had a four-foot area between the side of the small hootch and a duck pond to squeeze by this huge animal. I moved slowly, very slowly, until I was around the hootch. I yelled for my guys to get out of the way. A PRU came to me and I pointed to the hootch and he went around to check it out. The PRU was in his element, so he shot the buffalo. I felt sorry for the animal, this wasn't his war. We had a body count of eighteen VC KIA, eight VC WIA probable, and three VC captured. No friendly casualties except for the buffalo. I remember thinking, "All these dead men and here I am feeling sorry for the animal. Who is the animal here?"

We returned to the YRBM and in a few days Mr. Lyon met me at our SEAL office and handed me the following message:

BT
UNCLAS
SEAL OPS
A. YOUR 280907Z NOV 68
B. YOUR 202030Z SEP 68
C. YOUR 150710Z OCT 68
1. Results reported Ref A are outstanding. Sound intelligence, careful planning, and flexible employment of the tactics which you and your Vietnamese counterparts perform so well have once again hurt the enemy in his own backyard.
2. Ref B and its follow-up report. Ref C, also document a highly effective operation by your platoon.

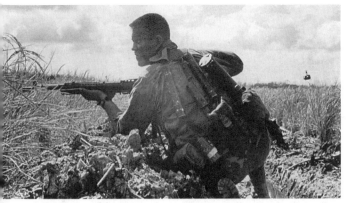

Mission to liberate Vietnamese civilian captives of the Vietcong, Ca Mau Peninsula, ALFA platoon. The author with his ever present Stoner carbine pulls security on landing zone as helicopters arrive. *(Credit: Chip Maury)*

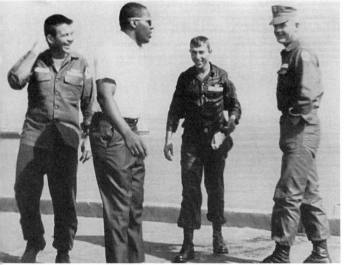

New chief hits the bay. *From left to right:* author, Dick Allen, Chief Roy Adams, and Bud Jurick. *(Credit: Jim LaVore)*

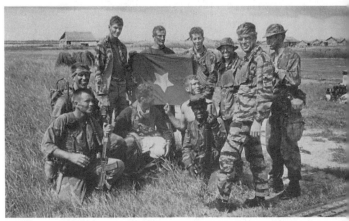

Operation Bold Dragon, ALFA platoon with captured Vietcong flag. *(Credit: Chip Maury)*

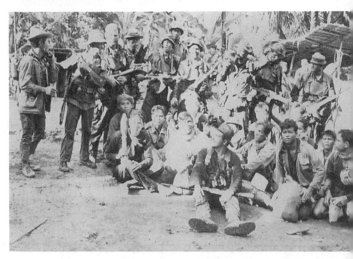

Scott Lyon *(third from left, standing)* led the first successful SEAL POW raid on Con Coc Island. *(Credit: John Ware)*

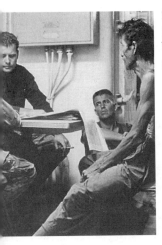

Scott Lyon *(left)* and author *(center)* debrief a Vietnamese fisherman. *(Credit: Chip Maury)*

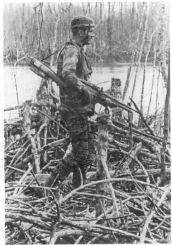

Agent Orange was dropped on Vietnam's jungles and forests. Note the mass destruction along the river as teammate Mike Beanan makes his way through tangled, dead mangrove roots. *(Credit: Chip Maury)*

Teammate Steve Frisk prepares for helicopter insertion. *(Credit: Chip Maury)*

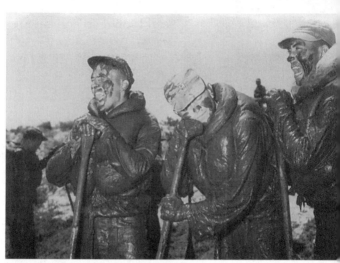

Some sing, some snooze. UDT training in San Diego Bay's mud flats. *(Credit: USN)*

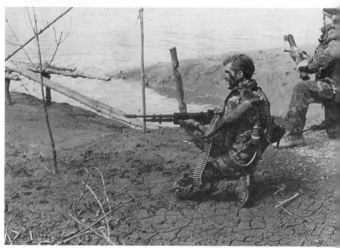

Teammates Beanan *(center)* and Frisk *(upper right)* engage VC attempting river crossing. *(Credit: Chip Maury)*

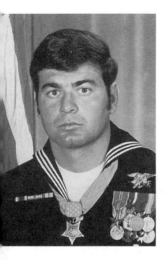

Medal of Honor recipient
"Big Mike" Thornton.
(Credit: USN)

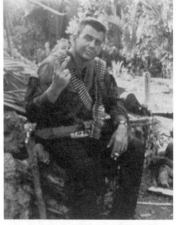

The author, carrying a
modified M60 LMG
and wearing Levi's,
throws a "V" for
victory after a
successful operation
with CHARLIE platoon
on Dung Island.
(Credit: Tom Boyhan)

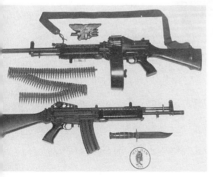

Tools of war. *(Top)*
Stoner 63A with 150-
round drum
magazine. *(Bottom)*
Stoner XM23
carbine, 30-round
magazine. *(Credit:
Ralph Stafford, Stoner
historian)*

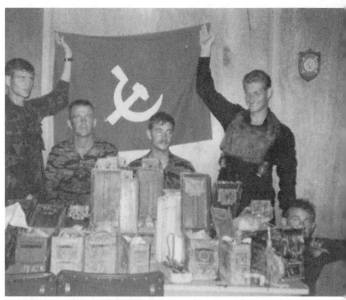

Members of ALFA platoon proudly display 150 kilos of NVA medical supplies and captured red communist flag. *(Credit: John Ware)*

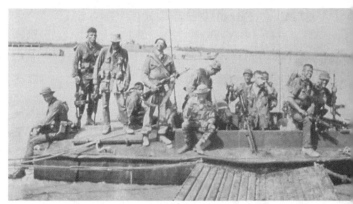

CHARLIE platoon aboard an LSSC, Coastal Group 36. *(Credit: Tom Boyhan)*

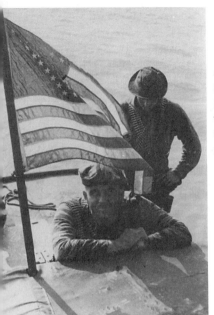

Author *(center)* aboard LCPL returning to base with ALFA platoon, Operation 101. *(Credit: John Ware)*

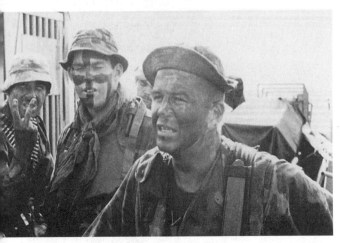

Author *(center)* returning with platoon to the USS *Weiss*, Operation Bold Dragon. *(Credit: John Ware)*

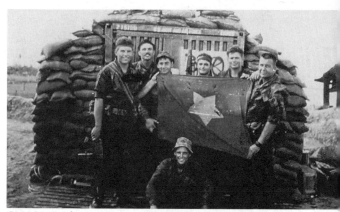

CHARLIE platoon teammates display VC flag after successful operation. *From left to right:* Solano, Doyle, DiCroce, Boyhan, Thornton, Enoch, and Tvrdik *(seated)*. *(Credit: Tom Boyhan)*

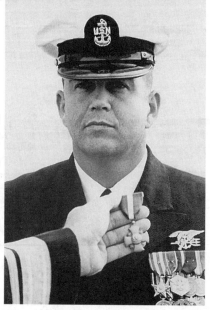

The big, the bad, and the ugly. The author receiving the Navy Cross on December 31, 1970. *(Credit: Chip Maury)*

3. The squads which participated in both of the instances were led by senior petty officers. The leadership and professionalism displayed by SFP2 Gardner and GMGI Enoch in the successful performance of these combat missions was superior.

4. My personal congratulations to the men of ALFA platoon, SEAL Team Detachment Golf, for another dangerous job well-done. Vice Admiral Zumwalt.

I didn't know what to say. I read it again and looked at Mr. Lyon and he said, "This is really something."

"Yes, I know it is," I replied. I still have that old message today. I was so proud of ALFA platoon and the Kien Hoa PRU. It impressed us all to think as busy as he was Admiral Zumwalt took time out for ALFA to offer a "job well-done."

12

The Operators

Courage is fear that has said its prayers.

—Anonymous

ALFA platoon was above all else made up of operators. Not only on combined SEAL and PRU operations but when functioning as a platoon and in squads carrying out complicated and dangerous combat missions apart from the PHOENIX program. The camaraderie between teammates was the highest I'd seen. They wanted to learn their business and to do so they needed to be on patrol. At that time ALFA may have been the most aggressive SEAL platoon ever deployed to Vietnam. ALFA spent one hundred and eighty days in-country and ran a record one hundred and one combat operations. Their results may not have matched other platoons that I'm aware of, but not because they didn't go to the field.

If you didn't count Scott Lyon, Harlen Funkhouser, and myself, the average age of a SEAL in the platoon was nineteen. Youth gave them strength and energy, however they were mature beyond their age. If the military service taught me anything about young SEALs, it was that they are ageless in combat and can always be counted upon to do what is asked of them. That's what operators do. They beat the odds because they are not alone when facing those odds. A SEAL operator tends to be a risk taker and his teammates are there to take the same risks. They have all learned from Hell Week that we're in the same boat, "So grab a paddle, teammate!"

In a letter from John Ware I received there was a story about geese that John felt best describes how we depended upon each other. "Geese create an uplift for the bird immediately following. By flying in a V formation, the whole flock adds at least seventy-one percent greater flying range than if each bird was flying on its own.

"Teammates who share a common direction and sense of team can get where they are going more quickly and easily because they are traveling on the energy of one another. When the lead goose gets tired, it rotates back in the wing and another goose flies point.

"Finally, and this is critical, when a goose gets sick, or is wounded by gunshots, and falls out of formation, two other geese fall out with the stricken bird until it is able to fly. Only then do they launch out on their own, to catch up with their group."

I agree with John, every man needs a swim buddy and requires trust from each other. This is what being a teammate is all about in the teams.

The platoon went on canal ambush, trail ambush, hootch searches, area reconnaissance, village sweeps, and to blow up bunkers deep in enemy territory. Night after night during September 1968 we went on patrol and sometimes both squads went out to conduct different missions on different objectives in the same night. Sooner or later something had to give. As odds would have it the something in this case was me. I became a sick goose. For about three days I had not been feeling well and was developing a cough. A cough is not something to take on an ambush but I don't always do the smart thing. One of the PRU showed me how to cough underwater so I went out on an operation despite being ill. We were on a canal ambush and I positioned myself in the water so I could, if necessary, cough below its surface.

Well, the longer we sat in ambush the more coughing I had to do. After a while the technique stopped working and once we were back home safe Mr. Lyon ordered me to sick bay. The next morning I checked in with a hundred and five degree fever. The corpsman put me in a cold shower to bring my temperature down and then I went to bed. The doctor wanted me to drink fruit juice every hour because I was dehydrated. The only juice they had onboard was prune juice. Within three days my original problem was gone but I had one great case of the "rice paddy two-step" or diarrhea from so much prune juice. All the time the platoon members checked in on me and offered encouragement. Never the less, I felt like a dummy for not taking care of the problem myself.

The next few days I took some time off and spent it on the beer barge getting to know the PBR sailors better. I found them to be very professional and full of stories about VC sightings on the river. I took my newfound information to Mr. Bliss and we began to interview the sailors after their patrols. Our operational contact with the Vietcong began to pick up as a result.

One area that came up time and time again was the Thi Cam Canal. This canal separated Banana Island from the south bank of the Ham Luong River. The river traffic kept to the north side of the river because of the island being a free fire zone. At night sampans were sighted moving into the canal from the north end. The PBRs didn't leave the main river and follow the sampans because the canal was very narrow and dangerous. Also, they had observed tracer rounds from the area during night patrols. Warning shots were fired when the PBRs were moving down the river which might be alerting the VC as to our presence. This was the area that we were headed into the night the PRU was bitten by the snake. I knew the VC were in there and we could make some good contacts if we ran an operation in there once again.

Each time I talked to the PBR sailors I made note of their sightings. When I spoke to Mr. Bliss, he said, "Why don't you take our squad on an operation in there and set up an ambush after dark?" It sounded good to me.

A search for more intelligence didn't turn up anything other than what we already knew. This was enemy held territory that no one had been in. On September 25, I decided it was time to go. We felt two boats might give us away on the canal so a platoon operation was out of the question. Mr. Lyon was going to run a recon operation with the second squad on the north end of Banana Island. This would happen after the first squad had inserted from the Thi Cam Canal. If the first squad ran into trouble the second squad would be able to respond within minutes. Seawolves, our gunships, were placed on standby for the operations.

The patrol order went down early and the platoon acted as if they were looking forward to the operation. Mr. Bliss and I exchanged positions in the order or march and he went with us. We had a full seven-man squad. Just after dark we loaded aboard the LCPL while the second squad loaded the LSSC. We were on our way. Just before we arrived at the head of the canal I ordered the crew to cut the engine. The boat drifted into the canal without a sound. There was no moon and it was dark, and I mean really dark. Hot too. You could feel the beads of sweat popping out of your pores underneath your camouflage face paint.

The LCPL began to move again, just enough to maintain steerageway. The tide was low and the banks on either side were almost ten feet high. Before long I pointed to a depression in the riverbank ahead of us. The bow swung toward the bank and Mike Beanan and I took our places on the bow for the insertion, the squad following our lead. Mike and I were off the boat before it came to rest against the muddy bank. We fanned out along the bank and waited, listening intently for any sign or sound that the VC had detected us, or if we'd just inserted into an ambush zone ourselves. The LCPL slipped back and out of sight without a sound.

We held our position the standard twenty minutes before moving out. It was quiet, too quiet. There was a *lai day* heard, which was Vietnamese for "surrender" and then Abe's Stoner split the night apart with its furious hammering. Abe had just busted a VC coming down the trail on our right flank. I yelled for Abe to cover me and I slipped out to check the body. He was carrying a grenade, otherwise there was nothing else worth anything to us. You don't find a rice farmer or fisherman running around in the middle of the night with a Chinese grenade on him so we added one more confirmed VC to our body count.

Now it was time to make a decision and one that was quick. The VC knew we were here, that was for sure. Should I call in the boat and extract us or should we go on patrol and move out of the area? "Saddle up guys," I whispered, "we're going hunting." Beanan took point and we moved south away from the canal. After one hundred and fifty meters we began to hit thick brush. The jungle was hard on the squad and we moved slower and slower. Beanan was doing a great job at point. I had never watched him work before but Mike was clearly a natural pointman. He was always moving back to me to let me know what he was seeing, or what was in front of us at just about the time I wanted to know the answers to such questions. If I looked behind me I could touch my radioman, Steve Frisk. As I was thinking about how well they were working Mike came back and said the brush was getting too thick for him to move. We decided to move to a treeline fifty meters to our left. The treeline was even harder to move in and I was beginning to think this patrol couldn't get anything going in our favor. I told Mike to take us back to the canal.

Beanan took us to the trail where we'd left the dead VC. I passed the word to move off the trail so we could set up a stay-behind ambush. The best cover was to the left of our original insertion point, right where the dead VC was. We had a ditch with three feet of water in it to our rear and the canal. Suddenly we heard a shot about thirty meters from our right flank. It was followed by an answering shot from the left flank. The VC suspected our presence and were stealthily moving toward us. Well, I decided to help them along with their plan. I had Frisk radio for a false extraction. In came the LCPL, running down the canal with its engine wide-open. They flew past us and beached the boat, backing out swiftly and flying back up the river. It got real quiet again.

The plan worked. After ten minutes or so we had VC chatting quietly off our left flank down by the VC body. Then one man came running down the path in front of us. His bare feet passed so close to us I could have reached out and touched him. We didn't move, my men in perfect control and very still. They waited for me to initiate the ambush and I waited for more VC to show up. The Vietcong on our right lit a torch. The torch seemed to outline us as we waited in the ambush position. I asked Frisk to lower me into the ditch behind us. I could see Bourne clearly, only five feet from the VC. His weapon was pointed toward the trail and three VC behind him. The one in the middle was a woman and she held the torch. The other two held weapons slung over their shoulders. Now what?

One of the VC turned around and looked at Bourne lying motionless before him. The man instantly unslung his weapon and I moved into the middle of the ditch. My Stoner's barrel lined up on his right knee and I squeezed its trigger, walking the rounds up and to my right in the direction of the other two enemy troops. The torch went out and I emptied the Stoner's thirty-round magazine. That's how afraid I was, standing in water up to my waist in torchlight. Right away Bourne's M60 went into action and I knew he was all right. We moved to the right flank and took cover on the canal bank. Then the incoming fire started up.

The second squad had patrolled to the middle of the island and had gained a small patch of high ground. They were watching two VC digging when the first squad opened fire. Mr. Lyon scrambled the Seawolves and called for an extraction from the LSSC. Frisk told me the helicopters were on their way. I called for an extraction now. The firefight lasted for three minutes. The VC were close to us, so close you could see the flash of their muzzles as enemy fire sought us out. I sent a grenade their way and the blast caused them to drop back a little. After the grenade went off Beanan yelled, "Enoch! I've been hit!"

I came back with some dumb response like, "Stick your finger in it and shut up!" Mike had been working for me like a pro all night and he surely didn't deserve that. He didn't call for Mr. Bliss, or any of his other teammates, he called for his leading petty officer . . . me. I still carry a hole in my heart every time I recall that night and his cry for help.

Sorry, Mike.

The LCPL came in under us and we dropped onto the deck. I called out six names and got an answer from each man. "Let's get out of here!" I yelled to the boat crew. "And turn your gunner loose on that point-fifty caliber to cover us!" The squad let our weapons do the talking and they smoked all the way out of the canal. Frisk reported the Seawolves were overhead and I told him to have them work the south side of the canal. Steve got busy on the radio and helicopters lit up the night with their guns. We linked up with the LSSC and transferred Doc Hubbard to our boat to take a look at Mike's wound. It turned out there was a small hole about the size of a pencil eraser in him. I asked about the wound and Hubbard shot me a three-letter word indicating the wound was in the posterior part of Mike's anatomy.

Once in the middle of the river we thanked the Seawolves for a job well-done and released them to go home. Mr. Bliss told me we had conducted a good operation and that the stay-behind ambush had been a great idea. I needed to hear that and it came at the right time. Mr. Bliss was a good operator and he let me call the mission every step of the way. He gave me one hundred percent as did everyone in the squad. He liked the way I'd led the patrol, and later I would find out just how much when the decoration he put me in for came down.

Back at the YRBM the doctor dug a small piece of metal out of Beanan and put a two-inch dressing in place. Mike was fine. During the debriefing everyone was excited over the operation and its stay-behind ambush. It worked, but I wouldn't want to try it again on the Thi Cam Canal for a while. In fact, I started thinking we would stay out of the area and let things settle down before going hunting again. We didn't though. Harlen Funkhouser came back for a week or two and took his squad in . . . and the VC handed them their lunch. No one was hit during the fracas but no one could remember seeing so much firepower coming their way either.

Apparently ALFA had made the VC very angry with the SEALs.

In October we got some help from the Vietnamese navy. Two LDNN, South Vietnamese SEALs, were assigned to us. PO1 Tich and PO2 Thai were both good men and would be with me for two tours of the war. They were SEALs and proved quickly to be as good a teammate as you could ask for. Harlen went back to the PRU for the rest of his tour. This was hard on me. I needed someone I could count on, to complain to, to lean on, and to be my swim buddy in all other things. Now I felt I had the weight of the platoon on my shoulders alone.

Deep down in my heart I needed a teammate to lock arms with. I needed a friend at the end of the day I could open up to. Thankfully this feeling was short-lived. First, ALFA platoon was too busy to spend much time thinking about myself. Second, Bud Gardner picked up the slack and did a fine job with his squad. So much so the workload was shared in true teammate fashion.

As serious as combat is, sometimes something happens that is so funny that it lifts you up inside. On one operation Doc Hubbard fell in a hole up to his armpits. Doc couldn't get out of the hole regardless of how hard he tried. He asked Ware to help him and John turned around and went to the task as a good SEAL will do. Before John could pull Doc out, Hubbard was suddenly standing beside him. "There was a snake in the hole!" exclaimed Doc. John Ware has never forgotten that incident, nor has Doc Hubbard, I'm sure.

Courage or fear?

Fear is what a SEAL feels when he steps on a riverbank in enemy territory for the first time, or when he approaches a treeline on a moon-lit night not knowing what lies silently in the darkness ahead. Fear makes him wish the mission was over and he was back safely on his base. Courage, however, is a special strength within which causes all SEALs to get up and move forward. Courage is overcoming the natural fear all men have. It is the desire to want to be part of every mission, a volunteer even when the odds are great and you're already tired from the last operation run.

SEAL operators are filled with a strange mixture of both courage and fear. ALFA platoon to a man were operators. They would ask to go on every operation, every mission, even when they might have just returned from one only hours before. They didn't want to miss any action where they might have the chance to do what they were trained for. Filled with fear, yes. Filled with courage? Absolutely! They were the men of ALFA, they were SEALs, and they were OPERATORS.

And that's what being an operator in the teams is all about.

13

POW Raid

WO Scott R. Lyon was on his third tour to Vietnam. His first tour was with a combat action platoon from SEAL Team Two and his second began the same way. However, Mr. Lyon was selected to become one of the first SEAL advisors to the PRU under the PHOENIX program, a program under the command and control of an intelligence agency. His duties at PHOENIX were to train and operate with 167 *chieu hoi* PRU in the Chung Tien Province. When Scott returned to Little Creek, Virginia, (home for SEAL Team Two) he received his commission to warrant officer. It brought along a transfer to SEAL Team One in California where he linked up with ALFA platoon.

The Kien Hoa Province was located just to the northeast of Scott's old operating area, the Chung Tien. Being back in the same area as his previous tour with the PRU was an advantage to ALFA platoon as was the experience Mr. Lyon brought with him from SEAL Team Two. His reputation had followed him into ALFA platoon and it served as the spark to develop the enthusiasm we had for our job. We were SEALs and bonded together in many ways, but there was no question how all of us felt about Scott.

During Lyon's tour in 1967 with the PRU he began

hearing about POW sightings in the Four Corps area. He followed up on these sightings, checking numerous intelligence reports on camp locations but to no avail. On October 4, 1968, he learned from another SEAL advisor about two Vietnamese women whose ARVN husbands had been captured during the Tet Offensive earlier that year. The VC had allowed the women to visit their men and now the wives were willing to provide information which would free them. The women would lead the PRU to the camp.

Scott saw all of this as an opportunity to finally liberate some POWs. His enthusiasm was uncontainable for the mission and he immediately went to work planning the operation. At his disposal was his ALFA SEAL squad, the PRU, RS 551 with their PBRs, HAL DET-3 and their Seawolves, and the USS *Harnett County* (LST) which would serve as a floating support base for the PRBs and helicopter gunships. Mr. Lyon moved his squad to a compound at Tra Vinh in the Vinh Binh Province so further assignment could be more easily made. Meeting them there was PRU advisor Brian Rand from SEAL Team One.

There were problems to consider. Could Scott trust the women? The story could be a trap meant to wipe out an entire SEAL squad with all the propaganda value such a victory would have for the Vietcong. At the same time, the women were necessary because they were the only ones who knew how to get to the POW camp. Obviously precautions against betrayal would have to be made. Another challenge in the tactical planning involved the size of the troop lift. The forces providing direct support would have to be capable of moving over forty personnel (SEALs and PRU) undetected to an insertion point known only by two women. Insertion by helicopter was out because of the noise it would make, noise which would assure the camp being abandoned within minutes. Further, the women had only visited the camp during daylight hours and probably wouldn't be able to act as guides under the condition of darkness. The raid had to go off at sunrise and by other means than air infiltration.

The camp was located on Dung Island *(Cu Lao Dung)* at a VC complex at the mouth of the Bassac River. This complex had been abandoned by the South Vietnamese to the

Vietcong who were now making good use of it. Con Coc was one of nine islands in the inland complex which had many canals, a small civilian population, and a very dense treeline along the river and the canals. The tide affected the river in such a way that its banks rose from just a few feet in height to over ten feet. This had to be taken into consideration in case the raid turned into a trap. Vinh Binh Province lay between the Co Chiew River and the Bassac. This put Dung Island in the Ba Xuyen Province so it was decided the operation had to be launched from the sea.

In the aftermath of Scott's raid, South Vietnamese ARVN forces conducted a sweep of Con Coc Island. Intelligence developed because of their operation put the enemy strength at one to two main force battalions. In addition, a security force to protect an HF communications station was present as well as a small factory for the manufacture of explosive devices. This plus the guards for the previously unsuspected POW camp. All in all forty men were going up against much more than previously imagined.

Missions were broken down as follows:

PBRs—conduct a clandestine approach to the insertion point, to provide direct support to the SEALs, PRU, and POWs upon extraction.

Seawolves—conduct close air support of the raiders should they become heavily engaged with a superior enemy force and become unable to break contact.

USS *Harnett County*—provide a floating platform for the Seawolves, fuel for the PBRs, and serve as a communications link for additional forces if these should become necessary.

ARVN—provide a company of combat soldiers to be deployed near the area should they be called upon for support. This company was not told what the target was in the interest of security. It would make a sweep of the island the day following the raid.

PBRs patrolled the river on a daily basis and the plan was to maintain their patrol pattern throughout a thirty-five-mile area. At a predetermined time all nine PBRs would come together at the mouth of a small river, this done under the cover of darkness.

About 0215 on October 6, this fleet of PBRs started

across the Bassac River toward Con Coc Island. In mid-stream the boats cut their engines and began drifting toward their objective. Scott Lyon was in the lead PBR with his squad and the two women who would take them to the POW camp. Getting closer to the island the PBRs restarted their engines so they could stay on-line with each other and maneuver safely. One of the women was given a Starlight night vision scope so she could more easily locate the proper insertion point. She suddenly pointed to a small indentation in the brush along the riverbank. Mr. Lyon alerted all the support teams that the SEALs were preparing to go ashore and to stand by. He elected to insert the team while the PBR was still moving so as to not attract unnecessary attention and to maintain the element of surprise.

The PBRs continued downriver after Scott's team left their safety. The squad conducted its normal security procedures and then began patrolling up a ditch. Suddenly, within fifty meters, the ditch came to a dead end. Lyon thought he and his squad had been set up for sure and he radioed the boats to come back for them as quietly as possible, all the while keeping an eye on the two guides. Getting back aboard, Scott calmed everyone down and told the women they'd picked the wrong point. With the boats collected up again the raiding force moved farther down the canal.

Mr. Lyon didn't want to continue the mission due to the bad break on the first insertion. But, the thought of liberating a POW camp was a strong one and it won out. By now it was almost first light and everyone was getting nervous. Like so many operations that go sour when you depend on other people, the mission was beginning to take on a bad feeling. Sullenness set in with the SEALs. The PBR crew was obviously nervous and fearful because they'd lost a boat in this same area earlier. The two women were on edge now because of their first mistake. About eight hundred meters down the canal the two Vietnamese wives pointed out another ditch but this time they offered they were positive it was the right one. Scott's squad executed another insertion. This time while checking out the area they found no real evidence of high enemy traffic.

The terrain was very muddy and choked with reeds from

two- to four-feet tall. The stubs of these reeds were sharp and firm and they hindered Scott's platoon as everyone was barefoot. The SEALs crept through the reeds for about three hundred meters until coming upon a well-worn path. Neither they nor the other friendlies along had operated in this area before, so the path represented something of importance. Following it as well as they could and mindful of booby traps and trip wires they continued until coming to a security halt just below a slight rise. Mr. Lyon crept forward and peeked over the top of the rise and BINGO, there the camp lay.

The women had indeed been there as it was exactly as they described. Scott counted about thirty men, some in irons and a couple tied to poles. There were two locked in a cage. The guards were just getting up, with one starting a small cooking fire. Only between eight to ten had weapons in their possession and only three appeared to be automatic weapons. Lyon slipped back to his squad and briefed them about what he'd seen. He then deployed the PRU force to the left flank and instructed that they come in after the SEALs completed the first sweep of the camp. Mr. Lyon knew that if the PRU were first into the camp that they would be impossible to control once they spotted the condition of the POWs. He also knew the PRU tended to stray from set plans once the action began, and this could get someone needlessly killed.

Alerting the PBRs to move to the extraction point while the Seawolves were taking off, Scott told his squad they finally had found "a bonafide POW camp and would be the first to liberate same." It was light out by now and Scott knew it was now or never. The squad started over the rise with weapons at the ready.

The SEALs were inside the camp's perimeter defenses before anyone noticed them. Those guards they could see were dropped under accurate automatic weapons fire. Scott's interpreter and one other SEAL headed straight for the prisoners, yelling and motioning for them to get their heads down even as they were being released from bondage. The camp offered three hootches and one long overhang. Two SEALs entered the first hootch but only after sending a light antitank rocket (LAW) through its door. The second hootch was hit with 40mm grenades and both structures began burning as a result.

The guard force was taken by total surprise. Mr. Lyon and his SEALs received very little return fire as most of the guards were running for their lives into the cover of the jungle. One VC simply lay down on the ground and surrendered without firing a shot. A tax collector who turned out to be a VC lieutenant came out of a burning hootch with $240,000 dong (Vietnamese money) on him. The initial assault was over within three minutes. The PRU now moved in with a megaphone telling the former prisoners to stay together and to remain calm. So far, everything was working out just perfectly for our teammates.

Immediately after the sweep with the VC fleeing into the jungle and the POWs freed, things got emotional. It became difficult for the SEALs to get everyone together and moving so they could extract them as planned. The ex-prisoners were all over the SEALs and PRU, crying and kissing their legs and feet in gratitude. They continually clasped their hands together in a sign of homage until it became necessary to drag them out of the camp and onto the waiting boats. One can only imagine how proud the second squad was to free these people! The natural high continued when the SEALs returned to the YRBM the next day. The rest of the platoon was waiting for them, everyone equally as proud of this terrific accomplishment.

John Ware wrote to his sweetheart back home:

> *Dear Jimmie,*
>
> *I know you are about ready to kill me for not writing, but I've been on an operation. We left the boat Friday morning at 4:30 A.M. and got back today which is Monday.*
>
> *The operation was a complete success, in fact it was by far the best op I've been on. We worked with some Vietnamese and went in after a Vietcong prison camp. We were inserted first so the SEALs could lead the attack. It was as cool as could be. Some of the people had been POWs since Tet, which was seven months ago, needless to say they were glad to see us. A Vietnamese*

woman led us or showed us the right way to the camp. Her husband was in the camp, they weren't too happy to be back together. Not much!

You can't believe how happy we were. For the first time since I've been here I really felt that I was doing something to help these people. After we got the people on the boats and were taking them back to Tra Vinh where we were operating from, we gave them food (C rations). They acted like it was Thanksgiving dinner. All I could see all over the boat was smiles. I really felt good.

I love you!
John

A few days later we were notified that Scott Lyon and the two women were to be decorated by the president of South Vietnam. The second squad was put in for Silver Stars and Mr. Lyon for the Navy Cross. As it turned out the women and Scott were decorated by the commander of the ARVN forces; we were told the U.S. Navy under direction of the political side of the U.S. government downgraded the awards to a Bronze Star for Mr. Lyon and Navy Commendation Medals for the squad members. I have heard of company clerks who never left Saigon during their tours of duty who got Bronze Stars in recognition for their typing and filing abilities. To this day, I still feel and believe this manner of honoring Mr. Lyon and the second squad was in keeping with the highest traditions of the United States Navy.

Our teammates liberated twenty-six POWs with no friendly casualties among the SEALs, PRU, PBR sailors, air crews, or the prisoners themselves. As for the enemy, the VC lost two killed in action and two taken prisoner. One VC tax collector and his bank were taken intact and a major enemy base was destroyed. Personally, the platoon felt the professionalism and plain guts of our teammates deserved much more than what was finally acknowledged.

It is time the real story is made known about the courage and heroism of the following SEAL operators:

Scott R. Lyon—who planned and executed a perfect operation

John Ware—pointman, Stoner 63, frontal assault element

Larry Hubbard—radioman, frontal assault element

Donald Crawford—M60 gunner, frontal assault element

David "Bud" Gardner—Stoner 63, frontal assault element

Leonard Horst—Stoner 63, frontal assault element

Harlen Funkhouser—assistant patrol leader, Stoner 63, frontal assault element

If this 1968 POW mission had been run after 1970 it would have been termed a "Brightlight" operation and there is a good chance the recommended medals would have been upgraded rather than reduced in importance and merit. POW raids would continue with some successful and some not. On November 22, 1970, a large force of Army Green Berets attacked the Son Tay prison camp deep inside of North Vietnam; their mission to rescue American POWs. No prisoners were rescued although a large number of Chinese military advisors were killed by the raiding party with no friendly casualties taken. On the same night Navy SEAL Dick Couch led his platoon on a raid against a POW camp in the Delta and successfully freed nineteen captives. This raid raised to forty-eight the number of South Vietnamese POWs set free by Navy SEALs.

Now the world knows who set the first twenty-six captives free and their names. Long-overdue credit goes to Scott Lyon and his six Navy SEALs.

Well-done, teammates!

14

Operation Bold Dragon

On October 17, 1968, ALFA platoon left our floating base at YRBM-18 taking with us our boat support detachment (MST-2 DET. "F"). For the next two and a half months we would become a "Gypsy" platoon, operating without a home base and moving from one Navy ship to another. Since arriving in-country we'd been under the operational control of CTG 116.6. Now ALFA was going on the road.

By nightfall the platoon had moved down the Ham Luong River and transferred itself aboard a U.S. Coast Guard cutter. A few hours later and out at sea we again changed ships, this time coming aboard the USS *Weiss* APD-135. Once underway we were told we'd now be under operational control of CTG 115.5 and our operational code name of "Game Warden" would now become "Bold Dragon."

It was good to have the deck of a Navy ship under our feet again. A ship at sea gives a sailor a secure feeling which was welcomed by all of us. In fact, it was the first time we'd felt truly secure since arriving in Vietnam.

The only problem was with our boat support unit. The LSSC had to be towed behind the ship or run alongside the *Weiss* when it needed to increase its speed. When under tow the support boats had to be checked frequently and they needed to have seawater pumped out every four to six hours, depending upon the speed of the *Weiss* and how much water the smaller craft took on. The sea could become almost too much for the LSSC at high speed so it was necessary for them to drop back and follow at a discreet distance when the APD began to ring up the knots. When it was necessary for the LSSC to run under its own power they dropped so far behind it was all they could do to keep the *Weiss* on radar. I know this was hard on the MST sailors, however, they accepted their new duties and challenges without one complaint.

We linked up with SEAL Team One's HOTEL platoon aboard the *Weiss* and it was not only good to have them to operate with, but to see old teammates again. The platoon officer was Lt. (jg) Gary Parrott who was a fine operator and who held our respect from the start. His platoon, like ours, began their tour of Vietnam with new men fresh from UDT Class 42. Their new SEALs had done well and there was some kind of reunion with their classmates now in ALFA. Many war stories buzzed around the ship that night. The two platoons were close, and this led to their being competitive. Each morning the men from Class 42 would check the message board to see how the other platoon was doing and it wasn't long before all of us were caught up in friendly competition.

Naturally it was not all competition. Everyone wanted to make sure the others were all right after an operation, as well. The men from the two platoons not only had a special relationship with each other but in the days to come they would operate with each other as if they'd been together in Vietnam from the start.

ALFA and HOTEL platoons were the first to be deployed in the Delta that hadn't had operational experience in the Rung Sat Special Zone. The SEALs who'd worked in the zone the past three years had done an outstanding job and dealt the VC a devastating blow in what the enemy considered his backyard. Not having to worry about breaking old habits and change from well-established Rung Sat tactics may have worked to our advantage. True or not, our two kindred platoons were fresh out of training and action elsewhere and we adapted as necessary to the new tactical environment.

We arrived on station at Phu Quoc Island the next morning. The island was located east of Vietnam in the Gulf of Siam, three miles from the border between Vietnam and Cambodia. Phu Quoc Island was twenty-eight miles long and seventeen miles across at its widest point. The north end of the island was thick with double canopy jungle covering a mountain range which stretched south to the central part of the island. This jungle was much like the jungle we'd trained in while attending the Jungle Warfare School at Fort Sherman, Panama.

The South Vietnamese government maintained its POW camp at the south end of the island and there was an Army Special Forces "A" team at An Thoi. However, our area of operations was to be in the jungle in the north and central portions of the island.

Phu Quoc was like no other terrain I'd ever seen in Vietnam. It was the kind of jungle you expect to see in the movies, with both mountains and grasslands. The jungle's floor was filled with soft, wet, dead leaves which were covered with blood sucking leeches. The leeches were even different from the dark black ones we were used to in the Delta's rice paddies. Our new little friends were brown and small, but in some places the ground appeared to be actually moving because there were so many of them covering it. The trees were filled with monkeys and they were responsible for all the leaves which fell constantly to the ground because of their activity.

The two-canopy jungle kept the sunlight out and allowed moisture to stay. Where there was an opening in the jungle, the grass would be chest-high. This did make it easy for us to move quietly but the jungle itself was noisy. Monkeys kept the trees moving and birds of every variety were everywhere you looked. From time to time some small animal would break out in front of us and add even more excitement to our already pounding hearts. We were not used to such noise and movement while on patrol. At night the large fruit bats would come out just before dark. These would make great crash landings high in the treetops and that really got the monkeys going something fierce. Not even while stationed in Da Nang had I seen so much wildlife in the bush.

On our first patrol on Phu Quoc we loaded aboard the LSSC while at sea. Pulling away from the *Weiss* we began to lose the quiet and comforting rumble of her engines. She was at condition "Darken Ship" and presented only a huge black form on the water. When our boat had moved a short distance away from the *Weiss* we lost sight of her completely. The bow spray from the LSSC was a bit cold against our faces as we headed for the island. The night was dark and Mr. Lyon knelt beside the coxswain so both could keep an eye on the radar in order to pick up our insertion point. I remember thinking my own feeling of uneasiness must have mirrored that of a U.S. Marine preparing to make a combat beach landing.

Finally the coxswain cut the engines to a soft idle and we only heard the hum of the radar as it peered its electronic eyes into the darkness. We could see a small white line of beach sand to our front and soon the sound of surf breaking against the beach itself came to us. In back of the beach only darkness lay waiting. The gentle surf lifted the bow of the LSSC and we nosed onto the beach rather gracefully. As one we went over the side and began running across the sand for the safety of the jungle. I looked back for only a split second and saw the LSSC slip back into the surf without a sound. In an instant the night swallowed it up from view.

As we conducted our security halt I began thinking about our intelligence briefing for the mission. Twelve prisoners had escaped from the South Vietnamese camp. One was a North Vietnamese colonel whose left hand was missing. The colonel had been left on the island by his superiors to organize the VC. They were using Phu Quoc as a cache site and taxation point, with heavy taxes levied against the population. The actual strength of the Vietcong on the island was unknown and it was one of our jobs to gather intelligence on this. Another mission was to kill or capture the VC leadership. Somewhat odd was a high-speed boat our Swift boats had been picking up on their radar. This unknown craft would slip across the border from Cambodia to the island and it could outrun the Swifts. It was quite a story and I couldn't help but wonder how much of it was based on solid information.

We needed to move down the beach a short distance in order to penetrate the jungle. Our pointman stopped short as he'd just noticed footprints in the sand. They were not ours from the insertion and they were less than ten minutes old! We had company. Following the prints we found ourselves on a small jungle trail taking us away from the beach. Even moving on a trail our pace became slower and slower. The canopy overhead closed out what little light we had and it became very dark. First light wasn't for another hour so it was decided we would slip off the trail and set up an ambush.

Noise. There was insect noise and animal noise all around us. Something would cry out and then begin thrashing around, death and life occurring at the same time while we listened and waited. I crossed my legs and drew my pants tight behind my knees to try and keep the leeches from crawling up them. Not content with this I pulled my Army issue mosquito repellent out and coated my lower legs with the stuff, hoping the nasty little critters wouldn't like it. It worked, but only for a while. As the night faded and morning began creeping in I noticed a new smell. It was the jungle. The aroma was musky and rotten, much like the odor of a seasoned garden compost pile but one thousand times more pungent.

First light does not come like thunder in the jungle. It moves slowly and is filtered by hundreds of trees with their limbs and leaves splayed out to catch the fragile rays of light. You suddenly realize you can make out the form of the man next to you and fifteen minutes later his features are clear enough you can tell who he is. With more light came more noise and we knew it was time to move.

The path was hard-packed dirt and as smooth as if it had been recently swept. ALFA moved slowly, much more slowly than we would have moved in the Delta. Stop, then move, then stop again became the order of the day. Each man was straining to see more than he could, to smell more than was possible, to hear more than could be heard. We'd lost the keen edge where our hearing was concerned because of the island's sheer force of life. In the Delta it was deathly quiet and we liked it that way. Looking ahead of me I could see each man covering his assigned field of fire, every muzzle pointing in the proper direction and ready to send rounds downrange in an instant.

The platoon found itself on the edge of a clearing to our left. It was covered with tall grass and you could see the mountain reaching upward into the sky. The trees were moving as if battling a heavy windstorm yet there was no wind. Just monkeys. Big monkeys, little monkeys, and very, very noisy monkeys. The trail skirted around the mountain away from the clearing and overhead cover became heavier. But the foliage around the patrol was beginning to open up and that made us uneasy. We needed to put some distance between us and the monkeys as they were a natural alarm system for anyone listening to their banter. Moving out we soon began to parallel a small stream which we crossed using a small log bridge, which was known to us as a monkey bridge. These were normally only four to six inches in diameter and laid across the stream so one could carefully cross one way or the other. SEALs did not like falling off monkey bridges and very few ever did . . . or told anyone about it if they fell off!

After crossing we stopped and dropped down to one knee, a security check in progress. Our pointman's keen eyes had picked out a small structure about thirty feet in front of us. It was an aboveground lean-to without enclosing walls. The floor was made from small logs placed three to four feet above the wet ground. There was a hammock hanging above the floor with cooking pots and other personal gear beneath it.

First Squad came on-line and began to move carefully forward. The hammock moved and that told us someone was at home. Our LDNN challenged the suspected VC in a loud voice and the man leaped from the hammock and pulled a weapon down from the lean-to's roof. Mr. Stoner's light machine gun brought the jungle back to life with its insistent hammering and the enemy soldier never heard his weapon hit the wooden deck.

ALFA moved swiftly now. We set up security around the structure and the patrol leader, pointman, and LDNN began a body search. The lean-to and the equipment found was likewise searched. We took the dead man's web gear, weapon, and some documents. The jungle's earthy smell was now mixed with the bitter odor of burned gunpowder. I recall a light blue-gray skim of gun smoke lay heavy against the ground.

As quick at the action took place we formed up and moved out. The patrol made its way back down the trail we'd come in on until the clearing was reached. We then moved off the trail and followed the treeline toward the ocean. I could hardly believe how fast we reached the beach but suddenly we were there. The platoon fanned out in the chest-high grass and dropped to one knee. Our radioman called for extraction and the LSSC radioed back that it was on its way. Great news!

I looked down at where I was kneeling and then back up and out to sea. Sometimes you look at something and think, "No, that's not supposed to be here," but when you look again, it's there and as real as it can be. In the grass where I was kneeling was a chalk-white horn. The horn was from some kind of Asian stag like a red deer or perhaps a small elk. I had heard there were some big cats on the island but placed very little stock in the rumor until now. If the island had deer it could have cats too.

When the LSSC came in to pick us up I carefully hoisted my new trophy and climbed onboard with my teammates. ALFA had conducted its first operation on Phu Quoc Island and we'd made the first successful hit. We had a story to tell HOTEL platoon but of greater importance "Charlie" knew we were there and that we meant to hurt him.

As the LSSC approached the *Weiss* we saw our teammates from HOTEL platoon waiting for us on the fantail. All of us stood and give them a hearty thumbs-up. They then knew for sure we were all right and the smiles and good-natured yells filled the morning air. A "Mike" boat was alongside the *Weiss* unloading supplies and ammo for our operations. We climbed over the boat and up onto the deck of the ship. There was a flurry of back slapping and then we had to get to the debriefing. HOTEL platoon joined us and they were all ears. I remember them sitting quietly and listening to every word of what was discussed. Each of ALFA's SEALs had an opportunity to tell what he'd experienced on the patrol. Others asked questions and made recommendations. This was standard for SEALs returning from patrol. Fourteen pairs of eyes can make the difference the next time out. Every comment made was written down by the patrol leader, then HOTEL was given the chance to ask their own questions.

Afterward we took our weapons into the hot showers with us and cleaned off clothing, web gear, and our bodies. The weapons were carefully dried, cleaned, and then oiled. We constantly talked about the operation between ourselves. Dressed, refreshed, and weapons in working order we test fired each gun aft over the stern then went to chow.

ALFA had a mascot named "Twiggy" who was always delighted to see us return. Twiggy was a tiny female monkey that Mr. Lyon came up with sometime shortly after we'd reported aboard YRBM-18. She was little more than a handful of fur and was full-grown. Twiggy became as attached to the platoon as we did to her. I don't think the ship's company was very happy about her being onboard but they probably felt the same way about the SEALs. For a while she had the run of the ship, walking the lifelines topside even when the *Weiss* was underway. Many a time I woke up feeling this small furry ball snuggled up asleep under my arm. As soon as we would come aboard after a mission Twiggy made her way to someone's shoulder, loudly scolding us for leaving her behind.

Soon we began running port and starboard platoon operations. One platoon would operate in the field with the other staying onboard, ready to assist if necessary. The next day the platoons would rotate positions and duties. It was a good way of doing business and everyone stayed refreshed and eager for the next operation.

We received a detachment of LDNN aboard the *Weiss*. They were without an advisor so we incorporated them to augment the SEAL platoons. The senior LDNN was Chief Daeng who proved to be both a fine operator and platoon chief. On one operation Chief Daeng was working point for Lieutenant Parrott and his platoon. It was one of those dark island nights when the chief grabbed Mr. Parrott and said, "Let's go! Let's go!" Parrott didn't have time to let his platoon know where he was going nor did he know himself. The LDNN grabbed him by the collar and they were off.

The chief led him into a base camp of some sort. Lieutenant Parrott reported they could hear bare feet running away into the darkness (or maybe they were monkeys) and that there were small cooking fires all around them. If the VC had been there they had run away and Mr. Parrott said Chief Daeng was one brave little man. The South Vietnamese SEALs, or LDNN, were always an asset to our operations.

We and HOTEL platoon were hitting the island hard every night. There was little resistance met. Someone remarked Phu Quoc was a "turkey shoot" with the VC breaking up into groups of two or three and hiding themselves and their weapons in the jungle.

HOTEL platoon conducted an operation in the central part of the island and captured a VC walking down a trail with his weapon. They brought the unfortunate prisoner back to the *Weiss* to question him. He agreed to lead the SEALs to the VCI who had recruited him as a Vietcong. The SEALs returned with the POW the next night, the LDNN having written *"Sat Cong"* all over his shirt. *Sat Cong* means "Kill Communists" and our LDNN believed the defector would be less likely to try something with such an advertisement. Chief Daeng held the man by the shirt throughout the entire patrol so he couldn't try to slip away. The VCI wasn't home but the POW did lead the SEALs to the man's web gear and weapon.

Back aboard the ship the MST crews had pulled the LSSCs up to the stern of the *Weiss* to make them ready for a night operation. One of the crew was a sailor by the name of Von Essen. In my opinion Von Essen was one of the finest gunners mates in the brown water Navy. The sea was rolling the LSSC around and it was hard to keep your balance. I recall seeing Von Essen standing on the bow of one of the boats receiving ammo for the operation. One of the men dropped him a belt of 7.62mm ammo just as the boat took a dive into the sea. The belt hit the steel deck and the point of one round hit the primer of another round in the belt. This caused the struck round to fire with the bullet striking Von Essen in the calf of his leg.

The hardest part of the incident was getting Von Essen back aboard ship from the LSSC. He was a big man. When we did get him down to sick bay there was a circle of SEALs around Von Essen giving him a good-natured bad time even while the corpsman dug the bullet out. Within a week he was back on duty.

The Navy sent an LST to the Gulf of Siam in support of our operations. Army Cobra gunships used the LST as their base of operations. We'd had some experience working with the Cobras when operating off the YRBM on the Ham Luong, however, this was the first time HOTEL had worked with them. The Cobra was armed with a 7.62mm six-barrel machine gun, a 40mm grenade launcher, and a 2.75 inch rocket pods. The helicopter was faster than the Seawolves with only the lack of door gunners a drawback.

We were able to schedule Huey HU-1D helicopters out of Can Tho for our airborne insertions on the island. The Hueys would use the LST as a platform to launch from and give us a hit-and-run capability offering air support at any point on the island where a landing zone could be carved out of the jungle.

Lt. Gary Parrott planned and executed an operation to recon the northern end of the island. His platoon was inserted just before dark, taking Abe with them. Both Abe and Darryl Wilson from HOTEL platoon were best of friends and Mr. Parrott and Mr. Bliss had blessed his tagging along on the operation. With Abe and his Stoner the platoon was rounded out to fourteen men.

After the successful insertion the platoon settled down alongside a trail to allow for the jungle to get back to normal. The helicopters had kicked up quite a fuss and it would take a few minutes for things to resume an air of normality. Mr. Parrott didn't think the VC would be moving around so soon but he was proven incorrect almost immediately. A lone VC with a rifle over his shoulder came wandering down the trail, pretty as you please. When the man was well into the kill zone the platoon challenged him and he tried to bring his weapon to bear. Darryl and Abe opened fire and one more VC fell prey to their Stoners.

When they moved forward to search the body the SEALs discovered the VC was actually our one-handed NVA colonel! His left arm was missing below the elbow and he was armed with a Chinese communist 7.62mm SKS rifle. Lieutenant Parrott always wondered why the officer was armed with a rifle when, with only one good arm, he might have been better off with a pistol or submachine gun. In the end it didn't matter. HOTEL platoon bagged the colonel and made a heavy dent in the VC's command structure on Phu Quoc.

The platoon continued north and the trail they were on turned into a road. As the patrol moved up the road they found engineered bridges using large timbers. As the road climbed upward into the mountains the SEALs found well-built bunkers and new fighting trenches. The VC were very active and well organized!

The moon was full that night and it filtered through the jungle strong enough for the men to see quite well. From time to time the jungle opened up and there was knee-high grass running alongside it. At one point they found what looked like the tracks of either a man or animal moving off the path at an angle to the road. The grass was wet with dew and the tracks showed up just fine. The SEALs moved off the trail and circled back to be extracted by LSSC.

We worked Phu Quoc Island from October 17 until the 8 of November 1968. Our platoons killed or captured many VC and eliminated their NVA leadership, the escaped colonel. We added new light to intelligence about the island's VC presence by showing how much communist activity was indeed taking place at the north end of Phu Quoc. But, it was time to leave the island. HOTEL platoon had orders to Rach Gia and ALFA was going to Sa Dec via YRBM-18. Teammates said their good-byes and ALFA transferred from the *Weiss* to the LST.

15

Sa Dec

No one serving as a soldier gets involved in civilian affairs—he wants to please his commanding officer.

2 Timothy 2:4

ALFA platoon made its way back to our floating base camp, YRBM-18, where it was tethered at the headwaters of the Ham Luong River. We had earned a well-deserved rest after the operations on Phu Quoc Island. Even though we were tired the order came down to begin preparing our equipment for transfer to the navy base at Sa Dec. As an old SEAL adage goes, the only easy day was yesterday.

Back in the relative security of the YRBM the men and I bathed our leech scarred bodies under Vietnam's blistering sun. It felt wonderful drying out, just lying on the deck and chatting with each other about things other than the war. I directed each SEAL to assemble, check, and then store his personal gear while likewise packing up his footlocker for the move to Sa Dec. Weapons and combat harnesses were always kept an arm's length away, just in case we got the call to prepare for a mission.

The platoon's equipment and gun lockers were made ready for the trip upriver. Bud Gardner and I took responsibility for ensuring the extra weapons and spare parts were properly recorded and stored away. Our officers were busy cleaning out the platoon's office, either throwing out or packing everything they could get their hands on. The move to Sa Dec would be accomplished by Mike boat so there was plenty enough room for not only our assigned equipment, but anything else we could scrounge. None of us had ever been there so we had no idea what to expect in terms of facilities or logistic support. I made it a point to tell the men to pack everything they could think of, from gun cleaning solvent to olive drab duct tape. Nothing was to be left to chance.

Despite the frenzy of moving we managed to spend some time on the beer barge with our PBR crews. We hadn't missed much since being gone on the island, with most of the talk centering on how quiet the rivers had been for the PBRs and the coming Vietnamization program. It seemed the PBR divisions so carefully constructed and fielded by our forces were to be turned over to the South Vietnamese Navy. A few U.S. advisors would stay with the boats, which seemed to me like turning back the hands of time. No one believed the concept would ever work, and indeed it did not.

It was very disturbing to us to hear that the "Brown Water Navy" would be pulled off the rivers. The SEALs had become very comfortable having them at our back door, providing a way home and lots of firepower when we were in trouble. We could depend on our PBR sailors and I was personally concerned at the decay in their morale as we visited. They had stood up and done their jobs well, taking casualties as we all did. Their spirit was being tested with the news they were no longer considered important, and I felt bad for them.

Mail from home had piled up at the YRBM and the platoon tore into it with relish. The news wasn't very cheerful, with letter after letter describing the huge antiwar demonstrations taking place back in the States. Long-haired protesters were marching across the land from city to city, spewing their poison and sapping the nation's will. I can now admit to a great rage which began burning inside me, a rage directed against those who I could only consider to be anti-American. If there was a bright spot in all of this it was the SEALs' attitude about such demonstrations. We didn't take them personally, meaning we felt it was the policy, not the soldiers, sailors, airmen, and Marines, which was under fire back home.

The men of ALFA platoon never lost their faith about why they were in Vietnam. It is this team spirit which makes SEALs so special and SEALs so effective as war fighters. We only became unsettled when we couldn't get into an area of operations because someone at a higher command level offered such AOs were already neutralized. SEALs were in Vietnam to fight, and such proclamations were a burr under our collective saddles because we knew the Vietcong were never "neutral" about anything. As for the antiwar protests, we were sailors, warriors. As such we elected to leave civilian problems to the civilians.

Our job was to kill communists.

Soon we were loading heavy gun cabinets and footlockers aboard the Mike boat. Sa Dec, here we come, I thought to myself. With the final locker safely stowed onboard the platoon believed we were on our way until Mr. Bliss advised us otherwise. "I need a squad of volunteers," he announced. "We're going to conduct one more operation on Banana Island." Bliss then outlined the mission, which I became more and more uncomfortable about as the details flowed forth. It was to be a patrol, conducted during midday and there was no reason for it other than to add one more mission to the platoon stat board. There was no intelligence available to us about what might be happening on the island and when I heard this, I offered Bliss could count me out.

I was upset, to put it mildly. My objections to the mission fell on deaf ears. It would not be until I had more experience as a combat leader that I realized what our officer's objective for the mission was. We'd been out of the bush for over a week, lying around fat and sassy, getting laid back and comfortable. Bliss knew we'd be down for another week or so settling in at Sa Dec, with more time on our hands doing little more than admin chores and lazing about. To maintain our operational readiness at the high levels demanded by Vietnam—not to mention our morale—we needed that last mission to remind us who and where we were.

A full squad of volunteers was assembled, briefed, and inspected. They loaded a PBR from RIVSEC 534 and moved out into the Ham Luong River. The insertion onto the island went smoothly, but it was all that went right from that point on. What took place had nothing to do with my initial objections about the mission, whether they were right or wrong.

Banana Island was a free fire zone and no one lived there, or worked the land. The terrain was overgrown with hard scrub brush which made movement difficult. Even the one-time palm and banana plantations were clogged with thick jungle foliage. Even in daylight the patrol's movements were slow and strength-sapping.

Steve Frisk, the radioman, decided to use his long whip antenna on the PRC-25 that day. It was a last-minute thought on Steve's part as he normally relied on the more compact short antenna. The long whip didn't work well in the jungle, becoming caught up in the brush and whipping back and forth as it was either pulled or tugged free. Paul Bourne was carrying our modified M60 machine gun and was assigned to walk behind Frisk. It was not to be Paul's day.

At some point the long whip antenna made contact with a massive hornet nest hanging from a tree limb Frisk and the rest of the patrol had to pass under. No one noticed the nest until the antenna sliced its way through it. Naturally the occupants became enraged at this insult and thousands of angry hornets exploded onto the patrol, with Bourne taking the brunt of their fury as he was the first available target behind Steve. The squad evaporated into the surrounding jungle trying to evade the stinging creatures, but Paul was caught flat-footed and stung over nearly every inch of his body. His exposed hands took the worst beating, hornet after hornet diving in and taking its best shot.

My time in the jungles of Asia had taught me not to be surprised by much, but none of us had seen or heard about Vietnam's hornets before now. I was stunned when Paul was brought back to the YRBM after the mission, his hands blown up like eight-ounce red boxing gloves from the insects' attentions. Maybe he was allergic to their venom but there was no doubt how much pain our teammate was in.

Even so, the patrol reformed after the hornet attack and continued on with the mission. They'd only moved a short distance when two people broke from the jungle and began running toward a bunker. The squad surrounded the structure and ordered its occupants to come out. No dice. Beanan offered to throw a CS grenade into the bunker to encourage the suspected VC to surrender peacefully. Given the okay to do so he pulled the pin, heard the fuse pop, and then for some reason hesitated before throwing the round green ball inside. It was a bad move as when the grenade exploded it got both Beanan and the "VC" with its eye-tearing load of CS gas.

The bunker's occupants turned out to be two Vietnamese girls. With Beanan and the girls crying, and the gas affecting everyone else nearby almost as much, the patrol released the girls and told them to scram. Someone began pouring water into Beanan's face in an attempt to wash the CS out of his eyes, which didn't work all that well. In the end, Beanan had to be led by a teammate and Bourne was by now unable to either hold or operate his M60. A vote of sorts was taken and everyone agreed it was probably a good idea to end the patrol.

Calling for extraction the patrol spotted six water buffalo grazing near where they wanted to go out from. The buffalo were most likely abandoned some time ago by their owner, and anything on the island living was fair game by the rules of engagement. The platoon dropped all six of the animals before the PBR came in, taking away the VC's primary method of moving heavy guns and food. When the "stumble and trip" squad got back aboard the YRBM and filed their after action report, they reported destroying "six VC cargo carriers." It quickly became a private joke among the platoon for obvious reasons.

The next day a message from DET GOLF reached us. It read "Interrogative VC cargo carrier." We sent back one word. "Buffalo." Nothing else was ever heard about our explanation until nearly a year later when someone read SEAL Team One's Presidential Unit Citation. Right in the middle of the official document's description of all the weapons and supplies we'd been responsible for capturing or destroying was our platoon's "six destroyed VC cargo carriers."

We got quite a chuckle out of that one.

The morning after the Banana Island debacle the platoon loaded the Mike boat and we headed for Sa Dec. By river it was only about twenty miles travel, but we were going against the current in a flat-bottomed boat so it made for a long and lazy trip. The sun was extremely ferocious that day and we stripped down to our khaki-colored UDT trunks and sacked out, lying atop our gear on the deck. The Mike boat held center line in the river, a move meant to allow us the maximum in security from anyone perhaps lurking along either riverbank with bad intentions. As the Mike boat droned its way into the entrance to the Co Chien River, ALFA platoon said good-bye to YRBM-18 and "hello" to our new digs at Sa Dec.

The coxswain carefully walked the big Mike in along the side of the pier just after midafternoon. Myself and the rest of the SEALs stepped onto dry land, our weapons in hand and our well-worn combat harnesses draped across our upper bodies like old friends. Work stopped as we began moving inland. Even in clean camouflage fatigues we appeared worn, albeit seasoned veterans. I remembered thinking to myself how we were wearing our Sunday best, and if it wasn't good enough for the locals they'd just have to get used to us.

Mr. Bliss and Mr. Lyon went scouting for quarters, with Scott coming back in an hour or so with news of our new home. ALFA took the top floor of a two-story barracks, which became a combination of sleeping quarters and platoon office. Mr. Bliss was likewise busy having scrounged a truck and driver to assist us in moving our gear off the dock and up to the barracks area. By the time we returned to the Mike boat it had moved to a boat landing, lowered its bow ramp, and begun unloading. The truck driver backed his vehicle onto the ramp itself and the work went quickly after that. I was pleased to see the platoon settled in with all equipment accounted for before the evening meal.

For the next several days we were busy finding our way around Sa Dec. At the same time the platoon as a whole was studying the maps we were given of the surrounding area, our new AO. We discovered we could communicate through the Navy Operations Center (NOC) on base and that our PBRs would be coming from RIVSEC 573, also stationed at

Sa Dec. Air support in the form of Seawolve gunships were available from HAL DET-3, and our PRUs were stationed in town. Their advisor was a member of the Australian Special Air Services, or SAS. Overall, we were pretty happy campers with Sa Dec and all it had to offer.

Finally, there was a platoon meeting called. Just like the military, plans changed. ALFA was to move south and operate on the Ca Mau Peninsula. This was the home of the Nam Cam Forest, which the Vietcong had owned since fighting the French years ago. We were once again part of Operation Bold Dragon. Helicopters would be transporting us so we could take only what could be carried on our backs and in our war bags. I didn't like the sound of this sudden shift in the program. Once again, there wouldn't be much mail for what was now being called the "Gypsy Platoon."

16

Ca Mau Peninsula

ALFA platoon flew from Sa Dec to the southern end of Vietnam in two HU-1D "Huey" helicopters which we called "slicks" for short. As the coast came into view we could also see the Nam Cam Forest below us, the mangrove jungle looking like the aftermath of a terrible forest fire. It was the first time we'd seen the severe effects of the defoliation program being carried out along the rivers of Vietnam.

As the slicks reached the ocean we discovered our LST, the USS *Terrell County,* was anchored off "Square Bay" (Cua Song Bay Hap) where the mouth of the Cua Lon River empties into the Gulf of Siam. The bay was so named because of its unique shape and it was a very large body of water. This area of operations would later become the home of Sea Float, a floating base in the middle of the river much like YRBM-18 was on the Ham Luong. But for now ALFA would live aboard and operate from the LST.

Landing a helicopter on the deck of a ship was old stuff for our Army pilots. However, this time around we were low on fuel and it took some doing to get us in safely. The pilots brought us in low on the water, popping the Huey up and onto the ship's deck at the last instant. Our crew then "walked" the helicopter across the pad so as to make room for the second one to land. Before anyone left the bird the crew chief jumped out and secured the huge overhead rotor so it would clear the second Huey now just landing.

Just before we left Sa Dec an old friend, Chip Maury, from UDT 11 dropped in to visit with us. Chip was a combat photographer with Team Eleven and possessed a unique set of orders. In short, Chip's open orders allowed him to travel from SEAL platoon to SEAL platoon anywhere in the country for the express purpose of logging a visual record of UDT/SEAL combat operations. This had not been an easy assignment for Chip because SEALs normally operate at night, a time and place where flashbulbs are normally frowned upon. We could and did change this for Chip's sake. He was an operator and well respected by the platoon so we said, "Grab your gear and climb aboard." With this invitation Chip Maury was on his way to Nam Cam with ALFA.

Our support people from MST-2 DET "F" were already aboard the LST so it was they who led us to our living quarters below decks. They had been enroute to the Ham Luong and were turned around and directed to report to Square Bay a few days before we ourselves got the word to move out. Outside of being in a new area of operations they didn't know anything more than we did about why any of us were now in the Nam Cam.

Onboard the LST were two men from CHARLIE platoon. Lt. (jg) Moses and his leading petty officer (LPO) David Wilson. They had only been in-country for a short time and were the advance party for their platoon. CHARLIE platoon would follow them in a few days and until then both Moses and Wilson would operate with us.

At our first patrol order we were informed we'd been ordered to the Ca Mau Peninsula to start running recon operations in the area of the Cua Lon River. Naval Intelligence was reporting that the real estate in and around the Nam Cam Forest was controlled by the Vietcong, however, unit size and strength was unknown. We felt like we were being asked to step into the darkness in order to bring daylight to someone else. No friendly forces had been in the Nam Cam so ALFA elected to go in quickly so we could fully exploit the element of surprise so necessary for SEAL combat operations. By hitting fast and hard the VC might not have time to get their act together before we had our intelligence gathered and were long gone.

We loaded the LSSCs in the early morning hours and slipped unseen into the mouth of the Cua Lon River, located at the southwest end of Square Bay. It was a short boat ride upriver to where we inserted on its north side. As was our practice we waited ashore for between twenty to thirty minutes before saddling up and moving out on patrol. So far, so good.

Once again the jungle was different from what we were used to previously. Now it was more like a forest with tall trees and only one canopy above us which the sun's rays broke through right away. The undergrowth varied from good thick cover to openings in the forest floor that offered no cover at all. One good thing was how quiet it was . . . no monkeys or other animals to distract us.

After a half hour we came to an opening along the river which was covered with tall trees. There were two big brick structures under the trees, each building about two stories in height. They were dome shaped and reminded me of two wardroom coffee mugs turned upside down. There were broken bricks all around each dome. We noted the structures had small arch shaped doors which were the only apparent openings to the inside. What we were looking at had to be some kind of kilns used for brick making. There was no one about and it looked like the place had been deserted for some period of time.

The patrol moved upriver checking old bunkers and "L" shaped fighting positions. We found a sampan pulled up on the riverbank too. While reconning the area John Ware discovered a nearby bunker which he entered. Later on he told us he was back outside before he realized someone had been hiding in the corner. Ware slipped back into the bunker's darkness and called out, *"Lai day! Lai day!"* The VC responded by coming out with his hands held high in the air. Mr. Lyon and the LDNN began to question the man and he ended up taking them back to the river where he'd hid his weapon under the sampan.

We were feeling pretty good right about now. ALFA had

inserted and patrolled deep in enemy territory without being detected and now we had a captured VC who was telling us about anything we asked. We gathered up his weapon and called for "Blacksheep" which was the LSSC call sign. It was time to extract and head for the LST. As the LSSC came upriver we heard automatic weapons fire which caused immediate concern. The LSSC crew radioed they were all right and on their way. The patrol leader pulled out a smoke grenade and threw it, the LSSC properly identifying the right color and coming in for our extraction.

Once onboard we all asked what the shooting was about. There was a South Vietnamese outpost just inside the mouth of the river and when our LSSC came by the guards ran out and began firing at the boat! Our gunners sent return fire over the guards' heads and they ran back to the protection of their outpost. The LSSC was flying an American flag so it should have been very easy to identify. A few rounds hit the boat but the ceramic armor did its job and no damage was done.

As we moved back downriver we were ready for our allies. But upon our arrival at the outpost they were nowhere to be found. Returning to the LST the incident was duly reported and we heard nothing about it again. Everyone figured the outpost was in such a remote area that maybe its occupants had never seen an American flag, or LSSC for that matter. Or, perhaps for their own survival they'd cut a deal with the VC in the area and we'd suffered because of it.

Our POW told us about a VC village upriver where he and twenty other Vietcong lived along with some civilians. He said the civilians were made to work in the rice fields and to cook for the VC. Mr. Bliss began planning an operation to hit the village.

It was December 19, 1968, when Lieutenant Bliss issued the patrol order. Our objective was to destroy the VC village and to bring back its civilians for questioning and then relocation to a safe area under government control. The platoon was inserted by two Army slicks with an additional two Cobra gunships flying support. This would be a daylight operation with time on target set for 1200 hours, or noon straight up. Mr. Bliss had conducted a helicopter reconnaissance flight of the target area and told us to expect it to be completely defoliated.

Twelve SEALs would participate in the operation. This would include Mr. Moses, David Wilson, and Chip Maury. The first Huey was to take Mr. Bliss, Frisk, Beanan, Crawford, Chip, and myself. Our squad would be the strike force tasked with taking out any armed or evading VC. The second helicopter's personnel was tasked to round up the civilians after searching/destroying the village. Mr. Lyon was in charge of Second Squad which included John Ware, Bud Gardner, Hubbard, Wilson, and Mr. Moses.

After the patrol order was given I told Chip this was his big chance to take pictures. I added, however, that any time I looked behind me when we were on the ground I wanted to be able to see and touch him. It wasn't that I didn't trust Chip as an operator because I did. Rather, he hadn't operated with ALFA platoon until now and didn't know our standard operating procedures (SOPs). So, I wanted and needed him close by.

The only problem with my decision and his compliance was that every time I turned around I got my picture taken.

The platoon checked their equipment and mustered on the flight deck by our helicopters. During our inspection I noticed that Chip was wearing the same type of life jacket I was. These jackets were actually a camouflaged load bearing vest which consisted of two CO_2 cartridges meant to inflate rubber lungs on either side of the vest. There were magazine and utility pockets on the outside of the vests for just such ammo and gear. Chip was carrying a standard ammo load for his CAR-15 plus cameras and film. The SEALs were carrying an extra hundred rounds or so for the automatic weapons and every other man carried an LAAW (light antiarmor weapon) to use on any bunkers we might find.

ALFA loaded up on the Hueys even as their engines began to whine and the rotors began spinning. I've always enjoyed the exit our helicopters made when leaving the deck of a ship and today was no exception. The nose seemed to drop and the tail would lift, giving you the impression you were going to take a dive into the sea below. It was a great feeling and soon enough we were on our way.

Our Huey flew just off the water's surface until we reached Square Bay, then it climbed for altitude. We were glad to see the two Cobra gunships had joined us by now. Passing over the chemically scarred forest below us the helicopters came down to treetop level. Not one green leaf had survived. It was like losing the color on your television. Huge mangrove trees were dead, still standing on their exposed roots like withered giant octopus. Operation Ranch Hand and its herbicides had done some kind of job. It had been said Agent Orange would kill an entire forest in a month and now I believed it.

Mr. Bliss was watching every turn on the river below us and following our route on his map. He had positioned himself on his knees between the pilot and copilot so he could communicate with them and point out the village as it came into view. When the target was sighted we knew we were going in hot. Chip smiled at me and I slung my legs out of the Huey's open door and pushed the safety of my Stoner forward. There was a large Vietcong flag flying in the breeze over the center hootch in the village and we could see armed VC running swiftly below us as the choppers rushed over them. Our door gunners with their M60s opened up on the enemy troops and we SEALs joined in the fray too.

Our pilot set us down in the middle of the village. The second Huey was right behind us and everyone was out of the helicopters and on the ground firing and running before their skids actually touched the earth! We claimed targets of opportunity and moved on them. I heard Steve Frisk fire an LAAW and a hootch went up in flames right in front of us. Two VC ran for the river with Beanan in hot pursuit. Frisk went to join him in the chase. When the two SEALs reached the riverbank the Vietcong were already halfway across, swimming like crazy. Beanan let off with a long burst from his M60 and the two enemy soldiers dove underwater. Frisk fired another LAAW, this time into the river, and our two divers never surfaced after its explosion.

I spotted movement ahead of me and went to investigate its source. There was a small canal with a sampan moving on it but no one was onboard. When I reached the stern of the boat I noted something strange in the water. It looked like some kind of muddy seaweed. A closer look revealed what I was seeing was the top of someone's head all covered up with mud! I called out to whoever was below the surface and a young boy of about fourteen years came up out of the water. Taking him prisoner I asked why he was where he had been hiding. He told me the VC had ordered him to hide in the river until we left and then to bring the sampan across to get them. There were two boxes of ammo and a case of canned milk under a canvas in the sampan. We sank the boat and took the boy with us.

The bunkers in the village were large and made up from six- to eight-inch thick logs and mud. They were built outside the hootches and camouflaged with dead tree limbs. The hootches themselves were elevated aboveground to keep the water out when high tide came in. The entire village was filled with deadwood and uprooted trees from Operation Ranch Hand.

We checked out some of the larger bunkers and then called for extraction. Our young boy was joined by a Vietnamese woman, and a little girl and boy. The boy was only about three years old. We loaded them into our helicopter. A quick head count and we were out of there! As soon as the Huey lifted off the little boy grabbed me around the neck and didn't let go until the flight was over. The woman kept her eyes shut the entire time but the young girl seemed to enjoy the ride very much.

As we lifted free from the ground and gained altitude I could see all the hootches were burning. We were still taking light arms fire from the VC who'd hidden or gotten away, but the Cobras went to work and soon suppressed their newfound courage. The raid had only taken fifteen minutes to conduct. We captured documents, destroyed a VC village, captured a VC flag, and removed civilians to what would hopefully be a better environment. A good day's work.

The civilians were flown to a Chinese settlement called Ha Tien. It was located up by the Cambodian border and there was a small runway from which our folks could be flown out to a government controlled settlement. The woman kept pointing to her wedding band, which made me wonder what the VC might have told her about Americans. The people we'd just liberated explained the Vietcong had kidnapped them and forced them to work the rice fields for food meant for the VC. We waited until they were safely aboard their aircraft before returning to the LST.

The ship was underway when our helicopters rendezvoused with it. As we unloaded Chip was taking pictures. He asked us to pose for a group shot with the captured VC flag. Giving his camera to a nearby sailor Chip asked him to shoot the photo and joined us. Years later this picture would appear in a Time-Life series titled "The Vietnam Experience." It was used to advertise the books and a new handle was hung on us as a result. The caption read "The Dirty Dozen—Vietnam Style." Part of the nickname remains with us today as our old teammates now refer to ALFA platoon as THE DIRTY DOZEN.

17

Return to Phu Quoc Island

Something woke me up and I wasn't sure what. My bare feet hit the cold deck of our berthing compartment and I stumbled to the head. I needed cold water in my face something awful. Quiet. That was what had brought me out of a deep sleep. The ship was quiet except for the ever-present humming noise common aboard Navy ships at sea. I dressed after my shower and went to the mess deck for a cup of hot, black coffee.

Topside it was daylight, the fresh salty smell of the sea refreshing after a long night below decks. Sipping at my coffee, I began going over yesterday's operation in my mind. It was then I noted we were dead in the water. That's why it was so quiet. Walking over to the starboard side of the ship I could see mountains in the distance. Where were we, I wondered?

Scott Lyon sidled up next to me and as if reading my thoughts he answered, "Phu Quoc."

"We're going back, I'll bet." Scott nodded in the affirmative.

"CHARLIE platoon arrives today," he continued, "and we're going to do it all over again."

I asked Scott what kind of support we could expect and he

mentioned a guided missile cruiser was at sea somewhere nearby. Cobra gunships were on call, and we'd be operating off an LST. "Scott," I asked, "have you ever called in guided missiles?" Mr. Lyon just smiled and I decided not to push for an answer. Together, we went back below to wake the platoon up.

The day before while returning from Ha Tien by helo we'd flown over the southern end of Phu Quoc Island. Below us I'd viewed an immense Vietnamese POW camp. Its size impressed me to no end. There were rows upon rows of hootches, surrounded by double strand barb wire fences and evil-looking guard towers. The scene reminded me of pictures I'd seen of the POW camps of WWII, but they were nothing compared to the sheer enormity of what was flashing swiftly past me as the helicopter continued on. Phu Quoc was an important area for us and it could ill afford to host a strong VC presence. We were back to make sure such a movement couldn't be birthed and take hold.

It wasn't until after we'd eaten that CHARLIE platoon showed up, arriving by Mike boat. We helped them unload and get squared away in their new quarters. It was good seeing so many friends again, and everyone was sharing stories about where they'd been and been up to. Mr. Bliss and Mr. Lyon flew over to the cruiser to coordinate fire support for our operations on the island. In the meantime I wanted everyone to begin checking their equipment and weapons. I shared my conversation with the platoon, with our frogman photographer, Chip, saying his good-byes and heading off for who knew where.

That afternoon Naval Intelligence told us that when we'd been operating with HOTEL platoon the Vietcong had sent out a message to all the VC on Phu Quoc. It said we (the SEALs) were actually an entire U.S. Army division which had been sent to the island to kill them all. The Vietcong had been ordered to bury their weapons and to take their hammocks into the jungle and hide there until we left. John Ware said, "They must have dug their guns up," because our "division" was back operating on Phu Quoc for a second time. I thought it was more like the VC hadn't learned their lesson the first time around.

After we'd pulled out the first time the enemy had become very bold and aggressive. They'd lost face running off like they'd been ordered to, and to save whatever face they had left they were hard on the civilians who lived on the island. Heavy taxes were levied against the populace, and brutal treatment for not complying with VC orders and directives became commonplace. That's why we were back in town, and with this knowledge our two platoons were eager to go to work.

Our first mission was to secure a small VC village located in the northern central portion of the island. The people were helpless against the armed VC, and the government was going to airlift them south to a new village at An Thoi. Our platoon loaded into helicopters early the next morning and it was a short flight across the water to the dense jungle on Phu Quoc.

We'd selected a landing zone on high ground just a short distance from the village. ALFA moved on line, using the trees as cover for our movement. Breaking into the open we immediately began taking small arms fire from the VC living in the village. Steve Frisk dropped a 40mm grenade atop the hootches where the most fire was coming from and kept a steady barrage of the deadly little bombs coming from the barrel of his MK 148 launcher. Myself and the rest of the platoon were leapfrogging forward, taking cover when possible and laying down a wall of hot steel from our weapons.

Beanan was hit in the forearm with grenade shrapnel. Not serious enough to slow him down he continued the assault. We sent him out afterward to an Army field hospital for treatment. When Mike returned to ALFA his scar was bigger than the wound itself had ever been. He wasn't too pleased about the doctor's ability in patching him up.

ALFA swept through the village, our firepower suppressing the VC defenders. Cobra gunships were called in and worked the perimeter of the village, turning it into a death trap for any escaping Vietcong. Some SEALs popped smoke grenades so our Hueys, or slicks, could locate the landing zone we'd secured. The village's populace was rounded up in the aftermath of the battle, loaded aboard the waiting helos, and sent onward to An Thoi. When it was all said and done, ALFA flew back to its LST to celebrate one more successful mission.

Our two platoons began running port and starboard operations on the island, mirroring the same effort made during our first tour of duty. But this time things were, as Ware had predicted, different. The VC had indeed dug their guns out of caches all over the island and we were engaging in running firefights during nearly every operation. Our Cobras always gave us the upper hand, but I believe the concentration of automatic firepower our patrols could muster caused the Vietcong to stand down once the war started in earnest. Still, we had people shooting back at us more and more often, and they were moving in larger units than we'd experienced earlier.

It was nearing Christmas 1968. Time was slipping past more quickly than I realized and our platoons had been working harder than ever before. Almost as if it were a common thought we noted our mail was weeks behind, and Mr. Lyon asked if I'd take an administrative helo ride one afternoon to pick up any letters from home being held for us. As long as I was back for Christmas, Scott told me, he'd be happy.

The flight to Can Tho went off without a hitch. From there I scrounged a ride to Sa Dec after less than an hour on the ground. Our living area at Sa Dec was filled with huge red mail sacks. Breaking these down I made sure each of my teammates had two packages and ten letters apiece. Finished, and satisfied with my work, I sat down and read my own ten letters, these from my wife and mother. The letter from Mom was bad news. My grandfather had passed away in November and this was the first I'd learned of it. I immediately wrote my mother and asked her to move to San Diego to be with us. That way she'd have family around her.

The next morning I filled three of the red sacks with the platoon's mail, sent my letter off, and went to chow. My flight back to the war took off soon after and in Can Tho luck was on my side. I ran into one of our four slick pilots just as he was preparing to return to the LST. I guess I looked like Santa Claus when I climbed off the helo on

December 24, my three red mailbags hanging off my shoulders and a grin on my face. Needless to say, ALFA was glad to see me back.

And it was good for me to be back with my teammates. I'd had all the time to myself I wanted, and enjoyed the companionship of my friends and fellow SEALs. Christmas that year was good.

Despite the Vietcong being more active on the island they didn't seem to be making any effort to conceal their activities from us. It was not uncommon to hear them coming long before they marched into our ambushes, their voices chattering away like jungle monkeys. They'd had free reign of the northern end of the island for so long it had given them a false sense of security. This is always a fatal mistake, regardless of whose side you're on.

On the other side of the coin we'd become used to the enemy's operating procedures. It was just after the first of the new year and ALFA was running a patrol in the mountains when we heard voices. A hasty ambush was put in place, meaning we simply melted into the jungle on one side of the trail and lay down. Weapons were slipped off safety and gun barrels trained to our front. We were so heavily camouflaged that no one could spot us once we went to ground. The first time the enemy knew of a SEAL platoon's presence was when the firing started and dying— on their side—began.

Five VC with weapons came walking down the trail, all of them talking as if they were taking a stroll through a park in downtown Hanoi. When they were well inside our kill zone they were challenged by our Vietnamese SEAL. The VC pointman swung around hard, his weapon going off in our general direction. We opened up with everything we had, aiming accurate fire into the tiny strip of trail. Three of the five VC dropped dead where they stood. The remaining two ran into the jungle opposite our ambush. As we rushed across the kill zone in pursuit we found one of the two dead just inside the treeline. He hadn't made it far. A blood trail was discovered belonging to the remaining VC, whose sandals we also found. He'd run clear out of them in his haste to avoid dying with his friends!

As was our habit security around the perimeter of the

bodies was set up and selected teams began searching the dead. Weapons were recovered and any papers or documents—to include personal letters or diaries—were scarfed up, as well. While this grisly but necessary chore was being conducted we began taking fire from the direction the VC had come. Mr. Lyon requested the Cobras put down a base of fire to cover our withdrawal. Slicks were scrambled off the LST, and once again the heat was on.

Racing for the extraction point we found ourselves facing one minor problem. An old tree was standing in such a way it was blocking the tiny clearing which the helo would use as a landing zone. The main force VC unit, whose point element we'd evidently hit, was tracking us with great zeal. Bullets were slicing through the jungle around us, the hard *snap* of each round cleaving what cover was available. Beanan and Ware took on the challenge of removing the tree while the rest of us provided cover fire. A gunship came in low and fast, its rockets impacting in one of the areas where the heaviest of the enemy fire was coming from. By radio we informed the pilots of their direct hit, and in response they came in again, this time at treetop level with miniguns blazing. Hot, empty, brass shell casings by the hundreds came cascading out of the sky as the helo passed over our position. Beanan and Ware took direct hits from the casings, exposed as they were in the clearing. Thinking they were under enemy fire both SEALs jumped over to the enemy side of the tree, where they were now indeed in mortal danger.

The platoon pulled back and popped smoke for the inbound slicks. Our Cobras made one final run and then broke free of the firefight so the Hueys could get to us without fear of a midair collision. As the slicks came barreling in for us the VC opened up with everything they had knowing the Cobras could not engage them. Second Squad laid down a strong base of fire so First Squad could break for the clearing and board the first Huey. I was with the Second and when our helo came in there was no question as to how fast we could move under fire! The bird came in hot, its rotor wash slamming the foliage around us into the soft earth as it flared above the LZ. We dove inside, colliding with each other's bodies as man after man thudded into the cramped open compartment. Grabbing what we could of the deck we pointed our barrels outward and joined the door gunners in searing the LZ and surrounding jungle with our combined firepower. All the time I remember us yelling at the top of our lungs, "GO! GO! GO!" to the pilots, as if they needed our encouragement.

Upon our return to the LST we began giving Beanan and Ware a hard time. Their reaction to the hot brass from the Cobra wasn't funny at the time, but it became so in lieu of our successful escape from the VC. In truth, any one of us would have done the same thing but you couldn't find a SEAL who'd admit so that day. All of us were keyed up, the frenzy of battle roaring through us as one collective being. We were all talking at the same time, cutting off conversations and starting new ones, laughing, slapping each other on the backs as if to assure one another we were all alive and well. Scott Lyon came over and asked if we'd seen the helicopter that had brought us in. From the door gunner's mount to the tail rotor there were no less than nine bullet holes. The rounds had passed through the Huey's thin skin, just missing the tail rotor's drive shaft.

This confirmed to me the VC weren't duck hunters. They clearly didn't know anything about leading a target in flight.

ALFA took the next day off to let our nerves return to normal. I knew we needed a rest and it was welcomed by all. However, the platoon knew it wouldn't last. Mr. Bliss was preparing to take a platoon patrol on the Cua Can Canal. This canal's head waters began in the mountains on the east side of Phu Quoc and ran across the island at its widest northern portion. From here it turned south, dumping its waters into the Gulf of Siam on the northwest shore. It was believed the VC were using the Cua Can as a waterway to move supplies and men and ALFA was going to check it out for this reason.

The platoon would load aboard two LSSCs which would take us up the canal as far as possible. From here we'd begin searching for any evidence of the Vietcong. Our officer put the Cobras and missile cruiser on standby, in case we needed fire support. The plan was to hit the mouth of the Cua Can at daybreak. I supervised the platoon checking its gear and weapons, then we tried to turn in early after the patrol order was given. It didn't do us much good as we must have stayed up talking until midnight before finally going to sleep.

Too soon we were awake again. The men were inspected before loading the LSSCs, which bobbed in the dark sea like empty shoe boxes. I remember the air on the deck being chilly with no sign of the sun in evidence any time soon. It would be an hour's boat ride before the dawn would greet us. Once aboard, ALFA hunkered down and nodded into a half-sleep, the rolling of the waves lulling us into a state of suspended anticipation.

Our heavily armed force slipped into the mouth of the canal without a sound. The banks of the canal were so close I could reach out and touch them from where I was positioned in the LSSC. We were sitting ducks for anyone up early and armed, with no way for the boats to turn around in the canal if enemy fire came our way. It was spooky, and very, very scary.

Without warning an M60 LMG began roaring behind us, its red tracers bouncing off the trees and ground as bullets chewed up the surrounding jungle. Two hundred lethal beats per minute screamed into an unseen target, alerting ALFA that the jig was up. A lone VC soldier, taking his predawn bath in the canal, was responsible for spotting the bow of an LSSC coming around a bend in the waterway. He'd apparently ducked under the water, only surfacing after we'd passed him by. Coming up for air he'd also gone for his rifle which was lying atop his clothes on the nearby shore. The VC's mistake was in watching only the first LSSC. Armed with the '60 Mike Beanan spotted the spotter and busted him with nearly a full belt of 7.62mm ball ammunition.

Mike's display of firepower gave our position and intentions away, but it was surely for a good cause. Mr. Bliss decided to continue the mission, so we prepared to go ashore. The LSSCs would stand by until we returned.

For an hour we moved through the jungle, every sense and every nerve honed past a razor's keen edge. The VC knew we were in their backyard, and we knew they'd want to get even for the loss of their man. ALFA soon reached a concave arrangement of mountains we later called the Ox

Bowl. Bliss took Frisk, our radioman, and left us in a tight perimeter while the two of them scouted the surrounding terrain. We waited a long time, however, neither man returned.

Then I heard voices.

The platoon had selected its position well. We had good cover and could not be seen unless walked upon. No one moved. Our training in BUD/S paid off once again as each SEAL accepted his discomfort and fear, turning both into a weapon forged through sweat and pain on the Silver Strand in Coronado. We were transformed into hardened, capable hunters of men. Men hidden by the jungle which swallowed us up in her dense bosom, men whose frames were wrapped and laden with the instruments of death so necessary to ensure our survival. We were teammates, gathered together in a tight band of sodden green uniforms and sweat-streaked green faces whose eyes were rock hard and all-seeing.

Our LDNN whispered that the VC now swarming around us were going back to get their machine guns. We figured to be outnumbered by three to one from the number of voices and activity. That's a lot of people to consider engaging, even for SEALs.

Mr. Lyon felt we needed to move because of the superior force facing us. Ware took point and Scott directed him to duckwalk the platoon out of danger. Ware later told me he believed Scott Lyon had lost his mind when the order was given to move out. A platoon of SEALs duckwalking right through half the VC on Phu Quoc Island! Our pointman then decided he didn't have a better plan than Scott's and he'd just go for it. Holding our weapons out in front of us as much for balance as anything else we did just what Mr. Lyon asked.

ALFA duckwalked out from under the noses of our pursuers with nary a shot fired.

Now to link back up with Mr. Bliss and Frisk. We didn't know where our two teammates were and they didn't know where the VC were. If the two bumped into each other it would be big trouble for all involved. The VC solved part of the puzzle for us by starting to fire their weapons into the jungle. This was the classic recon-by-fire tactic which most often only ate up lots of ammunition for no good reason or result. Only the Vietcong weren't simply firing a round or two and then waiting to see if we'd react, they were firing on full automatic from multiple weapons and different positions around us. I figured this meant they were either very scared, very angry, or both.

Since Bliss had the radio we made for the LSSCs so we could make commo with him and Steve Frisk. As it turned out the two men had figured themselves to be downstream from the platoon when, in fact, they were someplace else entirely different. When Mr. Bliss heard the engines of the LSSCs start up he zeroed in and brought Frisk and himself out of the jungle.

Once clear of the canal and away from the island Scott Lyon contacted the cruiser and requested a missile strike on the area we'd just duckwalked out of. The Ox Bowl was saturated with guided missiles, the mountains protecting it also pounded by the cruiser's enormous firepower. Evidently we'd hit the main body of VC on Phu Quoc because after Mr. Lyon's display of skill with guided missiles, the Vietcong's resistance on the island melted away.

On January 14, 1969, we climbed aboard our Hueys and headed back to Sa Dec. Our job on Phu Quoc Island was over, mission accomplished. With the VC taken down several notches the Dirty Dozen was out of there.

18

Medical Cache

ALFA platoon began operations from their new home base at Sa Dec. Our intelligence came from as many sources as we could either find or generate ourselves. Even as the war continued not all SEAL missions were directed against the VCI. It was now 1969, and the VC were working hand in hand with the North Vietnamese Army, or NVA. They used the same modern Soviet or Chinese Communist weapons and uniforms, and even the same tactics in the field. The two enemy forces were nearly indistinguishable because of this. In addition, their logistics had improved along the northern supply routes but these too had their weaknesses.

We learned many of the VC who surrendered into the *chieu hoi* centers were sick and in need of medical attention. Their illnesses ranged from malaria to wounds received in combat. They reported they were satisfied with their own medical attention but that medical supplies for the enemy had become a critical item throughout the Delta since the 1968 Tet Offensive. In that offensive the VC were nearly destroyed as a combat force while the NVA took enormous casualties themselves. Somehow the media hailed Tet as a victory for the communists when truthfully U.S. forces had nearly crippled them in this single head-on clash of conventional forces.

Regardless of how motivated or well trained for combat a soldier might be, he cannot function when he is sick or wounded. Without adequate medical supplies to treat an army its leadership must stand down from combat operations or move their units back into areas considered as safe. We called these areas sanctuaries. The 857th VC Main Force Infantry Battalion had been active in and around Sa Dec since 1967. Their units had been using hit-and-run tactics since the Tet Offensive, an impressive indicator as to how extensively the VC had been hurt during that offensive.

Humanitarian principles, however correct, don't always find a place in war. The military objective is to stop the enemy, not to let him rest or become resupplied. Therefore a medical cache becomes a worthy target, that if captured, would be costly to the VC both physically as well as moralewise.

And the SEALs knew the importance of just such a target.

On January 17, 1969, the Sa Dec *chieu hoi* center informed Mr. Lyon that a *chieu hoi* VC had turned himself in and reported he had helped bury something of importance the night before. The VC said he'd overheard the cache's contents were destined for a medical hospital. Mr. Lyon assumed custody of the VC and was soon questioning him about the cache. Scott learned the VC had unloaded a large sampan during the night before and had then been forced to help carry the cargo to an underground site a short distance away from the Mekong River. The *chieu hoi* agreed to lead the SEALs to the medical cache which caused us great satisfaction. The target was on a small island northeast of the Sa Dec Naval Base on the north side of the river. The PBR sailors called the island "Football" because of its obvious shape. Football Island was located on the border of Sa Dec and Dinh Tuong Province.

The *chieu hoi* was not aware of the location of the VC hospital and we believed it was most likely located at a base camp to the north as opposed to being right under our noses. Football Island was where the fighting was taking place and therefore not a good place for the sick and wounded to recover in safety and peace. If we were correct it meant the cache would be moved very soon. Mr. Lyon believed we had to do likewise.

The VC almost always chose to operate after dark. There was a good chance they would seek to relocate the cache that very night, especially knowing one of their own had suddenly disappeared. Scott elected to kick the operation off before dark. He arranged for an ARVN soldier, who also knew the area, to go with us. HAL-3 gunships were put on standby and the platoon got its warning order. Afterward, Lyon contacted RS 573 and asked for two PBRs to insert the platoon on the island. During the patrol order we learned this was to be a daylight operation and we should be ready to move out when the order was over with.

We assembled at the pier by the PBRs and began our inspections even as we were loading aboard. The *chieu hoi,* Mr. Lyon, Bud Gardner, and Paul Bourne wore VC black pajama shirts while the rest of us were in camouflage. The M60 gunners and our radioman wore the standard UDT C02 life jacket with two M26 fragmentation grenades clipped into the chest straps. Life jackets were standard operating procedure for SEALs carrying heavy loads because in the Delta you had to be ready at any and all times to swim with your equipment. The men knew it would be a short walk so the Stoner 63 gunners took along an extra three hundred rounds of belted 5.56 ammo. I remember thinking to myself, "Who's going to carry the cache out?"

Lieutenant Dirkx was taking over as Detachment Golf was visiting his platoons in the field to become acquainted with his command. Mr. Lyon invited the officer to come along on the operation. We loaded thirteen SEALs, one ARVN soldier, and the *chieu hoi* aboard the two PBRs and started downriver. Two more PBRs already on patrol joined us as backup fire support. Our boats rendezvoused with them on the south side of the river. Overall, we had one fairly impressive force headed for Football Island.

The sun was bright and very, very hot. Even the fiberglass decks of the PBRs were nearly too hot to touch with one's bare hand. Loaded down with all of our weapons, ammunition, and equipment, we were soaked with sweat already. I felt as if my face camouflage were melting, running in tiny hot streams down my neck and into my fatigue shirt. The air was mixed with the smell of the muddy river, diesel from the boat engines, and our own odor. I must have smelled like an old hot army tent being unfolded for the first time in years. It is not a good smell.

As for me I couldn't wait to get off that boat! By now we felt very much at home in the jungle and under the protective cover of darkness. Now we were in the middle of a river at high noon and very much of a target for anyone sitting on the shore or hiding from view in the jungle. At least we were in our own environment when operating at night, but now we were truly fish out of water. We agreed with Mr. Lyon's decision to go during daylight hours and supported him completely. Still, I never felt secure operating in the daytime and was uneasy with what I considered a bold op-plan.

When the PBRs reached the middle of the river the SEALs moved forward to the bow, taking assigned positions around each side of the .50 caliber machine gun mounted up front. We lay as flat as possible against the deck. I felt almost a part of the PBR's olive drab paint job knowing all the time a bullet wouldn't be stopped by anything but me if the shooting started. The boat slowed and the breeze evaporated, leaving the air around us still and deathly quiet. It felt even hotter than before as I lay there with my teammates preparing to go ashore.

Some thirty-five meters from our insertion point we began taking automatic weapons fire from the shoreline. The PBR gunners opened fire, raking the hidden positions with everything they had. We joined in the firefight as well, trying to move aft of the twin .50 calibers even as they opened up. My ears felt like I had air hammers inside them. The hot brass shell casings from my teammate's M60 LMG were falling between my legs and that didn't help matters at all. Everyone was yelling, with the .50 caliber gunner wanting us out of his way and me wanting to help him for all I was worth. By now my M60 gunner was lying across my legs pinning me to the deck, his weapon laying down steady bursts at our attackers' positions.

Much to our advantage (and good fortune) the VC were not exactly good marksmen. Their rounds were falling short, landing in the water both to our front and flanks. The two support PBRs came roaring in now with all guns blazing. With the SEALs added firepower I imagine old "Charlie" felt he'd made a big mistake. True to their past tactics under such circumstances they broke contact within a few minutes and it was all over.

Our PBR began to turn out into the river when Mr. Lyon grabbed the wheel and said, "We're going in!"

The coxswain said something to the effect of "You guys are crazy!" but he followed his orders and moved the PBR back on line. The two support PBRs were still firing at the point of contact made with the VC and two Seawolves were now overhead sniffing for targets in the open. The Seawolves were equipped with a 7.62 minigun and seven-shot 2.75-inch rocket launcher on each side. They began to pound the VC position as we moved two hundred meters downriver to penetrate the island at our second insertion point.

The platoon inserted onto a firm riverbank covered in tropical foliage. Our *chieu hoi* and ARVN moved fast for a short distance and then stopped. The area was booby-trapped. We moved off the trail into an area covered with large leaf plants knee- to waist-high. The going was slow due to secondary growth which clung to us, making each step difficult. The booby traps didn't help either. From time to time we heard shots being fired, sometimes a single rifle and other times fully automatic bursts. The patrol never took any effective fire, however, the enemy's probing shooting did slow us down.

In a short while we came to a hootch and the ARVN offered to go inside to search the place. He came back out with an old man and woman in tow, the two Vietnamese had been hiding in a bunker built inside the hootch. The ARVN told us the two would take us through the booby traps. Mr. Lyon moved forward to share the point with John Ware. It was hard enough for John to control the ARVN and *chieu hoi,* not to mention adding the two old Vietnamese.

We soon reached a small clearing with knee-high grass covering its surface. The clearing was encircled with palm trees. East of the clearing was a slight rise also dotted with the same kind of tree. The *chieu hoi* pointed with certainty to a spot on the rise where the cache was. I moved my squad forward and set up security around the clearing and its cache. Mr. Lyon instructed the *chieu hoi* and the ARVN to dig out an opening in the ground over the cache and to check for any booby traps. The area appeared to be undisturbed. It had been camouflaged extremely well by the VC. We ended up lowering the ARVN and *chieu hoi* into the cache site itself, which looked like a small cistern. It was very dark inside. Scott took a look using his flashlight and said we'd need help. There was too much inside for just our platoon to move back to the river before darkness fell.

Mr. Lyon began talking with the Seawolves via radio and I moved half the platoon up to help begin cleaning out the cache. The *chieu hoi* began handing out metal ammunition containers. At first I thought our target may have ended up being an ammo cache but one look inside the steel boxes confirmed otherwise. It was indeed a medical site. Inside the metal containers were surgical prep pads, suture kits, forceps, tweezers, scalpels, and medicines. The latter included antibiotics. There were also needles, syringes, and nurses kits. Out from the depths of the hole even came a portable surgery table! In one ammo box was a red communist flag with a white hammer and scythe in its center. Another captured flag for ALFA.

The seven largest of the containers looked very much like the metal cans the Navy receives their coffee in. They were made of tin, four-sided, and in five-gallon lots. Inside each can were light green plastic containers with some kind of liquid inside. One of my teammates said each bag held a pint of human blood . . . meant for use during battlefield surgery most likely. The most interesting thing about the tins were the markings on the outside which I was able to read because they were in English: "To the people of Hanoi, Vietnam, from the people of the United States who care."

Under this pronouncement was a list of names of antiwar activists, most of whom I had never heard of nor did I care to know. There was one name, however, I did recognize. When I saw it I recall thinking to myself, ". . . Well, Jane, this stuff doesn't help Hanoi much by ending up in the Delta."

We carried the contents of the cache into the center of the clearing and our Seawolves came in for it one at a time. The platoon loaded the gunships and they left for the Navy base. It was time to get the patrol moving and out of the area before dark. *Move!*

ALFA had only met with light enemy resistance going in and we moved faster with the two old civilians leading the way to the river. We kept them with us until reaching our extraction point, and then let them return home. Pulling out a smoke grenade we tossed it, with the waiting PBRs identifying the proper color and coming in to pick us up. The extraction went off without any problems and ALFA was back safely in Sa Dec just as it was turning dark.

After the platoon cleaned its weapons and equipment we went to a building on base where the medical cache was being held. The Navy base medical personnel, both U.S. and South Vietnamese, were already there inventorying its contents. There were one hundred and fifty kilos of supplies in addition to ten kilos of enemy medical records and the single flag. The cache was valued at ten thousand dollars and represented sufficient supplies to adequately support two hundred fifty to three hundred VC for a period of ten months! The only items to be whisked off to Saigon were the tins of whole blood with their English markings as to who the source was back in our own country. We took some pictures of the cache contents along with the enemy flag, pictures which exist to this day. It was not a bad afternoon's work and another Scott Lyon operation where everything went right.

We took the night off and went to the enlisted mens club across the street from our barracks. It was time to simply relax and have some fun talking over the operation. Everyone wanted the captured communist flag so we settled on having it framed and giving it to the club we were in. The last time I saw the flag it was still on the wall alongside a captured AK47 rifle we'd brought back from Phu Quoc Island. We'd had a good operation and the platoon was proud of what they'd done. The rest of the night was filled with back slapping and John Ware kept us on our natural high with his jokes until midnight.

That next morning we began to settle down some. After chow we returned to the barracks and began working on our equipment. I dumped the ammo from my Stoner magazines and replaced their loads with fresh rounds. Then I cleaned my "H" harness and began putting a new edge on my KA-BAR combat knife when one of our boat support people called me. Mr. Lyon, it seemed, wanted to see me right away. Now what?

Scott told me to find as many of the platoon as I could, round them up, get them in a clean uniform, and hurry back. We were to fall into formation for an awards ceremony. As it turned out eight of us were able to make it. A Vietnamese colonel, his aide holding a big red pillow that was filled with medals, and a photographer met us outside our barracks. We were told Mr. Lyon, Mr. Dirkx, myself, and two PBR sailors were to receive the Vietnamese Cross of Gallantry with Bronze Star for participating in the recovery of the medical cache.

I fell in beside Mr. Lyon, then there was a PBR sailor, Mr. Dirkx, and the other PBR man. The platoon was at a right angle to me. As the colonel read the citation and presented the medals I could see my teammates out of the corner of my eye. Beanan, Bourne, Gardner, Crawford, and Ware who was taking pictures. This ceremony didn't feel right. There'd been thirteen SEALs on that operation, not just those getting the metals that day. Besides, if it hadn't been for the courage and planning of Scott Lyon, the operation wouldn't have gone off at all. If anyone should be decorated it should be Scott. No, it wasn't happening the way it ought to have.

Later I talked with Scott about how I felt. He told me that since I was the senior enlisted man on the operation and that was the way they had called it I shouldn't worry, or be as concerned as I still was. My emotions were mixed because we'd all done our jobs well. We'd walked behind but one hero that day and that SEAL had planned and executed another perfect operation. We were teammates, and I still believe even to this day every one of the men in ALFA should have been standing on line in front of that Vietnamese colonel, or we all should have been proudly watching Mr. Lyon accept his award for all of us in ALFA platoon.

19

Ben's PRU

The first time I saw Ben I was actually trying to find the Sa Dec PRU headquarters. Actually, I was looking for Ben to begin with. Following the directions given me at the Navy base I turned, in my borrowed jeep, in to the PRU compound. What I saw caused me to believe I'd made a wrong turn somewhere along the way.

There were five platoons of Vietnamese soldiers standing in ranks, and I mean formation perfect. Four of the platoons were dressed in regular Army issue olive drab uniforms complete with M16 rifles. The men in the fifth platoon were standing in formation also, but they were wearing VC uniforms. This meant standard black pants and loose-fitting shirt with NVA sandals. No M16s for these guys. They had AK47 assault rifles, standard Soviet infantry issue. They stood out for another reason; a black, red, and white scarf was worn around their throats. These were smartly tucked into their black shirts which had a white skull and crossbones imprinted on the chest pocket. Each platoon reported in Vietnamese to their team chief, and the chief reported to Ben, who would become my teammate.

Ben was around 5 feet 8 inches tall and possessed a stocky

build. He was dressed in regular olive green jungle fatigues with black boots. He wore no rank nor did he have any patches or unit insignia showing. I couldn't even find a name tag. He was much older than most soldiers found in Vietnam. The only item which made him stand out was a full brim hat with the left side pulled up and snapped in place, Australian style.

After Ben dismissed his troops he walked over and extended his hand in greeting. He introduced himself in an Australian accent with a broad smile creasing his face. Taking his hand I introduced myself, as well.

Ben appeared to be glad to meet me and I was invited to his villa for a cold beer. His place was small and furnished with rattan tables and chairs. He showed me where the kitchen was and asked that I bring him a beer too. When I opened the refrigerator its interior was filled with Australian beer! I asked Ben where he kept his food and he offered he ate with the PRU. For some reason as I studied Ben in his big rattan chair he reminded me of the actor William Holden.

I told Ben how we'd been operating with the Kien Hoa PRU and I felt we'd complemented each other and why. Ben let me go on for a while before asking if I knew Scott Lyon. Naturally, I replied I did and fairly well. The PRU advisor smiled and told me he and Scott had gone over the same ground and that our two units would be working together soon. I have to admit I felt a little silly at this point.

Sooner or later in the conversation—now that business was out of the way—we got around to who he was and what outfit he was with. Ben told me he was with the Australian SAS but he'd been a soldier most of his adult life. He was from Scotland and had retired from the Royal Commandos where he'd also served with the British SAS. His dream was to operate a small sheep ranch in Australia and he'd taken his family there upon retirement. But circumstances and being from England prevented him from making a go of it and the ranch didn't work out.

Ben continued. He'd run into some old mates of his from the Aussie SAS one night and they'd had enough in common that they became fast friends. One thing led to another and he was offered a warrant officer position should he join the Australian Army. He did, and six months later he was a PRU advisor in Vietnam. I was impressed to say the least. Ben told me he was forty-four years old and he wasn't sure just yet if he'd made the right decision.

We talked for two hours about SEAL and PRU operations. I knew I could learn a lot from Ben, and I did. His troops looked exceptionally sharp and I told their advisor so. "The only way to train men is to make them proud of themselves," he said. His best men were assigned to the strike team. They were the ones dressed in black, and it was this platoon which made contact with the VCI first. You had to be better than just good to make this team and Ben made sure they were well compensated when they made a good hit. The rest of his men worked hard to be considered as soon as possible for the elite platoon, the competition fierce but professional.

After a while Ben turned the conversation to why we were in Vietnam. First, he didn't feel you could fight a war with "bloody civilians" running things. Second, he told me the American military command had never been given the objective by Washington to win the war. Third, he believed the "bloody Vietnamization program" would ultimately cause us to lose the war. He seemed to know what he was talking about, however, I noted to myself he sounded bitter too. I wouldn't realize how sound this old soldier's opinions were until years later.

We swapped war stories for a while, he talking about what his PRU had been doing and me on ALFA platoon's exploits and operations. I finally thanked Ben for a great afternoon and mentioned in leaving I hoped we'd be working together soon. He assured me this would be the case and that he was looking forward to it.

A few days later I learned Ben was a man of his word. We checked with Scott Lyon and then made our way to the PRU compound. Ben and his PRU were ready to move out when we arrived. The first change for ALFA was loading aboard ARVN 6X6 trucks. My Stoner gunners were loaded into different trucks down the line and Ben told me to ride shotgun in the second truck with part of his strike team. Ben himself rode in the first truck with the lead element of the strike platoon. With a roar of engines and in a cloud of dust the convoy was off.

It was a long and dusty ride with the trucks arriving at our insertion point just before dark. We unloaded, stretched warily, and stood by the trucks waiting for the word to move out into the jungle. Ben informed me my SEALs were to join his security force so he could use them on the flanks. I was invited to go with Ben and his command element.

As soon as it was dark, most of the men I knew to be with the strike force began moving out. An hour or so later we received radio contact with them and Ben's two support elements split up and began moving. Two SEALs went with each element. Shortly thereafter the command element joined the operation on the march. Ben directed me to fall back in behind him with two PRU on point. Each was dressed in black and armed with AK47s. Four other PRU were behind me and dressed like their pointmen.

This was not like any other PRU operation I'd ever been on. The men neither smoked nor talked as had other PRU I'd worked with, and they carried their weapons at the ready, covering their assigned fields of fire with deadly intent. In the past I'd watched PRU soldiers carrying their weapons over their shoulders like squirrel hunters. I couldn't help but note Ben's PRU handled themselves more like American SEALs than Vietnamese troops.

We patrolled over easy ground for four klicks before reaching tall grass. From time to time one of the PRU with a radio would move past me to Ben and report the progress of the other elements. Very professional. When we began moving into the tall grass Ben told me we were closing in on the enemy and to keep the radioman between us. It was slower going now, and we were in water up to our knees. And it was hot. I was soaked from head to toe from the humidity alone.

Whenever we stopped the PRU moved into a circle and began bending the grass over by the armful. First they bent it one way, and then the other. Then each would climb on top of the folded mounds of grass to sit comfortably as we conducted our business. Ben instructed me to do the same so I could keep out of the water and away from the leeches. He passed along that the support elements were in position about four hundred meters to our right and left flanks. Three hundred meters to our immediate front was a treeline where a VCI tax collector lived.

We waited. The strike and support elements were moving into position at the treeline and it was a long wait for me. It was so hot I kept washing my face with water I scooped off the grass I was sitting on. Ben handed me a canteen and I gladly accepted it. A drink of water sounded good right then. I tilted the canteen up and rolled my head back in anticipation of my first big gulp. To my surprise the canteen was filled not with cool, refreshing water but straight rye whiskey! The deep gulp I'd taken burned all the way down to my equally surprised belly. I could see Ben's grin in the moonlight but I was having a little problem breathing to say anything.

Ben put his hand to his mouth. The team was going in. We could hear loud voices and then the firefight broke out in a crazy mix of whirling red and green tracers. Our radioman was on the hook, or handset, and talking to Ben at the same time. He suddenly shakes his head in the negative. They didn't get our target. I ask about casualties and again the PRU shakes his head. Our right flank opens up and I hear the distinct and welcome sound of our Stoner 63s. I looked over at Ben and said, "That's my guys!"

He turned back to the radioman and then said to me, "They got him, your boys are okay."

We went out as slowly as we'd come in. Ben maintains radio contact with all the elements of our attack group throughout the operation. Finally we come to a stop. Our two pointmen move forward cautiously and we could hear them talking quietly among themselves. Now we're moving again, forward to where the trucks are waiting for us. After we arrive the support elements join us. I went to check our guys noting along the way some of the PRU are holding captured weapons. Shortly afterward the strike element reaches us and they, too, are toting captured enemy weapons.

The PRU chief was successful in capturing both documents and tax money. Ben confirms to me it had been a "good hit." We loaded up on the trucks and settled in for the long ride back to the base. I didn't like the truck ride, especially when daylight came and I could feel an ambush coming around every corner. But there was no ambush and we made it back without incident.

I met with Ben and talked with him about how he could control so many men, and I mean fully coordinate their movements so we acted as one unit, while in the field. He told me it took a lot of time and training. He'd started out small and worked up to team-sized operations. Most of the PRU operations were platoon-sized but they went on team, or multiple platoon, operations once or twice a month.

A few days later the PRU invited us back for dinner. When we got there they had the yard filled with blankets which we sat on while preparing to eat. It was getting dark and that was probably a good thing. The PRU had used some of the captured tax money to fund an impressive feast. They cooked up two pigs in a pit dug into the ground and I admit those pigs looked (and smelled) good.

When the roasted pork was finally passed my way all I got was fat. I picked through the greasy mass looking for some lean meat and when no one was looking, I flicked the fat behind me. Not a good plan. When the PRU saw I was out of fat they insisted on giving me more! Pretty soon I'd attracted four or five dogs who were happily sitting behind me . . . eating all that cooked fat. I think it was the dogs that gave me away.

Ben came over and sat down beside me. I told him I couldn't get anything to eat but fat. He laughed and told me he could see that by the company I was keeping. Ben reached out for the closest pig and cut me off a hunk of good pork. He explained to me later on that night that the PRU gave the guest the fat as it was their custom. Then he said, "With the dogs packed up behind you, you must have been an honored guest!"

On February 1, Mr. Bliss received intelligence from a Lieutenant Rambo who was serving with RS 573 (that's right, his name was *Rambo*). The PBR division had an agent who was a local fisherman and he'd reported that three

VC were living in a hootch. The fisherman had pointed out the hootch to a PBR crew. Lt. (jg) Bliss put the First Squad on alert and issued an early afternoon warning order. Also going with us were two LDNNs, or Vietnamese SEALs. This would be Tich and Gong. We went about checking our equipment and test firing our weapons. The patrol order went down after evening chow.

Our mission was to capture the three VC. We'd get a 0300 wake-up call and insert by PBR at 0430 hours.

When the SEALs were woke the weather was clear and the moon full. At 0330 it was cool on the river and the PBR was waiting for us at the pier. We held a quick inspection as the men passed by me to load aboard. I reported the head count to the lieutenant and the PBR slid quietly out into the river.

The insertion went off without any hitches. We patrolled a short distance using the treelines along the canal as cover. Once the target was reached we set up around the hootch so we commanded a field of fire to its sides and rear. Lieutenant Bliss and Beanan conducted the hootch search along with Tich and Gong.

No one was home.

An ambush was set up from inside the hootch itself and our rear security set up between the hootch and the canal. At 0715 in the morning two VC were spotted approaching our position. One VC entered the hootch and was captured immediately. The second enemy soldier was detected trying to flee and was taken under fire. Our rear security dropped him in his tracks. We moved out after a swift body search and patrolled back down the canal. Warning shots suddenly rang out behind us and Lieutenant Bliss called for extraction by PBR. We pulled and threw a smoke grenade, requesting its ID. The PBR crew radioed back the correct color of smoke and headed in for us.

ALFA platoon's LDNNs interviewed the captured VC and he agreed to lead us to the VC chief's house. Our next move was to contact Ben about our latest intelligence on possible VCI and he was definitely interested. Ben agreed to bring eleven PRU along to join our operation. All three of the LDNNs would come too: Tich, Gong, and Gieng. We had a visiting corpsman, Homes from UDT-11, and he was likewise invited to operate with us as part of the platoon. ALFA was getting short in-country and this would be our ninety-eighth mission. Lieutenant Bliss would be patrol leader and I would be his assistant, or APO. I took this opportunity during the patrol order to remind my SEALs it was too close to the end of our tour to take any chances. I didn't know it then but this was the patrol that would keep me awake many a night in the year to come.

We rolled out of our bunks, dressed, gathered up our equipment and weapons, and made our way to the waiting PBRs. Only a short time passed before our PRU showed up, the only sound the quiet, powerful rumbling of the boats' engines. We loaded aboard and were underway.

It took four PBRs to insert the SEALs and PRU. It was a full moon and the tide was high. This made the insertion of such a large force easy and everything went smoothly. Having the POW leading us to the target made patrolling much faster. Soon we were set up around the VC village chief's house and the LDNNs made their search. He wasn't home.

The PRU went to work questioning everyone in the village. Some of the women were crying and I wasn't comfortable with all the noise the interrogations were causing. Finally, after all the civilians were put in their bunkers and told to stay inside, the noise stopped. Ben said the villagers had told the PRU the chief would be returning around 0700 in the morning. After talking with the lieutenant for a while it was decided to set up two ambushes. The PRU would take one trail leading into the village with the SEALs taking the trail at the other end.

Mr. Bliss set us up in an "L"-shaped ambush with the long leg of the ambush running parallel to the trail, the short leg extending across it. Every now and then I would carry a Stoner MK23 LMG on patrol and this was one of those days. Mr. Bliss put Don Crawford with his M60 LMG and myself with the MK23 on the short leg.

Daylight came and I found myself behind a small bush beside the trail. So small was the bush that it offered very little cover, but it was the only cover around. The lighter it got the less secure I became. I drew my legs in and crossed them, pointing my weapon through the bush to cover myself as best I could. The small trail ran right beside me making a sharp turn fifteen feet to my front.

We waited until around 0700 that morning when the voices reached us. Uncrossing my legs, I sat up on one knee. My legs were numb from sitting on them for so long. At that moment I wasn't sure if I could stand up on my own if it became necessary.

Around the turn in the trail came two men. They were looking down at the trail as they walked along it. The first man was wearing a white shirt and he had a grass mat rolled up underneath his arm. What happened next took only seconds but it was as if my mind were running at flank speed.

Remembering another VC, who only five months ago was dressed in a white shirt and carrying a rolled up bedroll that spit deadly rifle fire meant to kill me, I reacted to nerves alone. *"Lai day!"* came from somewhere deep inside me, yet it sounded like someone else's voice, not mine. I stood and the man's eyes became wide as he stepped back surprised. His bedroll began traversing in my direction even as he stopped dead still in his tracks and my Stoner began jumping in my hands. Not just a burst, but a long roll of at least thirty rounds left the muzzle before my finger broke from the fear which held it to the trigger. Don's M60 joined in and both men were dead before their bodies struck the ground.

The man in the white shirt was lying facedown atop his bedroll. The once white shirt was now stained red with blood. I rolled him over by the shoulder, at least I tried to as only the top half of him moved. The Stoner had cut him in two just below the chest. Grabbing the bedroll with a jerk I watched mutely as it unrolled. It was empty. I had just killed an unarmed man. Shock came over me and I was devastated.

The PRU came to us and their team chief checked the dead men out. I had killed the village chief, our target, and Don had taken out his assistant. The team chief found a note in the dead VCI's pocket that told us the story. The two men had been returning from a VCI province level meeting.

I had not killed an innocent man, however, I still didn't feel too good about it. The dead man would now never tell us anything, he'd just been eliminated.

Going up the river on the PBRs that morning I remember thinking to myself there was no glory in war. It was one of the darkest times in my life. I didn't like to think about that day very much and I put it behind me. This tour of duty wasn't over with yet.

20

Operation 101

*If destruction be our lot we must ourselves be its author
and finisher.*

—Abraham Lincoln, January 1838

When we returned to Sa Dec we began to sort the bags
of mail which had been piling up for the last two months.
Everyone wanted their mail and we needed to create some
space so we could at least get around our living quarters.
The bags covered most of the floor space so we sorted
letters and boxes onto each man's bunk. There were so
many packages we decided to have another Christmas
party.

Someone turned up Christmas decorations from the
enlisted men's club and we even found a tree to put up in
our quarters. That night we opened packages, many filled
with cookies and candies from home. Pictures were taken
and we had a great time. No doubt about it, SEALs do know
how to party!

The next morning, however, it was time to go back to
work. Mr. Bliss and Mr. Lyon began assigning operations to
those enlisted men who hadn't run any combat patrols yet.
Those selected went right at their assigned tasks and turned
in good performances. The experience was beneficial and
each man came back with ideas that changed the way we
operated that final month in-country. We noted the brush
and cane were so thick around the canals that we couldn't

move through it. When we found ourselves in the water—sometimes neck deep—we couldn't see to set up an ambush because the overhanging trees were so thick. One way around this was to begin setting up LSSC ambushes because the heavy foliage was perfect as cover for the boats despite it making life impossible for us as a patrol.

For an LSSC ambush the boat's crew would have four to six SEALs aboard. This gave the LSSC and its crew additional firepower. This team would slip into those areas possessing heavy undergrowth without making any noise, working their way under the heavy foliage which came down to touch the water's surface. We'd grab a limb or some grass and hold the boat in place while waiting for the VC to come by in their sampans. The LSSC crew found it necessary to take soundings of the water's depth so we didn't end up high and dry when the tide went out. We even camouflaged the radar dome of the boat so the moon's light wouldn't reflect off it. These canal ambushes worked well and were documented so others could use the techniques developed.

By far, not all of our operations revolved around the LSSC. Doc Hubbard ran an ambush on a large canal where he moved to the ambush site by LSSC. Our intelligence suspected this canal to be a VC battalion liaison route. As it turned out there was more to it than just that. The VC 502 Main Force Battalion was moving down from the north to relocate in the Delta and you can guess who ended up taking them on.

Doc selected Beanan as his pointman and John Ware to handle the radio. Crawford carried the M60 LMG, with Abe and White joining the squad with their Stoner 63s. Hubbard put the PBRs on standby to act as backup support on the main river. He then alerted the Seawolves from HAL DET 3 for air support. The plan was to insert from the LSSC using the armored LCPL for close support during the insertion and extraction phases. It was a well-planned operation for being a squad-sized ambush.

The LSSC moved silently into the canal in complete darkness. There was no moon. It was so quiet only the soft hum of the boat's radar could be heard by the SEALs onboard. As the insertion point was reached the men eased over the sides and into the water even as the LSSC was underway. The squad swam to the muddy bank and remained in the water, the tide high and the jungle's foliage so thick it masked the ambush team completely from view.

At around 2200 hours the SEALs began making out the sound of sampans behind them on the main river, with troop movement taking place on the riverbanks. Across the canal and one hundred meters upstream the squad observed enemy sampans landing on the bank. The men were so close they heard the VCs' voices as the enemy unloaded their boats.

Doc whispered to Ware that he should scramble the Seawolves and to alert the support boats they had company on the water. It was John's first time as radioman and he told me later that when he finished his transmission he tried to clip his handset back onto his combat harness and dropped it. The hard plastic handset struck his hard plastic M16 where it was lying in his lap. "It sounded just like a rock striking something hard," he offered. The enemy apparently didn't hear anything as their work continued without pause.

Soon two heavily loaded sampans began moving across the canal and into the SEALs' kill zone. The first boat passed so closely by the ambush team they could have touched its sides with their weapons. Doc initiated the ambush and automatic weapons fire cut the first sampan in half, sinking it with its cargo. The second sampan drifted out into the center of the canal even as the team illuminated the waterway with hand fired parachute flares. Ware scored a direct hit on this boat using his 40mm XM148 grenade launcher. A huge secondary explosion occurred as the grenade set off whatever the VC had stored aboard the now burning boat. Ware called for extraction and asked the LCPL to come in, providing fire support.

The LCPL was outfitted with a 7.62mm minigun on its stern. It roared down the canal with its .50 caliber heavy machine guns working the opposite bank. It then turned around to go back out and the minigun let loose on the VC position. The SEALs were quickly aboard the LSSC and making their extraction even as all of this was taking place.

Once back on the river the combined assault group went to work on the riverbank where the ambush squad had heard enemy troop movement. The gunships were now overhead and directing their weapons on the main body of the enemy battalion. By now the VC were getting their act together and as much firepower was being sent up into the sky as was coming down from it. It was one huge firefight to be started by nothing more than a single squad!

Doc Hubbard and his men were back at the Navy base just after midnight. They could claim a body count of five VC KIA. An additional two VC KIA were tallied from the second sampan, these probably due to the secondary explosion. In all, two sampans were sunk and one set of enemy web gear with personal effects recovered.

Hubbard had enjoyed a good operation that night because of prior planning and preparation. Everything had gone off like clockwork. The fast response of the MST support boats and the SEALs' command of the element of surprise allowed them to hit and then successfully evade a much superior enemy force.

And they were a little lucky too.

ALFA platoon continued to run LSSC ambush operations throughout January. Most of these were without significant results. There was an increase in civilian traffic on the river during this period which made targeting that much more difficult. Our patrols stopped sampan after sampan that were breaking the curfew. Each contact compromised our presence due to having to illuminate the area to conduct searches. We discovered the civilians to be fishermen or old women on their way to market. Everyone had to be questioned and present proper ID.

On January 26 I took a six-man squad and inserted by LSSC on the same canal where Doc Hubbard had hit the VC battalion. We were able to patrol for a hundred meters in thick brush before breaking out into tall grass. We'd just settled down in our ambush site when voices reached us on our side of the canal. It was a clear night and we enjoyed the presence of half a moon, making it easy to see for some distance up the canal. A large junk came drifting into our kill zone. Beanan elected to carry a shotgun that night and it proved to be an effective weapon. When we made contact he took three VC out with it immediately.

We called for extraction and the LSSC responded. The

captured junk was too much for the smaller boat to tow so a call was made to our PBRs and they took the junk in to Sa Dec. It was quite a prize.

At the end of the month we received intelligence that the VC 502 was on the move again. Lieutenant Bliss asked me to take a patrol out that night. I picked Lenny Horst to be my APO and we set about planning the operation. Horst made contact with our MST DET and arranged to have two PBRs at our disposal for support. I called the NOC and secured the area we'd be operating in that night.

For some time I had been observing "Puff the Magic Dragon" which was working out to the north of us. "Puff" as we called her was an AC-47 transport aircraft outfitted with 7.62mm miniguns. Watching Puff at night was unbelievable. Sometimes you could hardly hear the roar of the guns because she was so far away but the sky turned red from the solid streams of tracer coming from them. Puff's guns could fire six thousand rounds per minute with every fifth round fired a tracer.

At the NOC I was talking with a lieutenant about the operation and I guess I showed some concern about running into a full battalion of enemy main force soldiers. He suggested putting Puff on standby and he found she was to be airborne during my operational window that very night. "Yes," I said, "let's go for it!" The officer wanted a code name from me and we agreed on "Red Coats are coming."

Horst and I didn't want to be anywhere around when Puff made her left turn and dumped a lethal dose of dragon's breath into the jungle far below. We planned to insert by LSSC on the north side of Football Island. The LSSC was fast and we could be back in the middle of the river if we needed Puff on station and firing. The more we got into the operation the more excited we became about where we were going. The one weak link in our plan was we were not going to be able to get a VR, or visual recon of the patrol area before the op. Later we would find out just how much a VR would have meant to us. As preparations continued we went over our checklist several times to be sure we had covered all our options. I selected Tich as my pointman. He was an LDNN and had been with us the entire tour. Most importantly, I trusted him as an operator. Every question was covered at the patrol order meeting and we were as ready as we'd ever be at its conclusion.

On January 30 we inserted at midnight. The moon was full and weather clear. We had only begun patrolling when the team began running into hootches. The SEALs slipped past them as much as possible as they were not our objective. When we reached the ambush site we discovered there were hootches on it too! A VR would have been nice. Tich and I searched the hootches and questioned the elderly men living in them. The squad stayed in ambush until 0500 hours that morning without making contact. We extracted by LCPL and returned to base.

Either the intelligence was bad or we had simply missed our targets. It wasn't the first time we'd had negative contact and it wouldn't be the last. All our operations were well planned and a miss was just part of the game. Anyway, I felt that I needed an ace in my pocket and that ace had been the presence of Puff if we'd needed her.

ALFA's last operation was on February 9, 1969. Mr. Bliss was the patrol leader and he took ten of us out, to include two LDNNs, Tich and Gong. Our objective was to gather intelligence for a possible future break-in operation for the platoon relieving us. ALFA inserted by LCPL at 0300 hours and began searching hootches. We set up around the first hootch and took one VC into custody. Horst fired a long burst from his Stoner and we went back up the trail for three hundred meters to set up an ambush which would stay in place until 0900 hours.

Sometimes the Vietcong, if they heard gunfire, would wait for a while and then come out of hiding to investigate its source. This time, however, they weren't that curious.

While patrolling back to our extraction point we took three detainees and then went out by LCPL. Our detainees turned out to be draft dodgers and were taken into custody by the ARVN. The VC was held over for a SEAL operation.

ALFA platoon ran their first operation on August 18, 1968, and their last op on February 9, 1969. In this time we ran 101 combat patrols, a record at that time. ALFA's greatest accomplishment, however, was that we suffered no one killed in action and we were all together and going home.

On the tenth the men didn't waste any time packing our equipment. Most of us lightened our war bags by donating our worn-out camouflage uniforms to the rag barrel. We cleaned our quarters and loaded our footlockers on a truck. By midmorning we were on our way to Saigon.

The platoon stowed its gear and climbed aboard our aircraft at Tan Son Nhut airport. The plane gathered speed as it rolled swiftly down the runway and with a bump we were airborne. One last look at Saigon, for some the final time they'd see the city and for others, like myself, a reminder of what was to come on the next tour. For those who would come back to Vietnam it would be too soon. Time goes by fast in the States.

I remember when we slid out over the ocean, Vietnam now disappearing behind us in the jet stream, a cheer went up throughout the plane and everyone began clapping loudly. Up until then it had been fairly quiet but now we were all talking at once. The danger and insecurity we'd felt and lived with for the last six months was now just a fresh memory.

The men of ALFA platoon had done well. We were all veteran teammates and on our way home to wives, families, and sweethearts.

21

CHARLIE Platoon

The heat was almost unbearable in the desert at Niland, California. It was July. I had left as early as I could but the temperature was already climbing past the one hundred degree mark and it was only 0800 in the morning. Every part of the truck cab's interior was hot to the touch. I downshifted as we began climbing out of the desert and the truck slowed to a crawl when it turned to face the mountains ahead.

ALFA platoon was busted up soon after we arrived back in the States. Harlen and I were reassigned to SBI to help build a new training camp. The camp, later to be named Camp Kerrey, was located between the Chocolate Mountain Bombing Range and the Coachella Canal. There was an area of scrub trees along the canal which gave the camp some security from outsiders and the remote location also ensured an air of isolation. The opposite side of the compound was separated from the range by a twenty-foot sand berm. Nestled between the berm and the canal was a new "U"-shaped metal building featuring a single story. Harlen and I had been installing an underground septic system for the SEALs' new quarters. It was a hot and very hard way to spend the summer.

The main reason for the camp's location had to do with the bombing range. The SEALs could shoot any kind of weapon, of any caliber on or across the range without competition or complaint. We were also able to schedule aircraft from Yuma, Arizona, for air strike practice. For a SEAL to be able to talk to aircraft and have them deliver live ordnance on target would prove to be invaluable training when we returned to Vietnam.

The 6X6 truck labored through the mountains, finally rolling down into San Diego with its cool air coming off the Pacific Ocean. After we arrived at the SEAL Team One compound at Coronado, Harlen and I unloaded and then washed the truck. I turned in our trip ticket at the office and the master-at-arms told me the captain wanted to see me upon my return from Niland.

As I walked down the passageway to Captain Schaible's office I noted how dirty I was. My uniform certainly wasn't the proper one to wear calling on the captain. As I entered, Captain Schaible looked up from his desk. "I see we need to get you 'desert rats' a shower." I apologized for the way I looked and the captain waved me to an empty chair. Leaning back in his own he came right to the point.

"Enoch, are you tired of the desert yet?"

"Yes, sir. I sure am." And it was the truth.

"Are you ready to go back to Vietnam?"

I was. Captain Schaible informed me I was to become CHARLIE platoon's new leading petty officer, or LPO. The captain went on to explain MACV wanted more SEAL platoons in-country and the new CHARLIE platoon would be an augmented platoon in Vietnam. To increase the number of platoons, the Special Warfare Group was pulling men from the UDT teams. Lieutenant Boyhan from Team 13 was already onboard and Lieutenant (jg) Duggar would be joining us from Team 11.

The captain said he was giving us as many experienced SEALs as he could. We would have HM1 Doc Brown as our corpsman. Rich Solano, Lou DiCroce, Rich Doyle, and myself would be the combat veterans who'd served previously in Vietnam. Lieutenant Boyhan and Lieutenant Duggar had deployed with their UDT teams and the rest were new men, some who were attending jump school even as I was being briefed.

I was asked if I had any questions and I did. "How long before we leave?"

The captain replied, "About six months." He told me he didn't know what to expect so he could fill me in on what might be ahead for us. "Get to know your men well and what their talents are, you may need them."

I couldn't realize at the time just how important his advice was.

Monday morning I reported to Lieutenant Boyhan and fell in with CHARLIE platoon. It was time to change my mind-set as I was going back to the war. Septic tanks and peacetime duty were a thing of the recent past. We started predeployment training right away. Soon, four new men joined us and their addition to the platoon would prove to be of great benefit after we arrived back in-country. Mike Thornton, Hal Kuykendall, and Mike LaCaze came from BUDS Class 49 with Wayne "Bru" Hampton a Class 50 graduate. We were still short two men. Mike Sands and Ken Meir from Class 49 would link up with us as soon as they completed the Army's Raider school.

Tom Boyhan was a quiet man who drew my respect from the beginning. He was a Naval Academy graduate and a full lieutenant with time and experience in the service. He asked me what I thought about going out to the Navy Ordnance Test Station at China Lake to see what kind of new toys they had come up with for us. I liked the idea because there were a few things in the armory I wanted to talk with the China Lake staff about. We agreed to take the platoon with us, relying on the lieutenant's van and my car as transportation.

It was an uneventful trip filled with lighthearted conversation. The next morning we met with the civilian personnel who'd been working on SEAL projects for the past five years. They were as eager to talk with us as we were with them. Small groups broke off around tables and work-benches throughout the shop. I already believed the trip was worthwhile and so did my teammates.

I talked with two men about some ideas regarding the construction of an electronic controlled range at our camp in Niland. The range would involve a series of pop-up targets where the student would walk a trail, rifle and live ammunition in hand. An instructor would supervise the student whose job it would be to engage the targets when they presented themselves. A control panel would score all the hits automatically. Today such ranges are commonplace and of great training value to those who use them. Lieutenant Boyhan called for me to join him at another table so I wrapped up my conversation and went to visit.

He showed me a rifle grenade that had been developed to fire from an M16 rifle. Its purpose was to mark targets at night for air support. It was built with a bullet trap to allow the grenade to be propelled by the issue 5.56 ball round rather than a blank special round. This meant the grenade could be fired in an instant under combat conditions without having to fit a specially loaded magazine or round in the weapon. The staff called the munition a "TIARA" grenade and upon making contact it would deploy a green chemical gel on the target which glowed at night.

Tom Boyhan had some experience with naval aviation and he told me a pilot could see fifty miles in any direction from his position in a plane. The new grenade would allow quick identification of a target in darkness, making air support that much more swift and accurate for those SEALs needing it on the ground. We asked if we could try some of the grenades in training, calling in air support on the range at Niland. The staff was more than happy to send us grenades for our testing and evaluation.

Our SEALs in Vietnam had been having problems making contact with VC/NVA tax collectors. The PBRs knew where the enemy's tax men were working and had actually observed them working, calling out to sampans on the river when these were returning from a successful day at the market selling their goods. Most attempts to intercept tax collectors were unsuccessful as they either spotted us or had ample warning to escape. Whenever the boats came into range of its weapons the tax collector would just fade away into the jungle along with his security force.

China Lake had just built a .50 caliber sniper rifle which was proven accurate up to two thousand yards. It was just the weapon needed to eliminate the illegal taxing of the

Vietnamese people living and working on the rivers. The weapon was made from a turned down .50 caliber machine gun barrel fitted with a bipod and flash suppressor at the muzzle. A rolling block single action was machined at China Lake and completing the rifle was a twenty power telescopic scope. I had never fired this heavy a caliber rifle from the shoulder, and the staff agreed to let us take the weapon to the range the next morning.

On the range the staff provided a bench on which to rest the rifle without having to support its weight physically. The desert range had a rimrock at the two thousand yard mark. A large white circle had been painted on the rock as a target, this being about the size of a basketball. All of the SEALs got a turn to fire five or six rounds. The rifle's performance was excellent, delivering round after round into the white circle more than two thousand yards away from our bench. The men began discussing the recoil of the weapon. We were surprised it didn't kick all that hard. In fact, it had more of a push which moved your body back and down at the same time. One of the civilians with us said a Marine on the base fired the weapon thirty times and then did thirty push-ups.

That was too much for a platoon of SEALs to handle as they were not to be outdone by a Marine. That was fine but they picked me, the oldest SEAL, to erase the unknown Marine's record. I guess they figured if they were going to make a point they would rub it in real good.

After a lot of good-natured pressure I gave in. They were to be always ready to hand me a new round whenever the weapon was fired. I took a seat on the bench and began sending .50 caliber rounds downrange, deciding if I was going to participate I'd make every round hit the target, if possible. After twenty-five rounds my face began to feel a little hot. At thirty rounds it was numb. It was at around forty rounds I began to really feel the impact of the big gun as it slammed time after time into my shoulder. To allow for some relief I stood and fired the final five rounds off hand at the target. The men thought I was showing off and cheered me on until Round Fifty smacked into the rimrock. Now I had to do fifty push-ups and the platoon owed me big-time. They got their push-ups and notice dinner was on them that evening.

The base only had a Petty Officers Club which meant most of the men couldn't get in. However, the China Lake staff pulled some strings and made arrangements for everyone to enjoy the club's atmosphere. I gave the men a lecture about how to handle themselves at "my" club and then made sure I got there first. I positioned myself on a stool at the end of the bar, the club quiet with only a few sailors present.

Trouble started almost immediately after the SEALs entered the bar. As in most Navy clubs, there was a large, highly polished ship's bell hanging at the bar. The custom was if someone rang the bell it meant he was buying a round for everyone in the bar. Wouldn't you know it would be one of my guys who rang the bell? The bell ringer was none other than Mike Thornton, the biggest and loudest member of the platoon. The bartender served the bar and then presented Mike with the bill. That's when it hit the fan. Mike became unglued and refused to pay the bill. I was embarrassed and tried to hide my face behind my glass, but this didn't work. Mike saw me at the end of the bar and started my way, complaining loudly every step closer to where I sat. Mike's best friend was Hal Kuykendall and he was backing Mike up all the way, being careful to stand behind him at all times.

By the time Mike reached me he'd really pushed all my buttons. I lost it and spun around on the stool, hitting Thornton in the jaw as hard as I could. Even though I'd boxed with some success for the Navy I knew I'd made a mistake when the pain ran down my fist and arm, all fifty rounds of the rifle's earlier recoil causing my shoulder to announce just how sore it was. Mike's head popped back and struck Hal on the nose, which sent him to the floor screaming in pain. Thornton didn't drop. He just stood there looking like he'd lost his best friend. He didn't try to remove various parts of my body from their moorings, which he was fully capable of doing. Instead, he began apologizing and said he would leave after paying the bill.

Turning to do so he told Hal to "shut up!" paying the bill and taking his wounded teammate with him. The bartender thanked me and I went back to our quarters to let a cold shower work its magic on my sore neck and shoulder. I'd just gotten my first lesson about Mike Thornton. He had a head as hard as steel but his heart was soft, which made me happy.

After we returned to SEAL Team One, Lieutenant Boyhan and I got into a conversation about calling in fixed wing aircraft for fire support. I'd never had the experience of doing so and was willing to try. He told me the OV-10 Broncos were presently training at the Chocolate Mountain Bombing Range at Niland and he'd do what he could to set up some training with them and the platoon.

Word of what was taking place in Vietnam had a way of getting back to us. During the last six months the OV-10 Bronco had become one of the SEALs' main means of air support in some parts of the Delta. Our reports said they'd acquired an outstanding reputation with the platoons as a versatile light strike counterinsurgency aircraft. We discovered some of the OV-10 instructors training at Chocolate Mountain had flown for our platoons in Vietnam and were more than happy to train with us. I was looking forward to it.

CHARLIE platoon moved to Camp Kerrey and Mr. Boyhan worked out the details with the Bronco training unit. We began SEAL training at night and worked hard to fine-tune our effectiveness. Our training operations with the Broncos started out as daylight runs so we could see what it was they were doing. Our crew at the parachute loft had developed some silk magenta "Ts" for marking positions during the day. The "T" was twenty-four inches wide and five-feet long at the top. It also had a ten-foot leg and could be folded into a small square and carried in a plastic bag. We used the "T" to mark our own position on the ground for the pilots working overhead.

The radioman would lay the "T" out on the ground and have the pilot identify it. He'd then turn the top of the "T" toward the target while communicating to the aircraft what the target was and where. That little bit of colored silk worked like a dream. The Broncos could pick up our position immediately and be directed on target with a minimum of confusion or radio traffic. I was used to our gunships, the helos, being right there on the ground with us during a firefight. The OV-10s delivered their ordnance from altitude but with no less accuracy. I would learn later this was not always the case, and in training it took some getting used to for some of us.

When night operations began we used the new TIARA rifle grenades to mark the target, and a strobe light to mark our own position. They worked well for us in training. In combat, however, we discovered the enemy could see our strobe light as well as the pilot could see the grenade's green glow!

By mid-October CHARLIE platoon was as ready as it was going to be. Hal Kuykendall was the man who would maintain our morale by simply being himself. Thornton and Sands became our M60 LMG gunners and were certainly strong enough to handle them. Mike LaCaze and Hal were already becoming accomplished radiomen and there was no doubt Solano and Doyle would become our pointmen. As for the rest, you couldn't pry their Stoner LMGs out of their hands for any price.

Tom Boyhan was terrific at coming up with new ways to train the platoon. One such idea was to have his patrol leaders and radiomen go for a ride in an OV-10 so they could see how it worked from the cockpit's point of view. Before we could do so we had to attend the course at the Naval Air Station. The first thing they did was put us in a parachute harness and tell us how to make a parachute landing fall if we had to eject. It made no difference that some of us had over two hundred parachute jumps under our belts. This was their game and if we wanted a ride we'd have to do it their way. Part of the training did get my attention, like how to work the oxygen and radio . . . and what not to do. We were checked out and deemed ready to fly. That had been the easy part. But we never did get our courtesy flights before going to Vietnam although Tom did go up once we were back in-country.

Another thing Tom involved us with was the U.S. Border Patrol. On weekends there could be over twelve hundred illegal border crossings a night in the San Diego area alone! It proved to be no problem setting up a listening post and capturing "Old Jose" as he tried to slip from Mexico into the United States. It was good training in prisoner handling for the new men in the platoon and sometimes I would lay my hand on the back of a teammate as he was handcuffing an illegal and feel him trembling. It was good to get over the jitters in a training environment rather than work through them in 'Nam.

In mid-December 1969 we received our orders. CHARLIE platoon would deploy on December 22 to the Explosive Ordnance Disposal (EOD) school in Hawaii, reporting in on the twenty-sixth. From there we'd go on to Vietnam and begin our tour. We were ready to go, however, I had missed the last Christmas at home and was looking forward to being with my family this year. We did have an early Christmas of sorts, opening gifts on the twenty-first. My youngest son, Mike, had a great time but Eatsie and the two oldest children, Laura and Ken, could offer nothing but long faces. I understood.

As it turned out the EOD school was about booby traps found in Vietnam. Most of us felt we knew all about them but I'm sure we learned something new. Most of all we were unhappy about spending Christmas Day in an old barracks in Hawaii when we could have been with our families.

CHARLIE platoon arrived at Tan Son Nhut, Republic of Vietnam, at 1700 hours on December 31, 1969. Once again the intense heat was the first thing to greet us as we stepped onto the hard tarmac. It had only been ten short months since I'd flown out of Vietnam with ALFA. But it felt, and even smelled, like I had never left.

22

Ben Luc

It is fatal to enter any war without the will to win it.

—Douglas MacArthur, July 1952

Lieutenant Boyhan had been successful in getting orders cut in Hawaii for Doc Brown, Lou DiCroce, and himself to go on ahead of the platoon to Vietnam as an advance party. Once there they'd made contact with DET GOLF and discovered we were to report to Ben Luc, a small Navy base on the Van Co Dong River. Once at Ben Luc our teammates contacted Lieutenant Bumgartner from BRAVO platoon who was ready to show us the ropes. He'd escort CHARLIE platoon during their first break-in operation in our new AO.

When the aircraft's door was opened we were greeted by Tom and company. The truck was loaded and we were soon on our way to Ben Luc. The men were lighthearted and eager to get settled in and begin operating. Ben Luc was about twenty miles southwest of Saigon by road. Our truck bounced over a secondary road that was at times no more than a jeep trail. The countryside was laced with canals and small streams. It was likewise dotted with small rice farms and banana plantations, separated by high marsh grass and treelines.

Ben Luc was in the "Giant Slingshot" area of operations which we were to become a part of. There exists a section of Cambodia that juts down into Vietnam called the "Parrot's

223

Beak." It was located just west of Saigon. The Van Co Dong River slips down from the north along the Cambodian/Vietnamese border to the Parrot's Beak, then flows southeast through the Delta. Another river, the Van Co Tay, runs out of Cambodia along the south side of the Parrot's Beak only to converge with the Van Co Dong to form a giant "Y." This natural meeting of the two rivers gave birth to the term "Giant Slingshot" as that's what it looked like both on the map and in the air. These rivers dumped their waters into the Nha Be River bordering the south side of the Rung Sat Special Zone. This river complex had been a direct supply route for the VC/NVA and lay within striking distance of Saigon.

The Tan An Army base was located on the Van Co Tay River fifteen miles south of Ben Luc. The U.S. 143rd Ranger Company was stationed with the 9th Infantry Division in Tan An. MST-2 DET BRAVO was waiting on CHARLIE platoon in Ben Luc with an LCPL and LSSC to support us. HAL-3 DET SEVEN with Seawolves gunships was available for close air support. All we needed was to get an intelligence network going and we'd be in good shape.

After the platoon settled into our new quarters at Ben Luc we began preparing for our first break-in operation. Lieutenant Bumgardner had a KCS (Kit Carson Scout) with him. The KCS were ex-VC who had defected to the government side and worked with us in running missions against their former comrades. The scouts worked well when they were operating in areas they were familiar with. I had heard a lot about them, both good and bad. Still, I was looking forward to working with them.

The First Squad ran the operation. Lieutenant Bumgardner added Thai, an LDNN, and Ah, our KCS, to the patrol. We inserted when the tide was at the flood level and the night began wet and would end likewise. The operation was more or less a long walk in the swamp. We stopped and set up a trail ambush, having to halt the patrol several times due to illumination on the west side of the Van Co Try River. It was an uneventful mission and we extracted wet and tired. The Second Squad met with more of the same the next night, again without contact with the enemy. Mr.

Bumgardner took the KCS with him when he left Ben Luc but we kept the two LDNNs, Thai and Doan.

It was good to see and work with Thai again. We'd worked together for the entire six months that ALFA was in-country. A few days later I was trying unsuccessfully to grab some afternoon sleep when I heard my name called. Thai had brought Tich to see me and I was glad he had. I asked my LDNN about his wife and after some small talk he asked, "We shoot many VC together again?" It took only a minute for me to figure out he wanted to work with CHARLIE platoon. Thai just smiled and let us talk. After Tich left I asked Thai what it would take to get Tich assigned to us, then turned the request over to Lieutenant Boyhan.

We were just about to get serious about combat operations when we hit a snag. It became almost impossible to secure an area of operations. Most of the time if the Vietnamization program got in our way the Army would secure AOs just in case they wanted to operate in any given area. It was very clear the United States was not determined to win the war, better yet, our government was committed and willing to turn the war effort over to the South Vietnamese even as our own combat troops were still in-country and under arms.

SEALs have always known there is more than one way to skin a cat.

Tom knew there was an outfit in the U.S. Army that could help us out. He made contact with the 143rd Ranger Company and cut a deal where when we felt we had solid intelligence an AO would be worked through the rangers' command structure. It was a good plan and worked for us. However, I still had problems with the "don't rock the boat" talk while all the time offering they needed more of us to do the job. CHARLIE platoon was called an "augment platoon" because MACV wanted more SEAL combat action platoons in Vietnam. On the other side of the coin President Nixon was calling for troop withdrawals. I couldn't help but wonder if I'd had to leave my family before Christmas to rush over here, only to go in circles as to what our government wanted from one minute to the next. Rather than drag the SEALs down, this apparent indecision and confusion only made us more angry for action against the VC.

Working our own intelligence network the Second Squad ran an operation on January 13, 1970. It gave us our first contact. The squad inserted after dark by LSSC and patrolled fifteen hundred meters through the rice paddies and treelines. They came upon five large bunkers and soon they heard voices. There were approximately thirty VC in front of our teammates. The squad moved forward and observed nine armed Vietcong coming out of a hootch. The VC began using a bull horn, telling those who could hear them that they were going to be operating that night. It was pretty clear they felt totally secure in their own backyard.

Lieutenant (jg) Duggar called for the Seawolves and then initiated small arms fire on the enemy soldiers and their bull horn. With the gunships overhead Hal Kuykendall directed an air strike on the main body of VC. The Seawolves were also used to cover the squad's extraction by LSSC. CHARLIE platoon had drawn first blood that night with five VC KIA and at least five more accounted for in the same straits.

Now this was the way it was supposed to be.

Two days later the First Squad drew more blood from intelligence provided by a *chieu hoi*. We inserted by LSSC and the *chieu hoi* led us up a VC communications trail. Lieutenant Boyhan set a guard post at a fork in the trail and we settled in. Soon afterward we heard voices and saw two VC with weapons in their hands walking along the trail. The lieutenant opened fire with the rest of us joining in when the enemy soldiers were within four meters of the SEAL guard post. The count was two dead VC, with two recovered AK47 rifles and ninety rounds of ammunition. The dead mens' backpacks contained letters from North Vietnam to NVA in the field. Also, NVA money was found on both bodies. Recovered documents would lead us to other operations. It was a good hit.

On January 25 the platoon ran an operation meant to target a VC squad leader. Inserted by LSSC after darkness had fallen, CHARLIE patrolled only six hundred meters before sighting ten armed Vietcong. The VC appeared to have entered a hootch and Mike LaCaze scrambled gunships overhead as we moved on the hootch. Only one VC was spotted about fifteen meters from the large hut and he was taken out of the picture with two Stoners. We found a blood trail indicating a second man had been wounded and dragged or crawled away.

A search showed the VC had been moving to a weapons cache. Where the VC had fallen we uncovered three AK47s, two M-26 grenades, and one kilo of documents, all of these wrapped in plastic. During the search another VC was discovered lying dead, adding to our body count. We wrapped everything we could carry up and moved back to the river. An air strike was called in on the area where we'd spotted the ten VC and Seawolves covered our extraction by LSSC.

Thai told me the two VC we'd killed on the commo trail were actually NVA because of the mail and money they'd had on them. The documents were meant for a district level VCI and were important. I spoke to Lieutenant Boyhan about this, thinking all the time about our snatching a major VCI presence who was operating right under the noses of those who were trying to convince the world this bit of Vietnam had been neutralized of VC/NVA forces. We'd made contact with NVA mailmen and they weren't working for the rice farmers at Ben Luc!

Tom responded to my excitement and he carried the ball right to the NILO responsible for our area. The NILO did have reports of multiple district level VCI in an area due south of Ben Luc. This put such a presence halfway between Ben Luc and Tan An. The excitement was building. We needed a visual recon of the area and I went with Tom to the Tan An Army base to scrounge a helicopter and crew for the VR. What we found was two small canals between the two rivers which allowed for easy movement by sampan to both Tan An and Ben Luc.

The area our VC were probably holding up would be along the smallest of the two canals. It was too small for our boats to travel on and possessed good tree cover with thick nipa palm along the canal's banks. In addition, a small hamlet ran along the waterway with hootches located on both sides of the stream. As we flew over the target we marked the hootches we could see on our map.

Now it was time to put the operation together.

Lieutenant Boyhan told me he wanted me to take the operation. We went to work planning the mission, which had its operational problems. First, we didn't know which hootch our VCI were in or on what side of the canal. I wanted both the Vietcong cadre bad. The only way to effect a capture would be to split the platoon into its two squads, hitting both sides of the canal at the same time. This was a dangerous thing to do with an experienced platoon, and CHARLIE had only one month's combat under its belt. But it was a good platoon and I believed they could pull it off.

Next we had to decide what to do with the people once we searched a hootch and moved on to the next. Taking them with us was out of the question and we couldn't leave men behind to guard them either. Both squads would have to move together and maintain radio contact at all times. I decided we had to put the people to sleep without harming them and so I turned to Doc Brown. He solved the problem in the fashion all good SEAL corpsmen did, and still do.

On February 4 I briefed the platoon. We would keep the squads in their normal order of march except for Tom Boyhan and myself in First Squad. Mr. Duggar would load his squad aboard the LSSC with First Squad leading the way in the LCPL. There would be no moon and the tide was to be high. Using the advantage of the tide's height our radar could pick up the small canals' openings. It would be a clear night with stars filling the sky.

The first entrance to the canal complex was very close to the Navy base. We slowly and quietly slipped past it and went downriver for another five miles where we found another entrance. Turning into the canal the boats slowed so as to keep the engine noise down. Just before the LCPL made its turn into the second canal we made contact with two armed VC in a sampan. Their AK47s were no match for the LCPL's .50 caliber heavy machine gun and down they went! The LSSC came alongside and we debated briefly about going on or aborting. Lieutenant Boyhan said it was my call and I said, "Let's go."

We began moving up the canal and it was indeed small. At times, the gunners turned their barrels in to keep tree limbs from hitting or snagging them. A wide spot in the canal greeted us and the LCPL inserted our squad as the LSSC slipped by very, very slowly.

Moving across a large rice paddy we found ourselves dropping down and taking cover frequently because of friendly illumination in the vicinity. During one of these security stops we witnessed a firefight to our right front area. The LSSC had been ambushed at the insertion point and was taking fire from three sides. They were furiously returning fire while withdrawing, Seawolves enroute to support. The ambushed LSSC with our Second Squad still onboard linked back up with the LCPL, both boats now taking fire from both banks. I hoped none of our men had been hit.

We patrolled another five hundred meters and began taking probing fire at ten-minute intervals. The enemy figured we were on the ground but weren't quite sure where. I passed the word that no one was to return fire. Suddenly from the north/northeast we began taking small arms and B-40 rocket fire. "Don't fire back!" I ordered, assuming ground control of the circling Seawolves.

Mike LaCaze, my radioman, fired a TIARA grenade to mark the enemy's position and the gunships picked it right up. At the same time Lieutenant Boyhan activated his strobe light to mark our own position so friendly fire wouldn't become a reality. But the enemy spotted the strobe and Tom's position began attracting unfriendly fire to the degree he swiftly turned the blinking light off. Now the VC started dropping effective 82mm mortar fire in our direction. I directed the Seawolves onto the enemy mortar positions and there was a large secondary explosion complete with a seventy-five-foot-high fireball roaring upward into the dark night as mortar rounds exploded, killing their handlers.

One of the gunship pilots reported taking .50 caliber fire from the Vietnamese outpost located nearby. I figured the outpost had probably been overrun by what was proving to be a superior enemy force. "Blow it away!" I ordered and he did. As the gunships worked over the enemy positions the VC let up on us and we elected to get on our way. I told Rich

Solano to move down to where Tom was and take the point. "Get us out of here," I said.

During the extraction which took place in open rice paddies we periodically fired 40mm grenades and 2.5-inch LAAW rockets whenever an enemy mortar exploded nearby. The enemy's exploding ordnance would cover the sound of our own being fired back at him. One of the 82mm rounds impacted right behind me, picking me up and slamming my body into a nearby rice paddy dike. It took a minute to get my breath back, and my hearing was affected although it would come back in a day or two. We got back to the LCPL and its crew put the pedal to the metal.

Rich Doyle received some minor wounds on his hand and returned to duty after they were dressed. The LSSC was a little worse for wear, however. For what we'd just gone through we came out smelling like a rose.

But it wasn't over with yet.

Upon our return to the Navy base Tom took eight of us that same night to Tan An where we woke up the 143rd Ranger Company. We still had the AO and we needed help in reconning the location of the night's earlier activity. The rangers were glad to go along but we had problems getting helos to take us in. Finally, after daybreak, our force got underway. We were eight SEALs, one LDNN, and eight Army rangers. Navy gunships joined us for the insertion.

The slicks inserted us short of the planned LZ and we ended up making our way through open rice paddies again. We patrolled the area with both squads in visual and radio contact. Suddenly we tumbled upon a large base camp concealed by nipa palm. The enemy's cooking fires were still burning. Fresh trails led out of the camp which showed the VC had left their camp during our extraction. Also found were punji pits, and fighting holes and bunkers.

The results of the night/day operation were: CHARLIE platoon made contact with the 314th NVA Light Force Company. There were 22 NVA KIA, 12 NVA WIA to include the unit's commanding officer and his assistant, a platoon leader. We killed one district and one province level VCI. A motorized sampan with a squad of enemy soldiers and an M60 LMG was also accounted for.

In addition, the morning's sweep of the Tan Duc outpost

saw three POWs taken who were district level VCI, to include the hamlet finance cadre and agriculture committee. One LMG, three AK47s, and three dead VC were also added to the tally.

Intelligence received from a SEAL source reported we had hit the 314th NVA Company which was composed of 105 men, four 82mm mortars, two ChiCom RPD light machine guns, six B-40 rocket launchers, and numerous small arms. The source reported the unit had targeted Ben Luc and Tan An for the upcoming TET holiday.

It had not been a bad night's work for any SEAL platoon. I had an even greater respect for Lieutenant Boyhan as he had charged me with running the operation and had never done anything less than support me, regardless of its surprises. Coming back from Tan An by jeep that morning I realized I was completely exhausted. If it hadn't been for Tom I would have called it quits after we'd returned to the Navy base on the boats. He was going to be some kind of officer to work for.

I closed my eyes . . . I was hungry. The jeep bumped along the road and I didn't care.

Operating on NILO provided intelligence, Lieutenant (jg) Duggar ran a platoon recon patrol on February 6. The mission was to search for an NVA mortar squad reported to be within three kilometers of Ben Luc. SEAL intel from our operations on the fourth and fifth supported the NILO's information.

CHARLIE platoon inserted by LSSC and LCPL at high tide. The night was partially cloudy and there was no moon. The men were itching for more action. We turned south and patrolled five hundred meters from the insertion point. We were moving across a rice paddy and had just passed a graveyard when artillery illumination skylighted us against the darkness of the ground and night. At the same time the illumination went off I heard a *"clink"* ahead of me and someone yelled, *"Grenade!"* Tvrdik, who was the third man from the rear in our line of march, had just been struck in the chest by a thrown ChiCom stick grenade. The grenade then bounced off his Stoner and onto the ground.

Tvrdik picked up the grenade and threw it into the rice paddy where it detonated underwater. His quick action prevented injury to himself and possibly other members of the platoon. From that night onward we knew he was an operator who had it all together.

We swiftly moved another one hundred and fifty meters to the north and set up an ambush. While in the ambush position we spotted signs of our being approached from the south. Then there was nothing. We held the ambush in place all night but had no contact with the VC. Gathering everyone back up we patrolled out to our extraction point, called for the LCPL and were back on the river by 0600 that morning.

By February 10 CHARLIE platoon had run seventeen combat patrols and racked up quite a score. Our success must have raised some eyebrows as we were ordered to move to Coastal Group 36, in the Long Phu District, Ba Xuyen Province.

The word had come down for CHARLIE to "start packing."

23

Dung Island

CHARLIE platoon loaded its equipment onto a well-worn truck and prepared to leave Ben Luc. Oddly enough, we loaded more on the truck than what we'd come with. Mike Thornton, always thinking of his stomach, managed to secure a pallet's worth of C rations. Lieutenant Boyhan knew these didn't belong to us and he knew they'd be missed . . . and who would be accused of taking them so he ordered them unloaded at the last minute. He felt it would reflect on the next SEAL platoon coming to Ben Luc to operate. Afterward, when rations became an issue, Tom offered he'd probably made a bad call leaving the boxed meals behind. CHARLIE platoon agreed with him, especially Mike Thornton.

The drive back to Tan Son Nhut airport went by much faster than the trip down to Ben Luc, or so it seemed. But when we arrived it took another twenty-four hours before we could get a flight out. The men lay around the airport amusing themselves by playing Oh Hell and Pitch, two of their favorite card games. It seemed we were always being interrupted by U.S. military men wanting to see our equipment and weapons as they were passing through the airport. Most only wanted to talk to some SEALs, to see what we were all about. I guess they'd heard all sorts of tales floating around Vietnam about SEALs and their missions, most of these unrecognizable to us as they were often very bizarre.

Finally the cards were stowed away and the curious left behind. We loaded a C-47 transport plane and made ready for the short flight to Binh Thuy airport on the Bassac River. It was an uneventful trip and back on the ground we found another truck waiting for us and our gear. This time we headed downriver toward the Navy base at Can Tho where we settled in for the night.

Looking around for Detachment Golf we discovered he had moved to Seafloat on the Ca Mau Peninsula. Lieutenant Boyhan was not happy with this arrangement for our platoon. We would now be working with Detachment Alfa whose hands were already full supporting SEAL Team Two's platoons in-country. Problems started almost immediately and this trend haunted us for the rest of our tour. Here we were, a platoon from SEAL Team One, somehow dependent upon SEAL Team Two's resources and good graces when they were stretched just supporting their combat action platoons' needs. We would just have to make the best of a bad situation.

Morale was high. We were looking forward to moving to our new operating area and everyone jumped right in to help load our equipment aboard a Navy landing craft provided for just that purpose. Much of what we were taking was new to us, to say the least. First to go aboard was a large metal conex container which held the platoon's ammunition and explosives. Then there were six heavy wooden boxes containing port-a-tents which would become our quarters when we finally set up home. A field kitchen came next, with a generator and hundreds of empty sandbags which would have to be filled upon arrival. All of this was foreign to SEALs more inclined toward combat than construction. The last item aboard was a piece of heavy equipment which would be used to unload the cargo we'd just loaded. At the time we assumed most of everything was for some support unit downriver. Bad assumption. Finally the platoon, tired and sweating, joined its gear and the craft slipped out into the Bassac River.

We were on our way.

On most maps the river we were riding along is called the

Hau Giang. However, both Vietnamese and U.S. troops referred to her as the Bassac. The river broke through the Cambodian border and cut almost straight across South Vietnam's Delta region. Just above Can Tho it widens, turning into one of the largest rivers in the country before spilling her fresh water contents into the South China Sea. "Fresh" water is being kind. Her waters were actually muddy and vile, fed from the marsh lands of Cambodia and the hundreds of canals lacing the Delta in South Vietnam. The people of both Cambodia and Vietnam washed their buffalo, pigs, and themselves in the river. They used the water's currents to move their garbage and raw sewage away from the villages, and it was not uncommon to see dead human bodies mixed in with other flotsam and debris rolling and bobbing on the murky surface.

If one was thirsty you drank from your canteen . . . or lived with the thirst.

Our destination was the Long Phu District in the Ba Xuyen Province, IV Corps Tactical Zone. Home would be at Long Phu where Coastal Group 36 was hanging its hat these days. It was an old French outpost now housing a small Vietnamese navy force. CHARLIE platoon would be operating in conjunction with the Coastal Surveillance Task Force whose operational commanders designator was CTG 115.3 within the Blue Shark area of operations. Our platoon was assigned areas of operation, or AOs, in the Dung Island complex. Each mission had to be approved through U.S. advisors at Sub Sector and Sector. In truth, there were very few military units in the area and we would enjoy having to put out less effort to acquire clearance for AOs than we'd experienced before. For future SEAL missions this would work in our favor.

The Swift boats, or PCFs, were operating on the Bassac and could be called on to support us from time to time. In addition, there was a Coast Guard patrol boat (WPB) in the area which could provide us with naval gunfire support. Our air would come from Army COBRA gunships and HAL-4, which flew OV-10 Black Ponies out of either Binh Thuy or Vung Tau. The platoon found itself without MST support for the first five weeks but due to the aggressive and bold nature of Lieutenant Boyhan we never had to pass up an operation for the lack of the specially designed boats SEALs needed to go to war in.

Our arrival at Coastal Group 36 was not without its surprises. First off, we discovered all the cargo we'd loaded was indeed for us, not some support unit. The north end of the compound was separated from the Vietnamese troops and their families by at least one hundred yards of space. It was agreed between CG 36 and CHARLIE platoon that we'd set up our quarters on the north corner of the compound, down by the river.

The base was laid out in the shape of a triangle with .50 caliber machine guns positioned at each corner. A two-foot high dike ran between the defensive bunkers and a large open field bordered us to the north. This was cleared back another four hundred meters to give us as great and open a field of fire for the machine guns as possible. The perimeter was protected with double apron barbed wire, with command detonated claymore antipersonnel mines sprinkled in to blow huge gaps in any attacking enemy force when it attempted to scale the sharp wire enclosure.

We laid out our new living area and used the heavy equipment provided us to unload the landing craft. Then it was time to hustle if we were to get our new portable tents up by nightfall. Each tent came in a large wooden box. When the box was opened and its contents removed, it would be turned upside down and so become the floor for the tent. The first three feet of the tent's structure was sheet aluminum with a screen door at one end. A tent frame was attached and the tent's canvas slipped over this so as to form the final product. As far as tents go, these were adequate quarters for us.

By the time darkness was making its presence felt we'd put three tents up and put in metal bunk beds with mattresses. Lieutenant Boyhan, Mr. Duggar, and myself took the first tent and called it home. Taking two wooden mortar crates and a quarter sheet of plywood, we built a desk, making our tent the platoon office. Other members of the platoon moved into the remaining tents by squad.

The next morning started with a platoon meeting and it began with the fact we had no breakfast to greet us. In the haste to move, no arrangements had been made to feed

CHARLIE platoon at our new home and we were forced to take stock of what C rations were on hand. The pallet we'd left behind was mentioned—more than once—and Lieutenant Boyhan agreed it would be nice to have such a stockpile on hand right about now. We agreed it was important to conserve the rations we did have, and that we would pool our Vietnamese money to buy food at the market in Long Phu. With that out of the way we moved on.

Our second administrative blunder concerned shower facilities. There were none. We had drinking water but when it came to bathing we ended up in the "Big Muddy" just like everyone else living on the Bassac. After three or four weeks of this, some of my teammates began having large white spots develop on their skin. We couldn't help but figure it had to have something to do with the river water.

The men in CHARLIE platoon took the support problems in stride. We joked about being hungry and how good a hot shower would feel, however, no one really complained seriously about our living conditions. Lieutenant Boyhan wouldn't let it go without a fight, though. Tom contacted DETs GOLF and ALFA about our problems at least once a week. If nothing else they knew who and where we were. The men took one of the Swift boats to Can Tho on payday to try and buy food from the mess hall there. When they arrived they were told that no food could be sold without formal authorization. In true SEAL spirit two teammates kept the supply chief busy attempting to explain why he couldn't feed the Navy's best while the rest of the crew got busy clearing out his supply shed of chow! The Swift boat returned full and for the next few days so were our bellies.

Our plight did have its light moments. Mike Thornton located some eggs from somewhere and was busy cooking them up over at Coastal Group 36's quarters. Hal Kuykendall, his freshly cooked eggs on a paper plate, was coming back across the compound when Mike LaCaze (who'd spotted him) jumped out from behind a bunker with a great loud yell. Hal's eggs went flying into the air, landing hard in the dirt near the startled SEAL's feet. Kuykendall's heart rate must have been pegged at two hundred beats per minute and he was so mad he could have killed Mike.

Everyone who saw the prank was cracking up and soon Hal was laughing as hard as anyone else. The spirit of the men remained at the highest level despite our administrative obstacles.

Joe Tvrdik was our cook and to his credit he did the best he could. Sometimes what he brought back from the marketplace had a taste which resembled no food any of us had ever eaten. One time, in Long Phu, Joe bought a batch of purple waffles which were filled with cooked breadfruit. They were so rich our unstable stomachs could only handle two or three bites before we had to push the meal away.

Mike LaCaze was hit the worst from having to eat local food. First he got worms, and then diarrhea. When our corpsman treated him for one problem the other got worse. We finally MEDEVACed Mike out of Long Phu just to get him well.

There was plenty to do and combat operations began right away. All of the port-a-tents were up the day after we'd arrived so an operations office and quarters were immediately available for planning and preparation. Rich Solano was not only one of the best operators I've ever worked with but he could fix just about anything, and make most engines run regardless of age or problem. Rich took our generator and dug a hole for it in the ground, building a plywood structure around it to muffle the distinctive noise it made. He then wired each tent for lights at night, making reading and other pleasures that much easier during our off-time. Mike Sands took on the responsibility of establishing a gun cleaning station and in short time the place began looking like home.

There was one job the men did get tired of and their complaints were justified. Fifty meters from our tents, which we now called "hootches," was our huge olive drab steel conex container. It was filled with ammunition and explosives, all the necessary toys SEALs do their dirty little jobs with. I had nightmares about incoming mortar rounds making a direct hit on the thing. It became such a concern for me that I put out the word, and it was unpopular, that we would be sandbagging our powder magazine. As teammates we would all be involved in the process.

We secured every shovel in the compound and began

digging. We dug and dug, and then dug some more. Some would use shovels while others held the sandbags open for filling and tying. The remaining men carried the heavy bags to the magazine area and stacked them. Our hands grew wet with water and sweat. Everyone got blisters but I was stubborn about finishing the job and we continued on. Finally, the lethal conex was well protected by a wall and roof of sandbags. After all was said and done both Hal and Mike Thornton began calling me "Mama Knock Knock" behind my back. "Mama" came from being a mother hen and "Knock Knock" was a takeoff from my last name, Enoch. It didn't bother me and in fact I felt kinda good about the nickname. It meant the men knew I was looking out for them.

Food remained a problem. Once, while returning from an operation we went alongside a Coast Guard WPB and asked if they had anything to eat. When the crew heard about our plight they made everyone sandwiches. At the end of the month they were on their way upriver to Can Tho to resupply themselves and afterward stopped to look us up. They ran the bow of the boat up onto the riverbank and began throwing sandwich meat, bread, and fruit over the bow to us. Even a can of coffee came sailing our way! The Coast Guard chief apologized for not having more they could share but he had to "save some for the crews' dinner tonight." From that day on we had a soft spot for the U.S. Coast Guard in our hearts.

Upon our arrival at Coastal Group 36 we found target folders waiting for us. These had been prepared by Naval Special Warfare Group Vietnam (NSWGV) and concerned the Dung Island complex. I remember the stack of folders being over two inches thick. Not only did we have intelligence support for the platoon but LCDR Ron Mullen and PT2 Gardner from NSWGV Intelligence, who'd been involved in the prior planning of the folders, were now located at CG 36. As it turned out LCDR Mullen had been the prime mover for getting a SEAL platoon assigned to Dung Island.

PT2 Gardner was a photo analyst and he could read the aerial photography provided to us in the preparation of an operation. His skill proved to be a positive asset to the platoon in the days to come. Having these two intelligence personnel on hand allowed CHARLIE platoon to concentrate on planning, coordination, and the preparing and final execution of our SEAL missions.

The NILO, (Naval Intelligence Liaison Officer) Lieutenant Friedell was located at Soc Trang. It was a full day's drive round-trip but he was a great help to our intelligence effort. Friedell lined up a number of *chieu hoi*s who agreed to act as guides for our platoon operations. He also enjoyed a close working relationship with LCDR Mullen and Lieutenant Boyhan, which only benefited everyone. One unique asset enjoyed by our NILO was Mr. Loc, a Vietnamese interpreter. Mr. Loc made it his business to visit the *chieu hoi* centers daily. He became a trusted friend of the *chieu hoi*s by bringing them things they needed and spending time talking with them.

On the average our officers spent eight to ten hours a day when we were stationed at Ben Luc just driving, questioning, contacting various intelligence agencies, and meeting with other combat units in order to enhance our own operations. Dung Island was a welcome change for CHARLIE platoon as everything was more or less centralized. This accelerated our platoon's operational time as we could now spend more time in the field which was our bread and butter. Our intelligence network was above all, the most positive asset CHARLIE platoon enjoyed. I'm sure the reliability of the network protected our teammates while they were operating, while also providing the kind of information we needed to be successful.

By the first of March we received an LDNN platoon of Vietnamese SEALs. They arrived with their SEAL advisor, BM1 Ron Rogers. Ron was from SEAL Team Two and he drew our respect as a teammate from the start. We moved Ron into a command hootch with us, the LDNNs going to the spare port-a-tent. Their leading petty officer was my old friend, Tich. It was great to see him and Thai again, and I was happy we'd be operating together again soon.

It wasn't long before the LDNNs found out about our constant food problem. They ate in Long Phu most of the time, our understanding their food was paid for by the Vietnamese navy. One afternoon Ron Rogers showed up and invited us to eat with the LDNNs. We followed them to a hootch in Long Phu where we were all seated around a large round table sitting on the dirt floor. A large dishpan was placed in the center of the table, a block of ice in its middle. Several bottles of Vietnamese "33" beer were poured over the ice until the pan was filled with cold beer. A single china bowl was placed on the table. The custom was to dip the beer out of the dishpan with the bowl and drink, passing the bowl to the next man at the table. It didn't take long for the bowl to come back to you and then begin its journey once again around the table. The dishpan was always kept full of beer by one or another of the LDNNs.

After a sufficient social hour meant to adjust our attitudes most favorably, the food appeared. Each SEAL was given a metal plate filled with mounds of stir-fried meat, which to me tasted like some kind of BBQ. We were a hungry crew and the meal was good! We finished eating and sat back to relax, enjoying the satisfaction of a full belly. I got the big idea of asking what kind of meat we'd just been served. At first the LDNNs couldn't tell me because they couldn't figure out the English word for whatever animal it had once been. Finally, one of the Vietnamese SEALs found a solution.

"You know, Mickey . . ." he said with a smile. To help me figure it out he took a chop stick and drew a fair image of Mickey Mouse on the dirt floor of our dining room.

"Mouse!" I said. The LDNNs began laughing and shaking their heads in the affirmative.

"City mouse is Number Ten," Thai told me. "It eat garbage. Country mouse Number One, it eat rice. We eat country mouse!" Everyone seemed to agree with his assessment of what made for a fine mouse meal. I figured we'd just eaten Number One rice mice for dinner. At least we'd washed it down with enough beer to kill any germs that might have likewise been consumed. It was another experience we could chalk up to our Dung Island ordeal.

CHARLIE platoon had been operating on the island complex for over a month without an MST detachment. Lieutenant Boyhan was asking for help repeatedly without much success. Finally, as a last chance effort on our behalf he made a trip to Can Tho to see the MST officer there. He took Mike Thornton and Mike Sands with him. These were the two biggest and meanest looking SEALs in the platoon and Tom had a plan which included their presence.

Upon arriving in Can Tho the trio burst into the MST office unannounced, demanding to see the officer in charge. "We need an MST Det in Dung Island and these two men are going to camp out on your desk until it happens!" he told the stunned man. Standing there next to Mr. Boyhan was Thornton on one side and Sands on the other. Each was dressed in worn Levi's and a camouflage fatigue shirt, their M60 LMGs dangling from one hand as if they were no more than pool sticks.

We got our boat support in less than a week.

I never knew for sure whether the terrible twins were the motivating force which solved our transportation problem, or if it was LCDR Mullen's influence at NSWGV which did the trick. In any event, the boats provided us with excellent support for the remainder of our tour.

From the time we set foot on Coastal Group 36's turf we heard rumors that the Navy's Seabees were planning to visit the base for the purpose of improving it. We hoped that if the rumor were true their efforts would include our little bit of ground, as well. About two months after we'd begun operating on Dung Island, MCB-5 DET HOTEL indeed landed. From that moment on things improved for CHARLIE platoon at CG 36.

The Seabees brought freeze-dried rations with them. Their cook took our field kitchen under their wing, putting the rations together with onions and potatoes and serving up hot food that tasted nothing like "country mouse"! A mess hall was built and then a proper living quarters for the platoon. We had brand-new facilities and new friends, both which were deeply appreciated.

Along with all of this the Seabees built an impressive mortar pit for fire support and provided such support for us on several occasions. Their gunners were well trained on the tubes and hit the target whenever called upon to do so. We found out right away that the "Fighting Seabees" were still alive and kicking. Because of them, Dung Island had finally become home to CHARLIE platoon.

24

Skimmer Operations

Courage is resistance to fear, mastery of fear—not absence of fear.

—Mark Twain

SEAL—the term is derived from *sea, air,* and *land*—refers to Navy frogmen who have the capability of inserting from the sea, sky, or *terra firma* and conducting clandestine or covert missions. It may be an underwater infiltration involving a submarine and SCUBA gear, or a high-altitude parachute drop from a C 141 jet aircraft, or a fast trip across the dunes in a fast attack vehicle especially designed for SEAL ops. All of these are methods for the SEAL to be deployed in or near the target area. All three mediums of insertion usually require supporting elements of the military, such as those units and crews who operate the unique SEAL boats, aircraft, and helicopters necessary to deliver the goods.

At CG 36, CHARLIE platoon spent five weeks without reliable boat support. This made operating tough as our Dung Island AOs were completely surrounded by the waters of the Bassac River. At least fifteen hundred meters of water lay between CG 36 and the nearest point on the nine-island complex. Boats were mandatory for the platoon's operational success. After all, SEALs—contrary to popular belief—cannot walk on water.

A platoon commander could have laid low and waited

those five weeks until the Navy provided something but this wasn't the style of *our* Lieutenant Boyhan. Tom, to say the least, was an aggressive operator. From the moment we arrived he'd been looking at the available assets at CG 36. There was a Coast Guard WPB which was designed for seagoing operations, a boat too large for SEAL insertions or operations in small canals. Next were the Vietnamese navy junks. These, too, were overly large and not as maneuverable as we liked in the canals. Junks were also slow and there was the language barrier between SEALs and the junk crews. The PCFs, or Swift boats, were very fast but also too noisy and too large for canal work. All of these craft were good to excellent for gunfire support or as a floating platform to launch smaller boats from. Mr. Boyhan logged all of this and continued his search on our behalf.

CHARLIE platoon possessed two rubber IBS boats which were designed for UDT/SEAL operations. These had to be paddled into combat and offered no protection for the operators if it were detected or taken under fire. Sampans were also considered. These rode low in the water but could only handle three or four fully loaded SEALs. Sampans would have to be rented on the local economy and such a transaction could jeopardize an operation. Captured sampans were almost always in bad shape, mainly because we shot them up pretty good. Still, both the IBS boats and sampan options could be launched from the larger available craft, if necessary.

Coastal Group 36 also had a single Skimmer . . . and we found it. A Skimmer craft is made from fiberglass and it looks much like the many small fishing boats you find throughout the United States. The boat had two powerful outboard engines and was very fast in the water. It was well-built and could carry a heavily loaded SEAL squad without problem. It was the best option we had to conduct our operations on Dung Island.

The commander of CG 36 was none too happy about loaning us their only Skimmer. He just knew we'd end up getting the craft shot up or sunk and he didn't know if he could get another one if this happened. Rich Solano came up with the idea of making the Skimmer bulletproof and he went to work immediately. The Skimmer had a metal hand railing running around the gunnel. Rich lined the sides of the boat with flak jackets, doubling them over the railing. The end result wasn't very attractive but it made the Coastal Group commander feel better about his boat going into combat with us onboard. Thanks to Tom Boyhan and Rich, CHARLIE platoon had its insertion craft.

On February 18, we ran our first operation against Dung Island. It had been eight days since we'd done so since leaving Ben Luc and the men were more than ready to do what they now knew they did best. Finding the Vietcong and hitting him *hard*. Mr. Boyhan was going to pack twelve SEALs and one VN interpreter onto our newly armored Skimmer. CHARLIE platoon left CG 36 just after dark aboard a Swift boat, the Skimmer in tow. After what we felt was a long tow the Swift came to a slow stop on the dark water's surface, the Skimmer brought alongside.

It was a full moon that night and we had a high tide. There was no problem finding our tiny canal's mouth, the entrance point of our upcoming insertion onto Dung Island. To maintain the element of surprise we paddled the Skimmer up the canal until reaching the insertion point. Three SEALs had to be left behind to paddle the Skimmer back to the Swift boat after the rest of us slithered up onto the shore.

We were still a formidable force at nine heavily armed SEALs and our target was a VCI hamlet finance cadre. The terrain we were now slowly picking our way through was covered in nipa palm. After three hundred meters, Rich Solano halted the patrol from his position on point. Our teammate had just located a cache site. A quick search showed the site to be abandoned and we continued the patrol. Rich bumped into the jungle's secondary growth and it brought us to a standstill. We were unable to locate the target because this living mass of foliage was six to eight feet in height! It became quickly apparent we needed a guide if we were going to successfully operate in this terrain. We turned around and patrolled back to the canal for extraction. The Skimmer came down the narrow waterway at full power this time, returning us to the Swift boat by 0630 the next morning.

The patrol had missed their target but the mission was

not a total loss. We knew we could run good operations and wouldn't be sitting around on our hands. The abandoned cache point confirmed the enemy was active on Dung Island and our morale was high. The Skimmer had proved its worth and it felt good to be back in action as a combat platoon. Overall, CHARLIE platoon's operators felt pretty good and were ready for the next operation as soon as it could be mounted.

By the time we got back to CG 36 the command hootch was buzzing with activity. A mission was already in the works for that very night. After cleaning our weapons and equipment the men were alerted they should get some sleep before the heat of the day set in. Later on in the afternoon Mr. Duggar gave the patrol order and it was a good one.

The patrol would consist of twelve SEALs and our Vietnamese interpreter, just like the night before. The target was to be a live VCI as we wanted a prisoner for intelligence purposes. We'd be taken in by Swift boat with the Skimmer in tow, using it for the final leg or our insertion. Weapons and equipment were checked and rechecked, ammunition drawn, and inspections held. We were ready.

The weather was clear and the air still warm from the intense heat of the day. As darkness began creeping over us the men lay on the deck of the Swift boat, settled in as comfortable as possible for the long ride up the river. Again, we were blessed with a full moon and high tide. These elements would make finding the canal opening easier once we were ready to take the Skimmer in.

I worked my way forward to stand next to Mr. Duggar. He was studying the radar screen, finally spotting our canal and then discussing the drop point with me. I was surprised by how quickly we'd made the trip given the much slower trip taken the night before. Duggar sent me back to alert the men that we were nearly there and to get ready to go aboard the Skimmer. "Saddle up," I whispered, "lock and load, safeties on."

We quietly climbed aboard the Skimmer and then paddled the one hundred and fifty meters to the canal's entrance. All but three SEALs inserted onto the island, the men left behind charged to set up a waterborne guard post aboard the Skimmer. We found ourselves in waist-deep water surrounded by nipa palm. The patrol went another one hundred fifty meters until clear of the water. So far, so good.

Our pointman, Doyle, located the target and we carefully moved into position. The hootch was a VC restaurant and once the patrol was set in place we initiated our assault. One VC made a break for the jungle's safety but Doyle took him out with a well-aimed burst of gunfire. We searched the area and recovered one M1 .30 caliber carbine and two ChiCom grenades. In checking the dead man we discovered he was the VC village chief we were after. He could have been taken alive but his decision to run canceled out that option. Warning shots began to be fired by other VC in the area as we patrolled out toward the extraction point. The enemy was not happy with the SEALs showing up uninvited for dinner. We contacted our teammates on the Skimmer and they brought the boat up under full power, taking small arms fire from both banks of the canal. It was to be a hot extraction!

The Swift boat was called up to support us as we returned fire from the now moving Skimmer. The sheer volume of our return fire must have shaken the VC badly as their own dropped off to near nothing once our two forces engaged each other. As we broke out of the mouth of the canal the two Swift boats supporting the operation began working the canal over with their .50 caliber heavy machine guns.

The Skimmer roared up beside one of the Swifts and we hastily clambered aboard, our infiltration boat hooked back on its towline. As we broke contact and began heading back to CG 36 the men were obviously on a mission high. We'd made our first successful hit on Dung Island and he'd turned out to be VCI. Someone in the darkness offered, "The VC know we're here and they'll be ready the next time," but that turned out to be somewhat wrong. We would learn the next day from our NILO at Soc Trang the Vietcong were convinced it was a PRU, not SEAL patrol which had hit them that night. I suppose that was quite a compliment for us.

Our Skimmer operations continued to improve in quality and execution as we became more active on Dung Island. On February 21, Lieutenant Boyhan ran a Skimmer op with ten SEALs, an interpreter, and a Hoi Chanh from the *chieu hoi* center in Soc Trang. We used the Swifts for fire support and their excellent towing services. Three SEALs stayed with the Skimmer and put in a floating guard post after the main force slipped ashore. Rich Solano, again on point, began running into numerous booby traps set up along the trail. These slowed us down but the patrol moved forward until its target was in sight.

The hootch appeared as if from nowhere. Like jungle ghosts we slipped up on it hoping to find someone home, someone we could capture and spend some time questioning about VC operations on the island. But before the patrol was fully set up a VC broke from the tiny structure, running for the treeline for all he was worth. The enemy soldier was taken under fire and a quick, hard burst from a Stoner 63 ended his flight to freedom. Searching his body we discovered the man was Nguyen Van Chau, Hamlet Liberation Committee Chief. Bingo! We'd found our man.

On the way back to CG 36 the Hoi Chanh wanted to check more sampans and junks for VC. Under his guidance we began searching several such boats in the area. We discovered one female VC who turned out to be the wife of a VC tax collector. The woman offered she wanted to surrender to the *chieu hoi* program which was okay by us. In another boat we found a Vietnamese draft dodger. Bad luck for him. We detained both individuals and they were extracted by Swift boat. The sampan the woman had been in was taken for use in future operations.

It was decided that Nelson, our interpreter, would visit the Vietnamese sailors at their base and rent us a sampan large enough for SEALs to operate from. Mr. Boyhan put together an operation where we'd first travel by Swift boat, transferring to a Skimmer, and then to a sampan which would take the patrol up a small canal to a VC hamlet. Twelve men plus Nelson were selected to conduct the operation and preparations were made.

Things were moving along fairly well until we reached the point where the Skimmer was towing the sampan. Within three hundred meters we had to stop because the rented scow was leaking so badly it required on-site repair efforts. Suddenly we spotted another sampan with two people in it.

A hand-fired flare lit up the night and both men were seen to be holding weapons. The enemy sampan came under immediate fire from the Skimmer and its SEALs.

The patrol bore down on the VC under full power, weapons firing and tracers lacing the darkness like fine webs. The sampan, rapidly soaking up lead, began sinking fast. Mike Sands spotted a weapon in the boat even as the hull began slipping beneath the water's surface. Mike yelled, pointing at the weapon even as Lieutenant Boyhan leaped from the Skimmer into the water in an attempt to recover it. A VC soldier who'd been hiding in the sampan's stern area suddenly rose up out of the water right behind our platoon commander. Rich Solano yelled, "Tom!" even as he fired a two-round burst from his Stoner at the man. The bullets took the top of the Vietcong's head clean off before he could harm Tom in any way. The Skimmer keeled way over as six sets of arms heaved Boyhan out of the canal and into the fiberglass boat.

Due to the firefight's racket our original operation was compromised and we returned to the Swift boat. Still, we'd killed two VC and sunk one of their precious sampans. The lesson learned was we needed a sampan of our own which was maintained by the platoon. Perhaps the Vietnamese navy preferred old, leaky sampans for their operations but not CHARLIE platoon.

It was quite clear we were losing targets trying to use a combination of the Swift and Skimmer boats. Unless the intelligence we received or generated was new, and the target hot we held off until obtaining an LSSC to work from. Boyhan decided to run some waterborne guard posts with the Skimmer and based on SEAL intelligence gathered during a previous operation we knew of a VC river crossing point at the mouth of the Bassac.

Tom took a squad to conduct the operation. As the fiberglass boat moved south toward the river's mouth the Bassac became very wide and the water got choppy. Solano turned the Skimmer north across the river on a course toward Tron Island. We were now moving slowly back upriver and were in Vietcong territory. Without warning we encountered a sampan heading directly toward our own boat. There were two male Vietnamese in it and Lieutenant

Boyhan fired an illumination flare high above the river's surface. He hailed the sampan's crew, which immediately jumped overboard and began swimming like crazy for the shore. We laid down an effective base of fire and both VC were killed outright. The sampan was also shot up badly and it sank before we could reach and search it. Again a chance contact had compromised our original operation and we aborted the mission. Lieutenant Boyhan kept the Skimmer in the middle of the river during the return trip so as to avoid the hostile shorelines.

An LDNN platoon joined us on March 10, planning to conduct an operation with us the next night. Their SEAL advisor, Ron Rogers, invited us to come along. This was customary among SEALs operating in Vietnam and it made good sense in this case. We could support Ron by calling in direct naval gunfire and air support. Thornton, Doyle, DiCroce, and myself volunteered to accompany the LDNN.

At 0300 the platoon inserted by VN navy junk. The target was two VC females living in a nearby hamlet. We patrolled until daylight and were rewarded as the LDNN searched several hootches, detaining six males and one female. The woman was identified as Vothi Tuyen, Section Leader for the Liberation Committee. She and the six men were taken back with us in two motorized sampans also captured during the operation. Once linked back up with the VN junk it was time to return to base. It had been a good operation and we all enjoyed working with the LDNNs again. They were excellent at impact interrogation with their own people. Navy SEALs had formed up and trained the LDNN and we trusted them completely in combat.

You could feel change in the air. CHARLIE platoon began taking the LDNN on patrol and some of us began operating with them. We received MST-2 DET DELTA on March 11, the detachment made up of two men and another Skimmer. It was a long way from being an LSSC, however, we now had two Skimmers and no longer had to leave SEALs with the boats to either paddle them to safety or guard.

We interviewed a Hoi Chanh regarding a possible operation against the VC on Can Coc Island. When Tich stood up and began yelling at the man I could tell the interview was not going well. Lieutenant Boyhan asked Tich what was up and our LDNN said the VC informant had described there being "many VC on the island" but that they were laying an ambush for the SEALs. Tom shook his finger at the little Vietcong soldier and told him that we were taking him in on the island. We were going to ambush the ambush, according to our platoon commander.

Tich related Boyhan's instructions and the VC began shaking all over. We had no intention of going on such an operation because we knew we couldn't trust this source worth a lick. It was worth watching him shiver in fear and anticipation, though. But the platoon wasn't in on our secret and believed we were indeed going to mount an operation against a well-planned enemy ambush.

It was March 11, the day before Hal Kuykendall's birthday. Our teammate had been thinking about the ambush operation all day, really working it over in his mind. Someone back home had written him saying a soldier from his town had been killed in Vietnam on the man's birthday. That night, Hal dreamed about headlines in his local newspaper which read "Local Boy Killed in Vietnam on His Birthday!" The morning of March 12 found Hal Kuykendall not at all happy, the dream an unwelcome present on his birthday.

He told no one about what had taken place and what his concerns were. He vowed he was not superstitious and he determined he was going on the ambush-an-ambush operation with us. About the time Hal had convinced himself all was reasonably well Mike Thornton showed up.

"Cuz," Mike said to Hal, "I had a bad dream about you last night and I don't want you going out tonight with us."

Hal nearly lost it when he heard this from his close friend, Thornton. Naturally we didn't operate that night, much to Hal's private relief. It wouldn't be until much later that he would tell us this story, complete with both his and Mike's dreams.

The platoon did operate the next night, though. Rogers took his LDNN out and I went along with DiCroce, Brown, and Hampton. The mission was to capture a VCI and we had good intelligence on where to find him from NSWGV. The night was pitch-black, no moon offering the least amount of natural light. Ron briefed us and Tich briefed the LDNN platoon. We all loaded into both Skimmers and were off.

We inserted just after midnight and patrolled about three hundred meters to where our target hootch was said to be. The hootch was found and searched but no one was home. A second hootch was discovered and this time we detained two males, who were ordered to take us to the VC. Our new guides led the platoon to a third hootch where we successfully captured three Vietcong. As it turned out one of the men was actually a North Vietnamese army regular, with the other men a VC squad leader and regular foot soldier. Along with the prisoners we recovered two kilos of documents, another two kilos of medical supplies, and a transistor radio. Before leaving we burned the hootch to the ground and then extracted by Skimmer.

Doc Brown and Wayne Hampton were great SEALs and wonderful teammates. I found I could always count on both men regardless of the situation at hand. They were men of color and we never saw them as a "white man's black man" or "black man's black man," only as brother SEALs and operators. They were American fighting men that the whole nation can be proud of and that's how I remember them today. Doc was our corpsman but he was also a real mechanic when it came to the Stoner 63. Brown was also very accomplished with a mortar tube. No white man can know the pain in a black man's heart, however, both Doc and Wayne had come through the 1960s without showing the bitterness that cloaked much of the African-American community of that time. If our two teammates were ever affected by the negative movements of the time we never knew it. They didn't carry a chip on their shoulder or let the race issue drag them down.

And there is more to this story which deserves to be told. In fact, it wouldn't be complete without talking about Wayne Hampton. From the very beginning some in the platoon gave Wayne his nickname, which was "Bru." It stuck. First off, Bru didn't like snakes at all, not one bit. Secondly, one of the CG 36 personnel had killed a cobra on base and Bru knew about it. Thirdly, the Army used gunships called Cobras; and here is Bru's story.

252

We'd been inserted by two Skimmers carrying a total of ten SEALs, Nelson, and three LDNNs. We were looking hard for a VCI hamlet chief and when the hootches were found, our man was nowhere to be found. Lieutenant Boyhan saw that daylight was fast approaching and reasoned the VCI would likely come home soon. He took the LDNN, Nelson, and Rich Solano to the first hootch which was about fifty meters from where we were standing. I was to take the rest of the platoon with me and set up an ambush on the second hootch.

This proved to be no problem as we found a three-foot dike with heavy cover around it less than twenty feet from our hootch. It was the perfect spot for an ambush. Everyone was positioned and we settled in for a long wait. It was quiet and it was still dark. Everything was going along just fine, or so I thought.

My radioman, Hal, whispered to me, "Bru wants to scramble Cobras."

"Why?" I asked back. Nothing was happening and there was no reason I could see or hear to bring gunships in on our position.

"I don't know," replied Hal. "He just keeps saying 'Coooobras.'"

"Tell Bru I'm running this patrol and I'm not calling for Cobras!" I told Hal.

But before Hal could pass my message to Bru the powerful thumping sound of our teammate's M60 LMG shattered the early morning calm with what has to be the longest sustained burst on record. When the '60 went off the entire ambush cut loose, as well. Rounds smacked into every sector of fire assigned and when it was all over we'd racked up quite a body count. Moving forward our impressive tally included six ducks, three pigs, and one very large cobra . . . snake, that is.

The entire time I'd been worrying over Bru's air support request with Hal, Wayne had been face-to-face with a huge cobra whose interest in him had reached the point of preparing to strike. Bru blew the "VC" snake away at point blank range, all the while probably wondering what Hal and I were arguing about while he was looking death right in the eye.

One of the most interesting Skimmer operations run by CHARLIE platoon was against a VC junk construction yard. The intelligence for this mission came from the NILO at Soc Trang. He also had a Hoi Chanh who'd worked at the yard and had agreed to act as a guide for the SEALs to attack it.

The target was located on the north side of Tron Island. We could either walk across the island through a combination of mangrove, nipa palm, and open rice paddies . . . or we could take a twelve-kilometer daylight boat ride. We decided on the Skimmers, planning to make the hit in late afternoon at high tide. This was critical as at low tide the canal was so small and shallow that even the Skimmers couldn't negotiate it. The canal that separated Tron from Dung Island was named the "Tee Tee" canal by the SEALs because it was so small. The boats would have to go up the Bassac to the end of Tron Island, and then down the north side some six kilometers through the Tee Tee canal in order to reach our insertion point.

The Skimmers moved slowly and quietly through the Tee Tee. There was heavy nipa palm on one side and mangrove on the other. The foliage and undergrowth was so heavy it was unlikely we would be seen or heard from the sides of the canal as these were bankless at high tide. The water, as far as one could see, was slow-moving. It was still hot even at 1700 in the afternoon and we were thankful for the shade of the overhanging trees.

We arrived at our insertion point without being detected by the enemy. As we began moving up the small canal toward the junk yard Mike Thornton cut the power on one outboard, bringing the noise level down but forcing him to try and steer the boat with only one engine operating. It was hard steering this way and the boat zigzagged from bank to bank, which was not to our liking. Mike shut down the second engine and we pulled the boat along the water's surface by using the heavy foliage within our grasp. When the canal opened up again and became too wide for this method, Thornton started the engine up again and we began tacking to and fro.

The platoon never lost the element of surprise. When we

finally made contact the Vietcong were stunned into inaction by what they saw and heard at the same time. Hal was in the first boat, positioned up in its bow. He spotted one VC leaning out over the canal with both hands on his hips, a look of sheer disbelief straining his face as we materialized from nowhere. Another VC popped up with a weapon in hand and both men were introduced to a Stoner's incredible volume of accurate fire. Mike started the other engine and we went all the way in wide-open.

Mike Sands brought our demolition charges up with me. Tom Boyhan took one squad and the Hoi Chanh about one hundred fifty meters to the south to search three structures located there. Mr. Duggar led the other squad to secure the junk yard itself. Mike Thornton turned the Skimmers around and stayed with the boats, M60 in hand, as rear security. I began selecting targets for the demolition charges.

I found two large, nearly complete sampans under construction. We placed two-pound charges along the keels of both sampans, then took the woodworking tools we found in the boats so they would be destroyed as well. A firefight broke out where Boyhan and his squad were, and we started taking incoming small arms fire above us at tree level. I made a quick visual survey of the yard and what caught my attention was unbelievable! Setting high and dry on land was a huge seagoing junk. From keel to the main deck had to be at least fifteen feet. It had been more built between the trees as these flanked the junk by no more than four to six inches from its hull. Boards were nailed to the trees so they could be used as ladders to get on deck. It was impossible to see the boat from the air due to the natural camouflage surrounding and covering it.

I wanted to see the junk from its deck and began climbing aboard. Two rounds smacked into the side of the boat, convincing me I'd had a bad idea. Down I came and soon I found a hole in the stern. I began tying C-3 charges along the keel and midway up the ribs of the hull. I tied the detonating cord to the demolition trunkline. Quickly securing a three-minute time fuse I began yelling, "Fire in the hole!" while pulling the fuse lighter. Mike Sands pulled his fuses on the sampan charges when he heard me give the warning. Everyone began heading back to the boats where Mike Thornton was patiently waiting.

Before we got there Mike fired on ten VC who were trying to set an ambush in behind us. He knocked the first two down and the rest ran for the jungle. As Lieutenant Boyhan brought his squad up for the extraction another VC soldier jumped up with a weapon and Thornton wasted him outright.

For some reason we all had this urgent feeling to get out of there quick. Time was ticking away as our charges burned down and everyone felt we'd be ambushed on the way out. The Skimmers went out under full power, and I mean full bore. Every man aboard was firing at our flanks with everything he had available. Hal later told me I was cutting up, placing my KA-BAR between my teeth when we hit the Tee Tee canal. Guess something silly comes out in a gunners mate when he gets a chance to really work with demolitions.

As Rich Solano cut his boat hard into the Tee Tee it came up out of the water so hard the bottom was fully exposed to us. Just then small arms fire began heading our way from the Dung Island side. Everyone heard the round hit the speeding Skimmer but no one knew where. What was known was the boat began taking on water and continued to all the way home. It wasn't until we pulled the Skimmer out of the water that we found a bullet hole in the bottom, it striking the small craft as Rich brought it up on its side during his high-speed turn.

We heard all of the charges go off and saw the debris and smoke rising above the treeline. A dark column of smoke marked the three hootches destroyed by the First Squad. OV-10 Black Ponies were overhead by now, Tom calling for them when his squad began taking fire from the treeline by the hootches. The aircraft had to remain overhead for fifty-five minutes while they waited for clearance to fire from the tactical operations center in Soc Trang. During this entire time we were taking small arms fire from both Tron and Dung Island on our way out. We later found out the TOC wasn't manned during evening chow! Finally, at 1915 hours that night, the OVs did get to drop their ordnance on the junk yard for whatever good it did.

The platoon was all charged up about the operation and it was the only subject of conversation that night. I believe our morale was at its highest after this one operation. Solano patched the Coastal Group's Skimmer the next morning and they would never learn their boat had been hit. All's well that ends well.

What we learned was that Skimmers and teammates worked for CHARLIE platoon.

25

Dung Island Gets Its LSSC

It took five weeks before CHARLIE platoon got its LSSC. EM2 McCormic headed up a two-man detachment (MST DET DELTA) and they gave us outstanding support for the remainder of our tour at Dung Island. When the boat finally arrived we were excited, to say the least. Someone, somewhere, had finally figured out CHARLIE was in-country and needing urgent help.

During the first week the LSSC needed to be outfitted and completely checked out by its crew. A pier had to be built for the boat and that job fell to us. The Vietnamese had plenty of empty fifty-gallon drums which would serve as flotation for the pier, and we found some unguarded metal matting which we claimed ownership of. This became the deck. Everyone pitched in to help and the LSSC was tied up at its own pier in short order. We not only secured the boat to the pier but to the riverbank too. The current was fast and powerful when the tide was going out so we decided not to take any chances on losing the LSSC.

The crew mounted two M60 LMGs on the boat's port and starboard sides giving us plenty of firepower. Rich Solano came up with a 90mm recoilless rifle—who knew from where—and enough ammunition to last us the entire tour. The recoilless was stowed in the bow under the coxswain's feet for easy and quick access. Ammunition for the bunker buster was placed in the SEALs' set compartments on the boat. The engines and radar were worried over by the crew until they functioned like a Swiss watch and soon we were ready to use the LSSC on operations.

You never knew what you were going to see on the Bassac River. I remember one morning walking out to the LSSC after a mission to check on something long forgotten now. I sat down on one side of the LSSC with my feet on the metal pier, taking a moment to think and perhaps enjoy the view. Suddenly and without warning this monster came out of the water, climbing up onto the shoreline only feet from me.

The thing was big. At least five feet long and it looked more like a lizard than anything else. It was without a doubt the biggest lizard I'd ever laid eyes on. I didn't move, not even an eyelash. It was one of those times to be still and quiet. The reptile had a long stout neck and a head shaped like a snake. It's tongue, bloodred, kept shooting in and out of its mouth as if testing the air for something to latch on to. He stood on four bowed legs which supported his body high off the ground. A long and thick tail rested on the muddy shore, much of it still in the water.

The lizard's head was the only thing that moved, and then very slowly. He finally looked right at me and just as suddenly as he'd appeared the river monster was back under the water's surface and gone. I stood up and waited for him to resurface, however, he never did. Must have been as much at home underwater as above.

When I told my trusty teammates about the big lizard they looked at me as if I'd lost all my marbles down by the LSSC. So I went and told the LDNN and they laughed like crazy, rubbing their stomachs while doing so. Apparently they ate lizards as well as mice. It wasn't until I returned to the States that I looked the reptile up in a book and found my friend was an old-world Asian lizard called a "monitor." If I'd had a gun with me that morning I know I would have shot it. In reading the description on the monitor I learned they live off the eggs and young of saltwater crocodiles. So, I'm glad I didn't shoot him as I'm for anything that keeps the crocodile population down.

However, for many a night afterward I had thoughts of that lizard being somewhere around when I was standing in water up to my armpits waiting for my own version of the crocodile, the VCI, to come by.

Shortly after the LSSC was placed in service we had three visitors from EOD (Explosives Ordnance Disposal) join us for an operation. The NILO in Soc Trang passed intelligence to CHARLIE platoon about a possible VC machine shop, as well as mine and grenade factory. Lieutenant Boyhan took the entire platoon with our interpreter and the three EOD men on the mission. We loaded seventeen men aboard the LSSC and linked up with a PCF just north of Coastal Group 36.

The insertion point we'd picked was on the north side of Con Coc Island. This meant we'd transfer to the PCF and tow the LSSC so as to conserve its fuel for the operation. It was a long and uneventful ride around the end of the Dung Island complex but by 0730 we'd transferred back aboard the LSSC and made our insertion.

The terrain was mostly nipa palm and palm groves. We started out wet until reaching some high ground, then found a well-used trail which ran along a dike. The patrol encountered a hootch and we set up on it, questioning the occupants about any VC activity in the area. Moving on, we finally reached our target area and right away took a running VC under fire as he burst from a bunker's dark doorway. We reconned the area and found four more bunkers, all of them large. The EOD men were brought up and they placed their charges, destroying all five bunkers. The platoon moved back to its rear security on guard post and extracted by LSSC by 1330 that afternoon. It had been a good mission.

The patrol ended up being as long as the boat ride. I never cared for daylight operations, which always seemed to include a long walk under a hot sun. For some reason I've always thought about the report of two VC main force battalions when Scott Lyon ran his POW operation on the same island only a year before. I wondered if one dead Vietcong and five destroyed bunkers were worth the effort, much less the chances we took.

Our thirty-fifth operation was successful but costly. We'd

had information from a past SEAL operation that a VC patrol was operating on Tron Island north of our base. Ron Rogers took a squad of six LDNNs and three SEALs after them. The SEALs were Hal Kuykendall, Lou DiCroce, and myself.

We inserted just after midnight and found ourselves in thick brush. The LDNNs located a well-worn path beside a small stream and this made it easier to patrol without making a whole lot of unwanted noise. It wasn't fifty meters later that we found a hootch with a large bunker alongside it. With security set up the structures were checked out. The bunker was empty. Three of the LDNNs moved forward to search the hootch. One rolled in to the right, the other to the left. They took fire the minute they entered and there was heavy close quarters combat going on from everything we could see and hear. Chuns went forward to help his comrades and was hit by gunfire as soon as he entered the doorway.

The perimeter began receiving heavy automatic weapons fire from three sides now. We returned fire and suppressed the VC attack for the moment. At three different locations in the jungle we could hear enemy soldiers calling for help because of their wounds. The hootch was quiet. Rogers and myself moved forward and entered the hut, finding four dead VC and one LDNN with a minor wound. Chuns was in critical condition with a head wound. The LDNNs swarmed into the hootch and began searching it as well as the bodies of the dead VC.

They ended up capturing one female VC and one Chi-Com rifle. There was also an M1 carbine, one set of web gear with 120 rounds of .30 caliber ammunition. A destroyed transistor radio was also found.

Ron and I carried Chuns to a sampan where we loaded him aboard. We'd just pushed it into the river when the patrol began returning fire and started moving back down the trail. The LSSC was waiting for us at our original insertion point and we swiftly loaded Chuns and everyone else aboard, calling for a MEDEVAC to meet us at CG 36.

Chuns was in the bow of the LSSC and we were trying to get an IV started when the boat hit a sandbar. It had been moving full out when we struck ground and everyone was thrown high into the air. I came down hard on the shin of my right leg but everyone was too busy to really take notice of any aches or pains. The LSSC was stuck, and I mean stuck high and dry. We all climbed out and used brute force to push the LSSC back into the river.

Ron decided to reinsert the squad in order to lighten the boat. The LDNNs were left on the riverbank with Hal and DiCroce. Kuykendall told me later they heard the VC behind them from the moment we'd left until returning to pick them up. He said the worst part was the mosquitoes, the thickest and most aggressive he'd ever seen in Vietnam. It was hard for me to leave them there but we needed to get Chuns back to CG 36 as fast as possible.

As the LSSC moved across the water I put a field dressing on the back of his head. He'd lost some brain tissue but was still breathing. It took only a short time to reach the base where we immediately took the wounded inside. Chuns was placed on his face atop an Army cot so we could take turns giving CPR, which was made awkward due to the wound in the back of his head. Doc Brown got an IV started and we were able to keep our LDNN alive. It took two hours and twenty minutes for the MEDEVAC to arrive and we never found out why it was so long a wait. Chuns died in the helicopter while enroute to the 3rd Surgical Hospital in Binh Thuy.

The next day Tom Boyhan ran an early morning operation acting on NSWGV intelligence about a reported VC repair facility on Tron Island. This was just across the river from CG 36 and literally in our own backyard. Mr. Boyhan put the Black Ponies on standby out of Binh Thuy and prearranged 81mm mortar support using the mortars at CG 36. Doc Brown was left to advise as the rest of the platoon squeezed aboard the LSSC, inserting on the island at 0645 hours.

We moved five hundred meters to the target. There were only empty bunkers in the area so we began to patrol back along a ditch line which offered tall grass along one of its sides. We'd moved very slowly for about two hundred meters when the pointman turned to the left, climbing up onto a bit of high ground to get us away from the leeches attacking us without mercy. I was on rear security and as I stepped up on the first bit of high ground a three-foot break in the tall grass exposed itself to myself and the rest of the patrol. Behind it was a twenty-foot opening, or clearing of sorts.

As I peered into the opening I spotted eight Vietcong with heavy weapons moving parallel to our patrol, but in the opposite direction! They were wearing white shirts and each had a red scarf around his neck. I could only contact the SEAL in front of me and by the time he realized what was happening the patrol had moved too far ahead for him to signal the situation forward.

There was only one thing to do.

I yelled, *"Ambush Left!"* even as I was pulling the trigger of my Stoner. My teammate did likewise and together we hit the VC pointman even as the rest of our patrol entered the fray on full automatic. The Vietcong ran for the high grass without ever firing a shot. The platoon mowed the grass down with its Stoners, just to make sure the enemy kept running. We then moved forward to search the area and began taking automatic weapons fire from four different positions in the treeline. Boyhan called for the mortars and within minutes the enemy fire was snuffed out.

We had no way of knowing that Doc Brown was having his hands full with the mortar tube back at CG 36. The Coastal Group had never used their mortar and therefore had never seated its base plate. This meant every time a round was launched the whole mechanism moved, completely altering Doc's aiming point. Brown was forced to constantly realign the gun after each round in order to keep it on target, all because the base plate didn't have a hard surface beneath it for support. Our training on mortars in the desert at Niland paid off and it was the only reason we had accurate and timely support that day.

The mortar having done its job was checked as the OV-10s radioed they were inbound to our location. Tom called for an air strike on the treeline and we continued our patrolling to the river. When we reached its waters we found a bunker used as an observation point, and it was obviously meant to target CG 36. The explosives charges meant for the repair facility were used instead on this bunker, and when it went up in smoke we called for our LSSC to extract us. Four VC were confirmed by the NILO at Soc Trang to have been killed, but enemy casualties due to the mortar and air strikes were unknown.

Moving up small canals by boat was now possible due to our new LSSC. Its armor gave us a degree of security which we'd come to respect since being ambushed at Ben Luc. At least it made us feel better about traveling exposed on the water like we did, the jungle always giving us enough to think about with its many, many surprises.

One such surprise took place when we began operating in the tight canals at night. As we were conducting an operation we began seeing strange lights in the foliage around us. Sometimes these lights would flash right beside a teammate, or in front of the boat as an entire bush would flash like a Christmas tree. The first time we experienced this everyone was sure the VC were up to no good, or that perhaps we were just seeing things. It never bothered the LDNN who just smiled at us, ignoring the lights totally. Much later and after we'd returned to the States Lieutenant Boyhan read an article in a science journal about a lightning bug that lived in Southeast Asia. The male bugs would gather in the bushes and they'd "spark" at the same time to attract the female bugs' attention during mating season.

Even years later now it's good to know myself and my teammates were not completely out of our minds.

The PCFs would sometimes run PSYOPS missions, cruising the main river and broadcasting recorded messages in Vietnamese. These were meant to encourage the VC to turn themselves in at the local *chieu hoi* center. One night CHARLIE platoon ran an LSSC mission under the cover of the three PCFs on PSYOPS patrol. Our target was a hootch a known VCI was using and we had a Hoi Chanh with us who'd made the original report.

The LSSC inserted us and the patrol moved about two hundred meters up a small canal at low tide. The undergrowth was too thick to move through and the canal was muddy, but the better choice. The patrol stopped and we began hearing a clicking noise. Once, twice, and then another. The Hoi Chanh pointed to the mud at our feet. In the moonlight we could see some kind of frog or tadpole about the size of a thumb poking its head up out of the goo. It would make a "clicking" sound like that when you snap your fingers and then disappear. Like I said, the jungle was full of surprises.

We climbed up out of the canal where a hootch was located and found no one at home. A rear guard was set in place and we moved on to another hootch. This time two VC made a break for it with weapons in hand and Rich Solano took them under fire from his position on point. We found one body which turned out to be the Hamlet Farmers Committee Section Chief. The second KIA of the evening was confirmed by an intelligence report.

The patrol moved back to the insertion point and we hailed a nearby PCF for extraction. The platoon later received intelligence indicating the Dung Island VC were calling for an increase in alertness since the SEALs had arrived in town. This news motivated us to no end. Not only were we hitting them hard and with great effect, they knew who we were!

During the debriefing that night we all talked about the clicking frogs. Someone brought up the idea we could use a finger snap to signal each other when next to, or in, a canal on patrol. It was also mentioned that if we'd thought of it the VC probably had too. The signal was used on a limited basis during our tour and with success.

It was now early April 1970. The First Squad was on their way upriver in the LSSC to conduct a recon when Coastal Group 36 contacted us. We were to proceed to the north end of Ong Cha Island to destroy a VC flag and large propaganda banner flying on the edge of the river. There was no problem finding the target as it turned out to be as big as one of those country fair banners I remember being strung across the streets back home. It was high in the trees for all to see and the squad wanted that flag.

I remember thinking to myself it was a crazy idea going after it. The thing just had to be booby-trapped. But I finally gave in. The deal was they would let me fire the 90mm recoilless at the bottom of the tree to set off any booby traps the enemy might have put in place. The squad happily agreed and my shot nearly blew the tree down. Mike

Thornton cut loose with his M60 and down came the banner. Solano and Doyle inserted and captured the flag. Mission completed!

This little diversion compromised our original operation so we returned to CG 36, burning the banner and having our picture taken with the flag. I've always believed we took a huge chance that day but the direct action and our success was a great morale builder. Sometimes you have to do these kinds of things just because they're there and the men need the lift.

One of the few problems we had with the LSSC, besides its limited boat design for SEAL ops, was its fuel consumption. In order for us to reach our targets many times we had to tow the LSSC behind a PFC. This was especially true when going after objectives around the north end of the Dung Island complex. The intelligence we received on VC movements and activities were now usually on the north side of Dung or across the Khem Bang Canal on Con Coc Island. If the LSSC were to travel this distance to insert us it wouldn't have enough fuel to return. Hence, the tow service provided by the PCFs.

Acting on intelligence from Soc Trang's NILO and the NSWGV we set out one afternoon to bag a VC extortionist and his security force. To do so we rented two sampans and their owner. Seven SEALs and LDNN Quang went by LSSC (in tow) to the south fork of the Bassac River. At the north end of the Khem Bang Canal the LSSC went under its own power, taking the two sampans in tow down the canal. At one point in their journey the SEAL squad transferred to the two rented sampans, preparing for the surprise we had in store for the VC target.

We proceeded south in the sampans until a very high-speed sampan was spotted also moving south with us. The owner of the rented sampans identified the men in the mystery boat as being Vietcong. We radioed for the LSSC to move up and then proceeded to take the VC boat under fire. When the LSSC came up we jumped aboard even as enemy fire began reaching out for us from Con Coc Island. The VC craft beached itself and also began firing on our LSSC.

Lieutenant Boyhan ordered an insertion south of the VC

position. We did so, setting up a guardpost for security. Ken Meier sighted three VC with weapons working their way toward our position and took the group under fire with his Stoner. Ken killed two of the VC outright, wounding the third. Normally a quiet man Meier was yelling, "I got them, I got them!" as loud as he could.

And he had.

We moved up and searched the bodies. One M1 rifle was captured, as well as a ChiCom 7.62mm carbine, 35 rounds of .30 caliber ammunition, and 10 rounds of 7.62mm long. And there was an M26 grenade, as well. We followed a blood trail belonging to the third VC for about a hundred meters until losing it in tall grass. Intelligence reported later he'd died of his wounds.

An extraction was called for. The LSSC was so low on fuel we decided to link up with another PCF at the south end of the canal for a tow back to CG 36. The LSSC couldn't have made it all the way back even if its tanks had been full, like when we'd left the base earlier that day.

When the Seabees showed up on base they'd set up their own 81mm mortar pit. Doc Brown kind of hung out with them for a while, reporting back to us that they really had their act together and wanted some action. Lieutenant Boyhan made contact with the Seabee folks and we began laying in prefire plans with their mortar crew. This would come in handy whenever we operated within the range of their 81.

April was winding down when we received intelligence about a VC sleeping station on Tron Island, just across the river from our own base. We set up a prefire plan with the 81mm crew and inserted on the island at 0100 using the LSSC.

The platoon patrolled alongside nipa palm to take advantage of its cover until we reached the hootches. The VC had posted a guard but he was sighted trying to sneak off by our pointman. Once again Eugene Stoner's fine weapons system accounted for another enemy soldier and we searched the dead man's body as well as the hootches. Our tally included one KIA, three kilos of medical drugs and supplies, one kilo of documents, and three M26 grenades.

Finished up we started moving back when effective small arms fire began heading in our direction. Mortar support was called in and the rounds came in right on target. The enemy fire was soon suppressed and Doc was proven right. The Seabees did have its act together. We extracted without any further interference from the VC.

The LSSC continued to provide good support on both long and short missions until the first of May. Then, to our disbelief, we were sent an MSSC, or Medium SEAL Support Craft. It came with its own officer and crew. This was a big but quiet boat with all the room we needed for personnel and fuel. We would continue to use the LSSC when working the tight canals and on squad-sized operations, but the MSSC's powerful engines were music to our ears.

By mid-May it was raining. The showers cut down on the heat and settled the dust and dirt at the base. We welcomed the rain for these reasons but didn't like how it affected our operating. The river and canals became swollen and left their banks. They began filling up with logs and debris of every kind. The boat's coxswain would have to keep a careful eye out during night operations to avoid striking the junk the rains brought with them. Sometimes it was difficult inserting without being in water up to your armpits. Oh, yes, and then there was the mud. The mud was something which you got tired of real fast.

On one operation we had trouble with the MSSC inserting us from the river. The water was so high that the trees prevented the bow of the boat from penetrating water shallow enough for us to get off in. It wasn't that we didn't want to get wet as wet is standard SEAL operating procedure. Rather, it was being placed in the water so far out from the bank that the current was too strong and fast to navigate in full combat equipment with weapons.

After moving to and fro a few times we finally found a sheltered cove which was free from the current's pull. The bow of the MSSC had a large web cargo net that hung down into the water for us to climb up and down on. When we slipped down the net and pointed our toes we could now just touch the bottom of the riverbed. Well, some of us could. Nelson, our interpreter, went right under. We ended up passing him from man to man, tree to tree, until he could put his feet down and keep his head above water.

Mike LaCaze told Tom Boyhan that something was in the water with us. Mr. Boyhan tried to convince Mike to keep moving, offering he was just feeling the tug of the current. Suddenly LaCaze screamed and I mean it was an unrecognizable sound! His Stoner went high in the air and Mike Thornton reached up, catching the precious weapon with as little effort as if he were playing first base back home.

We called the boat back for an emergency extraction with Mike all the time screaming in pain. Man by man we passed LaCaze back to the rear of the patrol and Mike Sands clambered up the net onto the bow in the wink of an eye. LaCaze was handed up to Sands who laid him on the bow while everyone else made their way aboard. There was a large bulge in Mike's Levi's pant leg and he was screaming, "Get it out! Get it *out!*"

Sands whipped his KA-BAR knife out of its sheath and cut the pant leg open. "I got it!" he yelled.

"Don't throw it back in the water with us!" said Thornton.

"It" turned out to be a fourteen-inch catfish which had swum up our teammate's leg and attached itself to his leg.

We were ready to go when I told Tom we were missing one man. Where was Nelson? We found him up in a tree where he'd climbed when LaCaze started screaming. It took some time to coax Nelson down from his perch and onto the boat. Once done, we headed back for CG 36 with Mike in so much pain that Doc gave him a shot of morphine in the other leg to ease his extreme discomfort. As it turned out one of the catfish's long pointed barbs, which protrude from both sides of a catfish's head, had run up under Mike's kneecap and broken off. Doc couldn't do much about it until we were back on dry land. LaCaze's leg began to swell and it was then I remembered studying submarine medicine and about Asian catfish. Their barbs, I recalled, were poison and capable of inflicting great pain. Well, Mike was certainly living proof of that course's information.

We took LaCaze to the mess hall and placed him on a table. Doc tried to remove the long spine from under Mike's kneecap but it was in too deep. Mike could hardly stand our corpsman's probing around, despite the morphine. A MED-EVAC was called for and Doc had to administer another shot before the helicopter arrived.

We were getting close to the end of our tour. After this, what would be next for CHARLIE platoon?

26

Brightlight Operation

June 1970. CHARLIE platoon was coming ever closer to the end of its tour of Vietnam. Coastal Group 36 was becoming a solid support base for SEAL operations. Target folders were being received in a steady stream from both NSWGV and NILO in Soc Trang. We had been hitting the VC hard, keeping the pressure on both day and night against his infrastructure. The men were tuned to the peak of combat readiness, and they were eager to operate even up until the last day we'd be in-country. Morale was likewise at its highest since our arrival.

Lieutenant (jg) Duggar had rotated back to the States to resume a place in civilian life. Lieutenant Boyhan submitted a request on my behalf for meritorious field advancement to chief gunners mate, the request approved in March. Tom decided to turn over Mr. Duggar's squad and duties to the platoon chief, which was now myself. Boyhan didn't feel it necessary to replace his second in command with only a little more than one month left in-country. Regardless if I were deserving or capable of the post, it struck me as the greatest possible compliment that a man I had developed the highest respect for, as both an officer and operator, would see me in this light.

We were both indirectly careful to keep the bond of friendship that developed between us well within the parameters of military respect expected between a chief petty officer and his platoon commander. Tom was always *Mr.* Boyhan and I was always the Chief. It made for a comfortable working relationship between us and made a good example for the men.

Lieutenant Boyhan was called to Saigon for a briefing by NSWGV. It concerned a possible mission which none of the platoon knew anything about. I continued to run operations in Tom's absence. The men wanted to operate and I knew they wanted their commander to be proud of them when he returned. We tried. . . .

One of our operations was a predawn recon mission in an area reported to have VC activity, our old friend Tron Island. We inserted by MSSC and patrolled for about three hundred meters when my rear security, Lou DiCroce, dislocated his shoulder. He'd been holding onto a tree to let himself down carefully into a canal and slipped. Lou twisted trying to keep his weapon above the water and when he did so his shoulder popped out of its socket. I attempted to put it back in place, but with no success. DiCroce wanted us to leave him behind but that was out of the question. We called for extraction and aborted the mission.

Back at the base Doc tried to put Lou's shoulder back in place but he, too, couldn't do it. A shot of morphine and a MEDEVAC call sent Lou to a more sophisticated medical facility. He returned the next day, a bit sore, but otherwise all right.

Boyhan soon returned with "big news." He acted surprised the platoon had continued to operate while he'd been gone but he was pleased we'd done so. CHARLIE platoon had been selected to mount an operation against a VC POW camp! The camp was supposed to have three American prisoners in it, and from that point on nothing else mattered to us but the rescue of these men. U.S. POWs were receiving greater attention from both our own military command and the world in general beginning in 1970. All of this affected us too, for it was a known fact American captives were enduring tremendous hardships in jungle camps throughout the Delta region of Vietnam.

In the States there was a public outcry over the cruel and primitive conditions our men were being held under by the VC and NVA. All this prompted a new intelligence effort which was directed at the release of these men by any means possible. Code named "Brightlight," the entire U.S. command was to convey their concern for the rescue of prisoners of war to its agents in the field. This included us, the Navy's SEAL platoons. Large amounts of money were rumored to have been set aside for any intelligence which led to the location and release of American POWs.

Our intelligence for this operation reported an Army VN agent possessed information on a POW camp near Thanh Phy in the Vinh Binh Province. The camp was reported to have both VN and American prisoners, and that these were housed in separate hootches. A third hootch was said to hold the VC guard force. All three hootches were under the cover of heavy jungle canopy and were situated beside a small canal. Lieutenant Boyhan had aerial photographs of the target in infrared overlays which were supposed to tell us where the hootches were. There was supposed to be two sampans tied up on the canal near the camp.

The photos were taken from high altitude and intelligence analysts in Saigon had "read" these for us. The one area of intelligence we questioned most was the Army's refusal to release the VN agent to us. We weren't even allowed to meet, much less talk with him. This was felt to be important as we all wanted any firsthand information he might pass on to us during the planning phase. It was common to request a reporting agent accompany SEALs as a guide on such high-priority missions. Still, we were told "absolutely no." The higher-ups were afraid the mission would compromise their agent, and their decision was final. Mr. Boyhan insisted on talking with the agent but no dice meant no dice. Although we couldn't accept this attitude we also believed there were Americans being held . . . so we would go without the precious mystery agent.

Our plan was to have the VN army sweep the day before we made the actual hit. The platoon would tag along with the Viets and at some point they would extract and we would stay behind. After darkness fell the platoon would patrol to the target area and make the assault at first light.

We had air support laid on with Hueys to lift both us and the POWs out.

LCDR Mullen gave the platoon a briefing on how to handle U.S. POWs. They were to be kept under strict discipline while in the hands of their liberators. We were not to give them any weapons or allow them to become involved in combat of any kind. This surprised some of the men in the platoon, but the officer went on to explain the dangers of POW handling and how it might interfere with our own effectiveness.

We went over and over the photo intelligence and made an in-depth map study of the area. Each teammate was more than just excited about this operation. The men checked and then double-checked their equipment and weapons. We were ready to go. That night was the longest I could remember in some time.

First we loaded aboard the MSSC, linking up with a WPB Coast Guard boat at sea, somewhere off the mouth of the Bassac River. When we transferred onboard we moved to a secure portion of the ship and were kept there for security reasons. Only select members of the Coast Guard crew could interface with us, and these were few in number. Sleep wasn't in the cards for the platoon. We were too keyed up and the lack of sleep simply went unnoticed.

Before daylight we transferred again, this time to a landing craft. Now it was up the Co Chien River and inserted with an ARVN company on the north bank of the river, south of Thanh Phu. The Viets began their sweep operation north of our target area as a diversion. We tagged along as rear security for them. It was a long walk before we SEALs found cover in a stand of trees which would do until night fell. The ARVN troops passed back through our position, each one smiling and waving as he went on.

Before long it was quiet. The sky became overcast and rain was sure to come. By dark, the rain was falling and we welcomed it as it would cover the sound of our movement. Our cover was good, provided as it was by the jungle's foliage. CHARLIE entered the canal, moving quietly and looking intently for any booby traps we fully expected to find in the target area. Every man was moving carefully, quietly, and with great concentration.

We patrolled to within five hundred meters of the suspected camp, moving all the while in the canal. It was waist-deep and fairly easy going except for the leeches. Hal Kuykendall was carrying a PRC 77 radio along with his web gear. He started to become uncomfortable because of something round and soft against his hip that felt like a large bulge. Hal couldn't do anything about it with all his gear on and being waist-deep in water. He believed it wasn't a leech because it was too big. So, what was it?

When the patrol finally stopped he unsnapped his web gear and dropped his pants. It *was* a leech! The biggest leech any of us had ever seen. This critter was at least five inches long and as thick as a big man's thumb. Hal dispatched the hitchhiker with his mosquito repellent. Better a leech than another catfish . . .

We were now as close to the target as we dared to be without risking detection. The platoon moved through an area of tall trees with little jungle foliage at ground level. The dirt was hard, and reddish in color. There wasn't any grass growing from it. We took what cover we could from the rain by hunkering down beneath the trees. Each teammate was about ten feet from his fellow SEAL, a tree providing both cover and concealment as we formed up in one big circle.

It began raining. And it rained so hard that night that most of the time you couldn't see the man next to you. Never before or since have I seen such a downpour. It felt like the water was being spilled over you by a bucket above your position, one after another. I remember it was cold, so cold I got the shakes. All night it went on like this. Hell Week couldn't have been worse for being wet, cold, and wishing for a break in the storm. Once the rain began to let up on us I saw some men standing beside their trees. I decided to try standing, just for the relief of stretching a bit. Water covered the ground around our positions and land crabs were rejoicing in it. They ran past us and each other sideways in what looked to be at least two inches of rainfall!

Mike Sands moved over to Doc Brown and said, "Doc, look at my hands." They were shriveled up and bleeding.

"Look at my hands," replied Doc. "They look like yours

and I'm supposed to be black." Sands just smiled at this and worked his way back to his tree. Teammates.

The rain finally stopped. We could see the signs of first light approaching. Boyhan gave the word to move out and I still remember wondering how a man could live in a bamboo cage in this kind of weather. Under my breath I recall saying to myself, "Boy! We've got to get these guys out of here!"

It was back to the canal. Its waters felt warm after the night's cold rain. There was only a short distance to go now. We reached an elbow in the canal. The photos had shown us two sampans, one heading straight into the canal's bank and the other boat at a thirty degree angle from the south. What we found instead made a hollow spot appear in my already empty stomach. Each man clearly felt the same pain without one word being uttered between us. Two long dead nipa palm branches in the shape of a sampan were lying in the water, just as pictured.

I told myself the nipa palm didn't matter. Anyone could have made a mistake looking at pictures taken from so high above the earth. But what about the infrared overlays? Something, or somebody, had to be in the hootches under the trees. "Keep sharp now," I told myself, "look for booby traps. Don't blow it now!"

We moved around the bend in the canal to a small rise in the trees. This placed us just behind the hootch that was supposed to be holding the Americans. We came on-line and moved to the top of the rise, weapons ready and fully alert. There was no longer any discomfort, any cold, any tiredness. We were a combat platoon of Navy SEALs, blooded and there to rescue our countrymen, if at all possible.

No hootch. No trails. No sign of any activity.

Quickly we crossed back and forth under the trees. Nothing— We rechecked the map and photos we'd brought with us. No chance of our being lost or off track. We were where we were supposed to be, where intelligence had sent us. We didn't want to give up, didn't want to believe what we were seeing. But the camp and its POWs weren't there. It was a dry hole, so to speak.

It was then we felt the letdown. The energy, once slowly

draining from us now rushed out. We'd been without sleep for forty-eight hours. We'd been hot, then cold. Chewed on by monster leeches and anything else with a taste for man in the jungle. We'd walked miles and miles, for no good apparent reason. CHARLIE platoon was dead tired. Worse, we'd been had by phony intelligence. The joke was on us and we began to feel crushed way down deep inside. Our morale slipped a notch or two, I can tell you that.

Lieutenant Boyhan called for the radio and gave the code word to extract SEALs only. We moved three hundred meters into the open and set up security around the landing zone. It was a good thing for the VC that they didn't show up as the platoon would have expended its frustration upon them with an anger I can only imagine today. When the two "slicks" were circling overhead we knew we'd been on target all along. The camp just wasn't there, period. We threw smoke and the pilots correctly identified it. The platoon extracted without incident, and without smiles.

The failure of the Brightlight mission caused great concern for not only us but for the NILO and NSWGV people, as well. We knew our men were still out there, cold and hungry . . . waiting. Our teammates would try again as failure was not a part of the SEAL vocabulary.

On the helicopter ride back to base someone said, "When we get back I'm going to sleep until it's time to go home." He was almost right. This had been our sixty-ninth operation.

CHARLIE would run seventy before calling it a day in Vietnam.

27

Our
"Green Angels"

The United States Navy has a precision flying team called the "Blue Angels." They are the pride of the Navy and rightly so. Every summer the Blue Angels streak through the sky at air shows across the United States. Crowds hold their breath with wide eyes and the Angels perform wing tip to wing tip maneuvers overhead. The Blue Angels are in every sense of the word, what little boys' dreams are made of. With all due respect to the talented, brave pilots who are selected to fly in this unit, they are not the only angels in the Navy's sky.

During the Vietnam war the OV-10 Bronco was a conventional representation of an angel from above for CHARLIE platoon's SEALs. In 1969 the Navy decided to deploy the North American OV-10 Bronco in lieu of obtaining additional helicopter gunships. The Bronco became one of the most versatile light strike and counterinsurgency aircraft to fly in Vietnam. It was ideally suited for Navy support needs in the Mekong Delta. The OV-10's qualities quickly developed an outstanding reputation for the plane's combat powers when working with the SEALs.

VAL-4 was commissioned to take the OV-10 into combat. The unit deployed to Vietnam in March 1969. The Broncos

278

swiftly adopted the nickname "Black Ponies" from their tactical call sign "Bronco." Throughout 1970 and 1971, the Ponies flew numerous sorties in support of the SEALs, working almost exclusively in the ground attack role. Many a SEAL owes the lives of his teammates—as well as his own—to the crews of these little fixed wing olive drab airplanes. I know this to be true because I am one of those SEALs. Today we reflect back on times when we were faced with overwhelming odds, fondly remembering the OV-10s as our "Green Angels" when it was truly too close to call. Let me tell you how they looked from down where I was in the brown water, mud, nipa palm, and green tracers of the VC.

Lieutenant Boyhan planned an operation against a VCI meeting site on the north side of Dung Island. To reach the target it was necessary to use the Khem Bang Canal between Dung and Con Coc island. Once again the platoon would have to move around the island complex to reach this canal. The only available resource which could put CHARLIE at the mouth of the Khem Bang was a VN Navy junk from Coastal Group 36. We would then transfer to our Skimmer as manned by MST personnel, which would also be towing two IBS rubber boats for the final leg of the trip to the target.

"Black Ponies" and Army "Viper" gunships were put on standby as air support. The operation was scheduled for the predawn hours of morning. This would put the platoon at the target by daylight. Based on sound intelligence we felt this could be a hot target if we were not detected during infiltration. Everyone believed Tom Boyhan had come up with a good plan and we were up for it. However, I was not very happy about using the rubber boats. They just didn't offer any protection from enemy gunfire. But it was time to keep my mouth shut and swallow my fear.

All went as planned until we transferred to the IBS boats. It was a clear morning and we had to paddle in close to the canal bank under the dark shadows of the trees. First, we missed the small canal that was to lead us to the target area. A less bold platoon commander would have called for the Skimmers and aborted the mission at this point. Not our

Lieutenant Boyhan. Even though it was getting light he turned us around and located the right canal.

The two rubber raiding craft slipped up the canal without making a sound. The narrow waterway got even narrower, with the foliage beginning to choke it off. Enemy barricades made things even worse. Lieutenant Boyhan entered the water and towed the boats by hand the last eight hundred meters. Tom had the bowline slung taut over his shoulder and was pulling the boats in chest-deep water as we maintained security. The scene reminded me of the Bogart movie *The African Queen*. It wasn't hard to turn the boats around and hide them beneath the nipa palm branches which lay all over the water's surface. With our camouflage job done, it was time to start patrolling.

We were hardly out of the water and moving when we came upon what appeared to be a deserted enemy base camp. Sleeping stations were built up off the ground, and there were numerous bunkers, fighting positions, and structures. Intelligence would later tell us the place was used as a medical field aid station. As we continued to explore the target area the jungle got thicker and harder to move through. Suddenly we found ourselves on the target before being prepared to be on the target. Talk about the element of surprise!

Six armed VC broke from a hootch and Solano and Boyhan took them under fire, killing three of the six. The rest of us moved forward and now we were taken under automatic fire from the north end of the target. We were unable to suppress the enemy's fire, which was coming from well-dug-in bunkers. The VC were moving swiftly down our flanks on both the east and west sides. They wanted to encircle us, and it looked like they just might. Lieutenant Boyhan scrambled the Black Ponies.

We found blood trails. We'd hit them hard. A search of the hootch and bodies recovered a .45 caliber pistol and fifty rounds of ammunition. There were also six grenades and one kilo of documents. Our guide identified the dead VCI as Muoi Law, a district level cadre. Hai Quyen and Thang Tre were district level medics. More infrastructure names to add to our list.

We used fire and maneuver tactics to get back to the

treeline as the enemy was really stirred up by now. Black Pony and Viper air assets were now overhead. Mr. Boyhan directed the Ponies on to the bunkers southwest of our present position. On their first run the Broncos took automatic fire and had to pull off his gun run. The second run saw them come in lower and the enemy fire was knocked out by rockets. The SEALs leapfrogged back to the deserted aid station, the enemy probing us with fire even as we moved. The planes continued their attacks on the target area to cover our extraction.

Our radioman called the MST Skimmers up and we paddled the rubber boats like crazy to meet them. Viper gunships covered us as the Skimmers moved at top speed across the water, the helicopters darting and bobbing like giant dragon flies above the Khem Bang Canal. The gunships were relieved by the Ponies when their fuel ran low. The planes now worked both sides of the canal until we were well out in the Bassac River, linking up with the VN junk.

It was a successful operation without any friendly casualties, thanks to our Angels. What impressed me the most about this operation was the Ponies' performance. First, there was their speed. They were called last but were over the target before the Vipers. Plus, the Ponies could stay with us until we were clear. Secondly, the aircraft had tremendous ordnance capacity. Because of this they were working the VC from the time we were on target until we were safely aboard the junk.

The Broncos flew in a two-plane formation and were on call twenty-four hours a day. They flew out of Binh Thuy and Vung Tau. Each airfield had an eight-plane section under VAL-4. After that day I always knew they were up there if I needed them, and the time came when I did.

CHARLIE platoon found the LDNNs to be an excellent combat unit. Not only could they fight, they did. In addition, they could plan and coordinate operations. An LDNN platoon under a SEAL platoon commander's operational command was an extremely good team. The LDNN had a number of personnel who had an impressive amount of operational experience. They only needed the SEALs for air and boat support to make them even more effective. Still, the addition of a small number of SEALs in their line of march helped to bond the US/VN relationship. Lieutenant Boyhan made a special effort to ensure our relationship with the LDNN wasn't overlooked. He always offered at least four men from CHARLIE platoon to operate with them.

On April 9, 1970, Lou DiCroce, MaCarthy (from SEAL Team Two), and myself agreed to join Ron Rogers and his LDNN platoon in an operation against a VCI target. The objective was located on the east side of Ong Cha Island. Except for a few very small canals the island was completely surrounded by nipa palm. The nipa palm and river were held back by a four-foot high dike which also encircled the island. It was high tide and we knew we were in for a wet patrol. But due to the nipa palm the enemy felt secure and the element of surprise was all ours. The swamp, clogged as it was with nipa, was four hundred meters thick at the target area. The plan was to insert on the south end of the island and to patrol northwest, right through the nipa palm forest!

We loaded aboard the LSSC and proceeded up the Bassac at 0330 hours. As we approached the north end of the Tee Tee canal, Ron and I moved onto the bow of the boat to try and locate our insertion point. We agreed on a spot at the bend of the canal and the coxswain slipped the LSSC under the overhanging nipa palm without a sound. Rogers and I slipped over the side of the LSSC into chest-deep water. The others followed close behind.

Even though the night was clear there was no moon. When we moved into the forest it got very dark. We had to zigzag around the nipa palm, lifting the branches and passing under them so they wouldn't make noise rubbing against us. You had to keep your eyes on the man in front of you all the time because it was so dark and easy to lose contact. The patrol made no noise when we were in the water but the patrolling was slow. At times the water level reached our necks and it was necessary to help the shorter Vietnamese along.

Daybreak found us still in waist-deep water. The patrol moved into tall trees growing out of the nipa palm. We stopped. I could see four or five men ahead of me. Thai was the next man to my front and I asked him why we had stopped.

"Tich is climbing a tree," he said.

Soon the men in front of me began smiling and talking low to each other. Thai told me he heard a chicken, which was what Tich had apparently climbed the tree for. We moved a short distance and came on-line under the cover of a four-foot dike.

Across the dike was a small clearing, no more than two acres or so. Smoke was drifting from a tiny hootch right in front of us. A VC guard was sitting against a tree with his weapon across his lap. He looked like he was sleeping. Two other weapons were leaning against another tree by the hootch. We began slipping over the dike, our weapons at the ready. The VC jumped up and went right back down, dropping his weapon and grabbing at the hole in his chest. He died. Then things began happening very quickly.

Small arms fire broke out as the LDNNs entered the hootch. I moved to the left of the hootch and saw six armed men running from the back of the structure. I cranked off an automatic burst from my Stoner carbine and two of the men fell. Flipping the selector switch to "semi" I fired again, with two more VC dropping in their tracks. One of the men started to get up and run when I felt a strong hand on my shoulder. Tich said, "You go to hootch and I get them!"

Thai was coming out of the hootch as I reached the door. He said, "Bib Cambo." In a pool of blood on the dirt floor lay a large Cambodian. He was dressed in a khaki uniform with NVA sandals on his feet. Lou DiCroce was already searching the hootch and had a handful of documents. I asked where Ron was but Lou didn't know. I felt Rogers needed my radio near him so I left to locate the SEAL advisor. Suddenly a heavy firefight began in the treeline to the right of us. Two LDNNs were firing their M60s down the trail in both directions. Their targets were VC trying to get into the nipa palm behind us. I started for the treeline when something hit me hard. I fell, striking the ground with a thump. My radio felt like it had gained fifty pounds. I got up and made it to the treeline, scrambling the Cobras.

Moving down the treeline I found VC fighting holes dug

every ten to fifteen feet apart. Ron came through the trees with someone over his shoulder. It was Tich. We stripped him of his uniform and found one bullet wound under his left arm. We couldn't help him. Tich was dead. I told Ron the gunships were on their way, and then called the PCFs' call sign, "Bureau" for mortar support. They responded but were too far away to reach our position.

Rogers asked me to move Tich's body back to the hootch while he brought the platoon back. We tied Tich's hands together and I put them over my head so I could carry him on my back. The LDNNs were right behind me firing as we moved. The radio antenna on my PRC 77 kept falling down in front of me and I thought Tich's body might have broken it. Wrong! When I took the radio off to see if I could fix it I found one bullet hole through the antenna and two in the battery pack. Now I knew what had knocked me down. I was carrying a large silk "T" we'd trained with at Niland. I spread the "T" out and began to direct gunship fire from the top of the ground panel. It didn't take a genius to realize we were surrounded and outnumbered. There was no doubt we'd take even more casualties if we tried to break out.

We called for the slicks to extract us and were told they were on their way. Keep in mind I was talking over a radio that had taken three rounds and was still working! Lieutenant Boyhan and CHARLIE platoon were aboard a PCF and they were enroute to support us. Viper was doing a good job keeping the VC in check, and we felt we could get out by slick. Then the gunships advised us they were low on fuel and had to break off their support. With the helos gone the enemy fire picked up on all sides.

I called for an ammo check. Most of the platoon was down to two magazines. Lou was still in the hootch and was in good shape ammunitionwise. I had him give the LDNN three hundred rounds of linked 5.56 ammo from his Stoner so they could refill their magazines. Things were real hot now.

It was then I began to hear Angels sing. Upriver the unmistakable whine of the OV-10 turbo-jet engines made themselves heard over the roar of gunfire. "Black Pony, this is Threadbare. Can you help us?"

"Threadbare, this is Black Pony one zero two and one zero four. We're overhead."

I went on to give them instructions about our "T," being careful to advise them to look out their starboard side so they would know we were Navy. The first strike came in fifty meters from our "T." The pilot asked me to confirm fifty meters and I said, "You better make it twenty!"

They did just that.

These guys were real pros. Their planes came in with guns roaring at treetop level. Never had I got such close Close Air Support. One run after another hit the enemy positions but the VC wanted us some kind of bad. They kept up the fight regardless of their losses and the Ponies' fearsome firepower. There was a hootch in the treeline that the Vietcong were running for. Black Pony 102 asked for permission to hit it and I told him to "blow it away." The first run on the hootch resulted in an overhead explosion behind us. I asked what it was and the pilot apologized for hitting the top of a palm tree with his five-inch rocket! We took some shrapnel from that one but his wingman hit the hootch dead-on. It was quite an air show.

All the time I was busy working with the Ponies the LDNNs were laying down a base of fire. First in one direction, and then in another. The battle went on and on. The Ponies would make a run in one direction and the VC would fire on us from another. We were always shifting fire but the OV-10s were extremely effective with their ordnance.

At one point during the action the slicks, code named "Warrior," advised us they couldn't get in because of the lack of air support. They said the fixed wing aircraft couldn't provide close enough support for them to work in tight. I couldn't believe what I was hearing but there wasn't any choice but to let them pass. When Lieutenant Boyhan heard the transmission from his perch on the PCF he was ready to come in after us with "guns blazing." I radioed back to him "Negative! Negative!" You just had to be there, I guess. Any direction they would have come from would have found them taking VC fire. To return that fire would have meant shooting at us too. For the minute we had enough stuff coming our way without adding a SEAL platoon's overbearing firepower. Our platoon commander understood the situation and they stayed on the PCF.

We called for a MEDEVAC as one LDNN was wounded in the face. The Black Ponies made a run on the north and south treelines and the helicopter came in for our dead and wounded. He was out of there as fast as he'd come in, green tracers chasing his tail rotor as he cleared the treetops. They were a great and gutsy crew. The chopper dropped our people off at CG 36 and stood by in case we needed them again.

Black Ponies 102 and 104 let us know they were now running low on fuel and ammo. They planned to stretch things out by mixing their runs with live and dummy attacks. The Marines, they said, were coming down from Vung Tau and the Ponies would stay with us until the Corps arrived overhead. The planes relieved each other on station and all I had to do was change the call signs to 106 and 108. The firing never stopped on our behalf. I asked the new pilots to save their five-inch rockets, which they did.

The weakest side of the encirclement was the nipa palm side to our east. If we were going to get out that was the only way to go. I directed air strikes between us and the river, telling the Ponies to blow us a hole in the nipa palm with their rockets. I asked Ron if he was ready to give it a try. He was. He led the LDNNs out to the river and I took rear security, still working with the OV-10s. However, when the chest-deep water hit the wounded radio my transmissions started to break up. I called for the LSSC and passed ground to air control over to Boyhan on the PCF. We took probing fire but moved fast through the water until we were aboard the LSSC. Our extraction was logged in at 1020 hours, putting us on the target for four straight hours. Most of this time the Black Ponies were with us.

Unknown to us the PCF and LSSC had been taking small arms fire from the Dung Island side of the canal. Boyhan was now having Black Pony 106 and 108 work both sides of the canal until we were clear of the islands and back in the middle of the Bassac. We released the Ponies and the MEDEVAC, then returned to Coastal Group 36.

Our body count numbered eighteen VC killed in action.

We'd captured weapons, grenades, and documents with a VC flag. Two days after the operation we got word from the NILO at Soc Trang that their intelligence indicated the VC had taken carpenters from Xom An Duc to Dung Island. They were to build forty coffins for their dead comrades, killed on April 9 by our combined force of LDNNs, SEALs, and Black Ponies/Vipers. We'd made a deadly team that day.

It should be said that the Black Ponies were the winged guardians with a like spirit of the Navy's SEALs. Together we had a grim determination to do the job we'd trained for . . . a job we did very, very well.

28

Farewell to Tich

Humility must always be the portion of any man who receives acclaim earned in the blood of his followers and sacrifices of his friends.

—Dwight D. Eisenhower, July 1945.

Tich was five feet, four inches tall. He weighed one hundred forty pounds and had light brown skin with straight black hair and high cheekbones that gave way to a round face. His piercing dark brown eyes appeared as black holes resting under Mongolian slanted eyelids. Tich's smile was seldom seen but when it was it was quick and, in some ways, very gentle. Always it was genuine. He had a stocky build and was respected by his fellow LDNNs and the SEALs he worked with for his courage and boldness in combat. Tich was a South Vietnamese jungle fighter.

He absolutely hated the VC and NVA. He was as loyal a patriot to South Vietnam as they come. He was not only proud to fight for the South, he was also very proud to be a Vietnamese frogman; *"Lien Doc Nguoi Nhia"* . . . the soldiers who fight under the sea. Tich told more than one Navy SEAL, "You fight and go home and some day come back to fight again. I stay and fight all the time and I will fight here until I die!" It was his country and Tich would not be free until it was, I remember him saying. South Vietnam was his obsession and he remained true to his convictions until the day he fell from a VC bullet.

When you plan to stock support items for a SEAL

platoon, body bags are not on the list. In a remote area such as Coastal Group 36 they weren't on anyone's list. Upon the platoon returning to base after Tich was killed Doc Brown came to me and said he'd done the best he could with Tich's body. When I asked where Tich was he said he had him over at the CG's headquarters. On the way over Doc told me we didn't have a body bag so he'd put Tich in an IBS cover.

The IBS cover was made of hard rubber and snapped closed for the entire length of the bag. It had carrying handles at both ends and was used to store our rubber boats in. Doc had cleaned Tich's body and bandaged the wound that killed him. I thanked Doc for the care he'd given our friend and we stood by him for a while without speaking, knowing we shared the same loss in that moment.

I found Ron Rogers writing his report in the platoon office. What Doc had done was satisfactory with Ron and he told me he was sending the LDNN back to Saigon for Tich's burial service. They would be going by PCF that morning. Rogers was taking the body back later that afternoon by PCF and I told Lieutenant Boyhan I wanted to go with Ron. He agreed to my request without hesitation or question. Ron was happy to have the company.

CHARLIE platoon left Ron and me to ourselves as much as possible. They must have known and shared the loss we were feeling because when I showed up at the gun cleaning table, the normal chatter stopped. I was very aware of the silence. Mike Thornton offered to clean my weapon for me, but I refused and went to work on my Stoner. To this day I remember how Mike reached out to me. I did appreciate his offer, but more so the big heart behind it.

Late that afternoon Ron and I loaded Tich's body aboard a PCF and headed up the Bassac to Can Tho. The trip was cool and we tried to get some rest. My thoughts were of Tich which was normal for the circumstances. It was time to remember when we first met in 1968 aboard YRBM-18. Tich and Thai were the first two LDNNs I'd met and worked with. I respected them and trusted them almost from the beginning.

When ALFA platoon moved to Sa Dec, Tich came in one night after a little bit too much celebrating. He'd cut his left hand to the bone and needed several stitches to close the wound. Gary Abrahamson wanted to sew him up and that's what Tich wanted too, so Abe did the needlework. The next day I learned from Thai that Tich was getting married and asked if I wanted to go. It was at the wedding I learned that Tich was a Vietnamese Catholic.

His wife was such a little thing in white Vietnamese pants with an overdress that was split up the side. She had long black hair down to her waist and looked like a little girl. I was surprised to learn that she was a school teacher. She didn't look to be that old to me, in fact, she looked more like a schoolgirl than teacher. First I was a friend who went to his wedding and now I was a friend who was going to his funeral. It occurred to me I had really developed a bond with these people whom I was fighting alongside of.

We arrived at Can Tho and reported in at the SEAL office on base. A ride was arranged which took us to the airport at Binh Thuy. It was dark out when we arrived at flight operations. Our plane was scheduled to take off at midnight so we located a spot out of everyone's way and told the desk where they could find us. The night air was taking on a chill but the metal matting of the runway was still warm from the heat of the day. We placed Tich on the cooler ground beside the matting and lay down on the warm surface, our heads resting against Tich in his IBS cover.

Just before midnight a young airman came out to tell us our plane would be an hour late. He asked if we wanted a sandwich and some coffee. Neither Ron nor I had eaten all day and we jumped at the offer. A short time later the airman returned with food and hot coffee. He sat down while we were eating and began asking questions about SEALs. Both of us had been through this routine before but we answered the airman's questions, if nothing else for his kindness to us.

Finally we'd had enough and Ron set the stage. "Enoch," he said, "Tich has such bony legs. Would you trade places with me?"

"Sure, Ron," I replied. We casually moved around so Ron was resting where I'd been and I was now lying up against Tich's lower body. The airman didn't say anything for a moment or two, and then asked what we had in the black bag. Ron stopped eating, and holding his sandwich in one hand he reached behind his head. With a single slow pull Rogers drew down the hard rubber cover, exposing Tich from the top of his head to his waist.

"This is our buddy, Tich," I told the airman. "We're taking him home."

The young man's eyes grew and grew as his mind took in the scene we were playing out. When they reached the size of a healthy quarter he suddenly rose and left. Ron smiled at me in the darkness. "Now Tich would have enjoyed that," he said.

I agreed. Soon we were in the air and on our way. The ride to Tan Son Nhut was a short one.

At the airport we found a soldier with a jeep who took us to the U.S. morgue. We contacted a master sergeant at the morgue and asked him to house Tich for the night. He explained to us he couldn't accept Vietnamese dead in a U.S. morgue. The sergeant was an understanding man and after some conversation he offered he had an overflow locker outside the morgue he could keep Tich in until morning. He checked the body in and filled out some paperwork. The locker itself was a long metal building filled with litter racks. We placed Tich on one of the racks and the sergeant locked the door behind us as we left.

Early the next morning Ron contacted the LDNN at their headquarters and informed them where they could pick up the body. We went to the morgue to meet them. With Tich turned over to his own people we headed for the Vietnamese Navy base and contacted the LDNN officer in charge. They had Tich's body in the middle of the office floor when we arrived. The officer looked up and came over to thank us for bringing their man back. We asked permission to attend the services and he approved.

I asked him about the protocol we should observe. The officer looked confused until I explained we had heard it was their custom to give the wife a sum of money. He confirmed this, but said we didn't have to abide by their customs. We told him that we considered the LDNNs as teammates and that Tich was special to us. The officer then said we could follow their custom at the grave site. He told us what to expect and when and where the funeral was to be held. I wanted to know what the appropriate sum of money was to give because we didn't want to embarrass anyone by giving too much or too little. At that he smiled and became more helpful.

If we wanted to each give 3,000 P it would be proper and he then asked if we wanted to ride with the men in the platoon that we knew. You bet we did. A short time later Thai came to get us and it was good to see him. He acted as if he were equally as happy to find us there.

Thai took us to an LDNN building on base and we met many of his teammates. There were some I didn't know but the brotherhood was the same. In two hours we loaded up in the back of a VN military 6X6 truck with Tich's platoon and started through the streets of Saigon. The truck finally stopped in front of the Notre Dame Catholic Cathedral.

It was full of Vietnamese people and they were having some kind of mass. Tich's casket was by the altar with a Republic of South Vietnam flag draped over it. Ron and I took a seat about halfway up the church with the LDNN. I didn't understand most of the service but sometimes I picked up the language. I think the priest must have been speaking in French. It didn't matter to Ron and me because we were there for Tich's family and the LDNN.

At the end of the service six men from the platoon carried the casket out on their shoulders. Tich's picture was in a frame on the front of the coffin with his new chief's hat on top. It was the custom of the Vietnamese Navy to promote their men who were killed in action to the next higher rank.

A hard way to make chief.

Behind the casket four other members of the platoon were acting as the escort for Tich's wife and another young woman. I found out later she was the wife's sister. We loaded into another 6X6 and worked our way through Saigon's traffic, our horns blowing all the way. As the truck broke out of the main part of the city I could hardly believe my eyes. We were now on a four-lane freeway! This was the work of the U.S. military, no doubt about it. The trip to the graveyard wasn't a short one and I was uneasy without my weapon.

Finally reaching the cemetery Ron and I were surprised at its size. It was the largest cemetery I'd ever seen, with gravestones stretching on and on. Tich was unloaded and we walked behind the LDNN to the grave. They lowered the casket into the ground and the flag was given to his wife. The officer we'd spoken to earlier said some words and then shook her hand. Each LDNN said something as they held her hand for just a moment. The sister held a basket and after each man filed past and took her hand she would drop whatever was given her into the basket without looking. When it was our turn we palmed the money we'd agreed on and took her hand. I told Tich's wife I was sorry in Vietnamese. She looked up at me and said, "I remember you . . ." then lowered her head.

I didn't know what else to say.

Back in Saigon the truck dropped us off on a small street and left. We followed the LDNNs to a small building with only one door and window in its front. Tich's chief's hat was on the top of the triangular folded RVN flag beside his picture in the front window. Once inside the group was seated at a long table. The only ones present were the members of his platoon with Ron and me. We were served a meal by Tich's wife and three other young women. Some custom, I felt like we should be serving her. The women didn't eat with us, only serving the food. I never saw them again. Each of us slipped a few hundred Ps under our plates as we left the table.

We followed the LDNNs through the streets of Saigon until coming to an outside cafe. Ron and I sat there for hours drinking Vietnamese 33 beer by the bottle. The LDNNs didn't talk much of Tich but rather they spoke of killing the Vietcong. Ron told me the platoon wasn't going back to Dung Island for a while and he'd be staying with them. They'd lost two men and had two more wounded. Their command felt they needed some time off and I agreed. I told Ron I'd paid my respects and it was time for me to get back to CHARLIE platoon.

Rogers offered to take me to Tan Son Nhut and I rose to leave. The LDNNs wanted to know where I was going and I just said, *"Sat Cong,"* which meant "Kill Communists." They shook my hand and thanked me for coming. Thai went with Ron and me to the airport that night and as I was boarding the plane he said, "You keep your head down."

In Can Tho I checked out my web gear and weapon, then

climbed aboard a Swift boat for the trip down the Bassac. It was good having my Stoner in hand again. For the first time in three days I felt somewhat secure. The trip downriver was uneventful and I had some time to enjoy looking back over the stern at the wake the boat rolled back behind her. Tich was always on my mind as was the grief that goes with the loss of a teammate. Part of me wanted to get back in the field as soon as possible. But another part of me was tired of all the killing. It was late afternoon when we arrived at CG 36 and I was just in time for chow.

The platoon was eager to hear about Tich's funeral and about the LDNNs. We sat in the chow hall for some time as I went over the trip, answering their questions one by one. It became quiet after that and the men filtered out to the club for a beer or two. The platoon wasn't operating that night and I was a little disappointed. I felt like I needed to get back on the horse that threw me.

I left the mess hall and walked down by the river, stopping to look over at Dung Island. The island looked the same as when I'd left, almost as if it were waiting for me to return to its muddy banks and narrow canals. The sun was almost down and the fruit bats were active over the trees. The island in the distance gave me an eerie feeling for some reason. Soon darkness stole the last remaining light away and the only sounds were the music and good-hearted noise coming from the club behind me. I turned and spoke aloud as if I wanted the island to hear each word, Tich's memory softly haunting me still.

"I'll be back!" The wind from the river carried my vow across the Bassac's waters to the island complex's mute and waiting darkness.

29

Big MIKE

Mike Thornton had many qualities that all SEALs carry inside them yet he was unlike any man I've known. He was brash and always ready for a good time, two attributes which sometimes made him a problem for his lieutenant and his chief. Mike could walk into a room and—if motivated by some one or some thing—simply tear the place up, almost always causing grief and misery for his platoon. He was big and he was strong, very strong. His teammates thought the world of him but he needed watching at all times when we were not operating.

On the other hand he was one of the best operators in the teams. Mike Thornton was the kind of man that you were thankful to have in any combat situation.

Hal Kuykendall was Mike's best friend and he describes his old teammate's heart and personality like this. "Mike has the biggest heart and is the most fun loving human being I've ever known." It didn't start out that way for Hal. When they first met they were checking in as late arrivals the night before UDT Training Class 49 began. As the two men walked to the unit Mike took advantage of Hal's Southern accent and began calling him "Cuz," a nickname that's stuck with Kuykendall for twenty-six years now.

The barracks were dark when they reached them and Hal made every effort to be quiet because the rest of the class was fast asleep. Not Mike's style. First, Thornton turned on the lights and then he began making all matter of noise like the proverbial bull in a china shop. Hal told him the students were complaining and Mike's response was "That's what God gave you eyelids for! You can turn off the lights anytime you want."

It was October and cold in the barracks. Hal was a bit apprehensive about what he'd gotten himself into, as many a student is when he first reports to BUDS. Without warning a 220-pound, buck naked, bull of a man jumped into his bunk with him. Before Hal could say or do anything Mike Thornton said, "Cuz, I'm cold. Let me in bed with you." Kuykendall began fighting the big lug off, all the time yelling for help with the whole barracks coming instantly awake. Everyone was in an uproar and Hal was thus introduced to the man who would become his best friend.

In fact, Thornton took an instant liking to Hal although he was always picking at him. In fact, he drove poor Hal crazy with his barbs and antics. Each day after training was over the students would head for the showers. Hal would have a face full of soap, his eyes shut tight, and Thornton would slip up behind him with yet another joke to play. Pinching Kuykendall on the butt he'd yell out for all to hear, "Cuz, you sure got a cute butt!"

This irritated Hal to no end. He would yell back, "Don't do that!" It went on to no end and finally Kuykendall devised a plan. Just as Mike was getting ready to pinch him Hal spun around and hit Thornton full in the head, expecting to drop him flat-out in the showers. He didn't. Mike just shook his head and said, "Cuz, what did you do that for?" It was then Hal realized Mike Thornton was different in that he had no fear, knew no pain, and sure could take a punch.

As the class continued its training Kuykendall discovered something else about his friend. Mike was a natural morale builder, not only for the class but for Hal too. Their bond of friendship grew, especially so at San Clemente Island. One of the classes they had was an IBS recovery by submarine. Two IBS boats and crews would paddle in two different directions with a line between them. The submarine's periscope would break the surface, cut between the two rubber boats and snag the line. This caused the two IBSs to swing in behind the sub's sail. As the submarine surfaced the boat crews would paddle like crazy so they would end up on the deck of the sub, and therefore be recovered.

The students were told beforehand that if they fell in the water while all this was taking place it was important to swim away from the sub. Its propellers were razor sharp and spinning, with the vessel actually creating a suction so that if someone fell in they would be dragged back and into the propellers, end of exercise. This was such a concern the instructors did everything possible to scare the students about this possibility for their own safety.

When Class 49 showed up to train with the submarine, it was Hal Kuykendall who fell into the water as the submarine surfaced. He remembered every word the instructors had said and began swimming for his life. Suddenly someone grabbed him. It was like he was hooked to a power winch and was being pulled without effort through the water back toward safety. Mike Thornton, without thinking about his own safety for a moment, had leaped into the ocean after his friend. He pulled Hal back aboard the surfacing submarine and that was simply that.

As big and powerful as Mike was he surprised everyone by being the strongest swimmer in his class. He was also very protective of his teammates. The submarine incident told Hal that Thornton would always risk his own safety to save someone else in trouble. It would always be so. After San Clemente Island the two men became real buddies and were transferred to SEAL Team One where they were assigned to CHARLIE platoon.

Orders came down and the platoon was heading for Vietnam. Hal called his father to say good-bye, and Mike was there. Thornton wanted to talk with Mr. Kuykendall so they got on the line together. Before Mike gave the phone back to Hal, the senior Kuykendall asked Mike to take care of his son in Vietnam. For the entire time we were overseas fighting the war, Mike Thornton believed it was his mission in life to watch out for Hal because he'd told Mr. Kuykendall he would. Hal carried the radio for our platoon and Mike was right there behind him in the line of march with his M60 LMG. Hal knew why, and he knew that was just the way Thornton was.

To have Mike as a friend is special. Hal told me that even today he could call Thornton wherever he might be and say, "I need you here," and Mike would be there the next day without asking why. That's the kind of heart and loyalty Thornton offers a teammate.

He was also the kind of athlete who was good at just about anything he did. Not only was he exceptionally strong but he was extremely coordinated, even when carrying a heavy load. Dung Island was laced with small streams and canals which could only be crossed using monkey bridges. These were no more than a small log about six inches in diameter. Once two or three SEALs had crossed a monkey bridge on patrol it became slick with mud. Thornton, who carried the M60 plus eight hundred extra rounds of ammunition and his other equipment, never slipped or fell off a monkey bridge. He walked like a cat, his sense of balance unbelievable.

The only time I saw Mike fall was when a monkey bridge broke under his weight. There was a loud cracking noise and then a huge splash and Mike was in the canal. Of course, this meant the rest of the platoon behind him had to wade through the water afterward. Only one monkey bridge per crossing.

If Mike Thornton knew fear we never knew it. All of us liked to operate but when it came to courage you just weren't in Mike's league. On October 31, 1972, he would prove this to all of his teammates as he became the third SEAL in history to be awarded the Congressional Medal of Honor. He received his MOH for saving the life of a teammate, Lieutenant Thomas Norris . . . the second SEAL in history to see this honor bestowed on him.

Here is their incredible story, heretofore untold by one who was there.

It was late March 1972 and the communists launched a massive attack south of the DMZ in I Corps. It became known as the Easter Offensive. Shortly after the shooting started a U.S. Air Force electronic warfare jet was struck hard by a SAM (Surface to Air Missile), its pilot radioing he was going down. Lt. Col. Iceal Hambleton parachuted from the doomed aircraft deep over NVA held territory. Where he landed was pinpointed by a spotter plane, but he was also likewise fixed in place by the NVA troops who were surrounding his position on the ground.

Because of the classified knowledge Hambleton had as an electronics warfare expert he would have been a real prize for the NVA if he could be captured alive. The Air Force knew this and launched what proved to be a very costly rescue mission to try and get Hambleton out before the NVA got to him. Several aircraft, both fixed wing and helicopter, were shot down in their attempts to reach the colonel.

On April 10, Lieutenant Tom Norris took a five-man team deep into NVA territory on a rescue mission. They were successful in locating and retrieving a missing OV-10 pilot but were unable to get to where Hambleton was working hard to evade his pursuers. On the eleventh, Norris led two three-man patrols into the same area but again was foiled where Colonel Hambleton's fate was concerned. Finally, on the night of the twelth, Tom Norris and a LDNN named Kiet made contact. They dressed in black and posed as Vietnamese fishermen, paddling a sampan up a river to the agreed upon rescue point. Once there they kept close to the treeline, finally linking up with a greatly relieved Colonel Hambleton. The two men, one U.S. Navy SEAL and one South Vietnamese Navy SEAL, placed the airman in the bottom of the sampan, covering him with banana leaves so as to hide him from prying eyes.

It was far from over.

After the successful linkup the men began the trip back downriver. From the start there were problems. Norris made one stop after another to hide the sampan under the riverbank's thick foliage. NVA patrols were thick, their objective no doubt to find the pilot before he could be safely brought out. From time to time the SEAL officer called in air strikes on enemy positions which were blocking their path to freedom. At one point, when it finally appeared they were in the clear, the NVA began pouring heavy automatic weapons fire toward them from the riverbank. Lieutenant

Norris requested an immediate air strike on the enemy position to cover their escape. Finally, just before daylight, they reached the forward operating base and safety.

Tom Norris stayed in Vietnam as an LDNN advisor and for the daring rescue mission he was awarded the Congressional Medal of Honor. His comrade-in-arms, LDNN Kiet, who volunteered to go with Norris became the only Vietnamese sailor in the war to be awarded the Navy Cross.

Later that same year Engineman Second Class Mike Thornton was given his chance to operate with Lieutenant Thomas Norris. No one could have predicted the outcome of this relationship, and what it would lead to. They were teammates. But they reached deeper under the Trident than most other teammates in order to excel at their jobs. Truthfully, they sought to achieve at superhuman levels and it was this drive which saw them through their darkest hour together.

In October 1972, Lieutenant Norris and Mike Thornton were operating as LDNN advisors out of Cat Lai, Vietnam. Tom Norris received a mission to gather intelligence on the Cua Viet Naval Base, previously owned and operated by the South Vietnamese prior to the Easter Offensive. Located on the Cua Viet River in Quang Tri Province, it was now believed to be under the control of the North Vietnamese Army. It was unknown if the NVA had taken prisoners or if all the RVN personnel were either scattered or dead. Lieutenant Norris was to put together a small team and infiltrate the area. Their mission was to locate and capture an NVA soldier for the purpose of interrogation.

Tom Norris had been working with a newly trained LDNN officer, trying to light a fire under him. He decided to take the new man along to see how he'd operate under pressure. Norris asked Thornton to handpick two LDNN enlisted men to join them on the operation. Mike knew exactly who he wanted, two combat hardened veterans he'd worked with on a previous tour.

The plan went into effect the night of October 30. The five-man team loaded aboard a Vietnamese Navy junk along with one other SEAL advisor, "Woody" Woodruff. Woody would handle communications from the junk during the operation. The vessel's captain assured the team he could insert them about eight kilometers south of the river. The junk stopped some distance offshore and launched the team in an IBS. Two other VN sailors from the junk went with the team as far as the beach, then returned to the junk in the IBS after Norris and Company were well on their way inland.

As it turned out their landing on the beach had gone undetected.

The team began to patrol inland across the sand dunes, then altered their course to move north to the river. Norris, a small SEAL, carried an AK47 on point because he could easily be taken as an NVA soldier if confronted by the enemy. That vital half second could mean the difference between life and death for the team. Mike was a big SEAL and he pulled rear security. He was armed with an assault rifle, which was mounted by a Starlight scope for night vision purposes. Tom Norris would say later that Mike made every effort to shrink himself that night, but that it was impossible. Thornton was just too big a man in every respect.

It wasn't long before Norris realized something wasn't right. As it turned out they were in the wrong place. From time to time Mike would move forward and confirm to Tom that he couldn't see the river, even when using the Starlight scope. Norris felt they should continue the mission because the young Vietnamese officer was showing initiative and wanted to operate. According to Lieutenant Norris, they could always come back the next night and go after an NVA prisoner.

Soon the team began passing platoon and company-sized encampments. Norris had never seen a bunker complex as large as what the recon team was now encountering. There were "major people" in the area, according to Tom. It turned out later the junk captain had dropped them north of the Cua Viet River instead of south. For all intents and purposes the team was dangerously close to being inside of North Vietnam proper.

At each security halt Mike came alongside his officer to confirm he'd seen and noted every detail of their patrol. At one point, Thornton picked out a Russian made tank sitting on a sand dune over one-thousand meters away using the

Starlight scope. There was no way of determining the size of the armor unit at the time, however, they now knew the enemy had moved some big guns up. Daylight was fast approaching and Norris knew it was time to get out while the getting was good. The team had to get back to the insertion point, plus they'd possibly already crossed over the dividing line between South and North Vietnam, which made things even more interesting. Daylight would not be the time to get caught over the border, smack dab in the middle of an NVA buildup!

The team was moving swiftly now, crossing the sand dunes and making for the insertion point. It was very hard to pinpoint their location because of the dunes and without clear reference points they couldn't call in accurate naval gunfire. Still, they almost made it but their luck ran out at the last possible second.

A two-man NVA beach patrol was spotted moving their way. The team froze and hoped this action would keep them undetected. But for some unknown reason the new LDNN officer called out to one of the NVA soldiers. The element of surprise evaporated and Mike knew he had to act quickly. Thornton moved around a sand dune and dropped the first NVA soldier with a horizontal butt stroke using his assault rifle. The second enemy soldier fired on the team, then dropped his weapon and ran. Mike was up and after him in a flash. Suddenly an entire NVA squad came running over the dunes and the firefight was on. Thornton gave up his chase and returned to the team's position. Together they killed or wounded all the NVA attempting to engage them. Lieutenant Norris spotted between fifty to sixty enemy soldiers rapidly moving forward to reinforce the shattered squad and he attempted to call in naval gunfire support.

For the next forty minutes heavy fighting took place between the SEALs and the NVA. Sporadic naval gunfire pummeled the beach from offshore. Tom recalls he had more than one Navy destroyer firing in support of his team. Every time he corrected the ships' fire a different voice would come up on the radio. The South Vietnamese junk had mortars onboard but it was refused permission to get close enough to participate in the action. It was later

302

learned one of the destroyers had taken incoming fire from an NVA shore battery.

The ground fighting reached a new level of intensity. The North Vietnamese now closed to within twenty-five meters of the team, well within grenade range. An NVA soldier rose up and threw a grenade at Mike, who scooped it up and threw it back. The grenade came flying back at Thornton who grabbed it up and threw it even harder back at the enemy. The third time around the grenade exploded behind Mike, its hot shrapnel striking him in both legs and also wounding one of the LDNNs in the hip. Thornton rolled onto his back and waited for the NVA grenadier to come running over the dune. When the man appeared Mike shot him.

Lieutenant Norris's next radio contact with the Navy was with the USS *Newport News*. He called in gunfire around the SEALs' position and remembers the rounds landed much closer than even he was comfortable with. So close, in fact, that every time one hit the beach the resulting explosion's power lifted a man as big as Thornton off the sand and well into the air! Still, the NVA kept coming. Norris knew he had no choice, no options left if they were to survive at all. He instructed the *Newport News* to give him five minutes then to commence firing directly on his position. With the coordinates given Tom ordered all of his men back to the last sand dune which might provide some kind of cover before all that was left to the SEALs was wide-open beach. Five minutes wasn't all that long but during this period a lot was to occur.

Mike and the wounded LDNN were the first two men to reach the dune. The last two LDNNs covered each other as they moved back, leapfrogging meter by meter toward their teammates. Norris raised up to fire his last LAAW rocket into the advancing NVA and was struck by a bullet in the left side of his skull. It was a critical wound and he only remained conscious for a few moments, then darkness fell. When the last LDNN reached Thornton he told Mike, "Mr. Norris shot in head. Dead now."

I suppose what happened next can only truly be understood by another SEAL. In training we are told time and time again that you will never leave a swim buddy, no matter what. It is drilled into each aspiring SEAL that no Navy frogman has ever been left behind, dead or wounded. None. Not one. Ever. Mike Thornton had learned this lesson loud and clear, and there was no other action he could take other than the one which now took place.

He moved. He not only moved he rose up and sprinted through one hundred twenty-five meters of deadly enemy gunfire to where his fallen teammate lay. Two NVA soldiers were nearly on top of Norris's body when Mike arrived. He killed both with his rifle. Bending over his officer, certain he was dead, Thornton was shocked when Tom regained consciousness long enough to say, "Mike, buddy . . ." and then he was lost in that long black tunnel again.

Thornton didn't hesitate. Lieutenant Norris was still alive! Slinging the wounded man over his shoulder Mike made the run one more time. Somehow he made it back to the sand dune despite the furious NVA gunfire aimed at the two SEALs. Now the LDNN asked Thornton what they were going to do. His answer was to fire his rifle into their radio so it wouldn't fall into the enemy's hands. "We swim," he told the astonished LDNN. He then headed for the water's edge with his teammate under tow. The LDNN provided accurate cover fire as Mike pulled and dragged and carried the now semiconscious lieutenant two hundred and fifty meters across the open beach. Wounded himself, and exhausted as well, Thornton turned time and again to fire his own rifle at the enemy even as they were trying to kill him and Tom Norris. The roar of the surf mixed with the roar of the gunfire was overwhelming. Still, the two men reached the surf zone. When they did the LDNNs followed, firing their weapons as they moved.

Mike dragged Norris into the four-foot surf and then inflated his CO_2 UDT life jacket. Using his powerful breaststroke Mike swam out to sea, pushing Lieutenant Norris ahead of him as both men bobbed in the water like tiny corks. He felt someone grab him and turning he found the LDNN who'd been wounded in the hip was having trouble swimming. Mike stopped, holding onto the man until the last two LDNNs reached them. Then he grabbed hold of his swim buddy, Tom Norris, and began heading out to sea again.

The NVA weren't through. Reaching the surf's edge the enemy soldiers fired everything they had at the swimmers. Bullets popped and squealed into the water around them. So close to freedom and safety but would they make it? Now several of the NVA waded into the water, firing their weapons in a last attempt to kill our teammates. Then the Navy spoke with authority. The *Newport News* sent a shrieking barrage of death onto the beach, right on time. Tom Norris had planned it just right, the NVA scattering and being scattered as salvo after salvo pounded into the beach. The NVA assault was broken up and brought to an end. Still, Mike Thornton led the way, swimming strongly farther and farther away from land.

Along the way Mike gave Tom what first aid he could under the circumstances. At times the wounded officer came to, but only for a moment or two and then he would black out again. He says he still remembers being in the water with Mike, once asking if everyone had made it out from the beach. For two hours the team swam, moving always out to sea, farther and farther from the beach.

On the junk, bouncing from wave to wave, all eyes were straining for anything that would indicate someone had survived the onslaught. From the sea it appeared the team had been overrun by the enemy. No one had heard from them since Norris had called in fire on his own position. To a man everybody in the crew save one man believed no one could have lived through what they'd just witnessed. It had been more than a firefight, it had been a war. Soon, the crew and its captain wanted to give up the search and head for the safety of the base. But Woody Woodruff was both a SEAL and onboard the junk that day and there was no "give-up" in him. You didn't leave a swim buddy, you never left a SEAL behind. Woody insisted on continuing the search.

And when a SEAL insists on something you had better listen up. In my heart I believe if our teammate had not forced the issue this story would not have had anything other than the ending it did. To my knowledge this is the first time Woody Woodruff's critical role in this event has been told.

After two long hours of searching, the junk's crew finally spotted the swimmers. At 1130 hours they pulled them aboard, the junk captain wasting no time in putting out to sea for a linkup with the *Newport News*. When Mike Thornton was pulled onto the junk's deck he was completely drained of his immense strength, strength that had once pulled Hal Kuykendall away from the jaws of death, strength that today had saved yet another teammate's life. All three wounded men received medical attention as soon as it was made available. Lt. Tom Norris survived and fully recovered from his head wound but only after many months of treatment and care. Mike Thornton became the only enlisted SEAL to receive the Congressional Medal of Honor, and he did so by being the only MOH winner to realize this honor by saving another Medal of Honor winner's life under enemy fire.

Men like Bob Kerrey, Tom Norris, and Mike Thornton march to a different drummer than most of us. They push themselves to the very limits of their abilities. Are they superhuman? Well, I don't know about that. What I do know is the effort and loyalty they demonstrated when most others would waiver sure comes close.

I am proud to have once been Mike Thornton's team chief. I'm proud to have had him in CHARLIE platoon. Most of all I'm proudest of having been "Big Mike's" teammate.

30

A Commando's Homecoming

It is well that war is so terrible, or we should grow too fond of it.

—Robert E. Lee, December 1882

CHARLIE platoon was preparing to end its tour of Vietnam. Soon we would be packing up and leaving Coastal Group 36, heading once again back to the States. Rich Solano wanted to visit some teammates at Seafloat whom he'd served with on a previous tour. Solano was the kind of man who could always be depended on in any situation and we saw no reason why he couldn't make his visit. In fact, he'd always operated with our platoon and had never asked for a break throughout the tour. Lieutenant Boyhan once told me, "Rich Solano is the All-American Boy." I thought about that and I haven't been able to come up with a better way to describe Rich. Now, he wasn't a boy at all, in fact, he was very much a man. But the term fit him as the compliment it was meant to be.

The rest of the platoon packed our equipment and nothing else was thought of or talked about but going home. Home to a wife and family, to a Mom and Dad, to a sweetheart. Home to the teams in Coronado and our teammates which made them up. Home to clean clothes, good food, and all the things we'd lacked, overlooked, done without, or taken for granted most of our lives. Most of all we were going home to security. The security of not having to look over one's shoulder day and night. It looked like CHARLIE was almost home free. Almost.

The platoon had done an outstanding job under the most adverse of conditions. We'd conducted seventy combat operations netting ninety-one VC/NVA KIAs by accurate body count. There were eleven VC/NVA KIAs probable, thirty VC/NVA WIAs confirmed by intelligence reports or blood trails, fifteen VC/NVAs captured and numerous weapons, documents, and supplies taken. Among the enemy accounted for were one province level and seven district level VCI chiefs. With a total of one hundred nineteen members of the Vietcong infrastructure either killed or captured, CHARLIE platoon had made its mark up high on the tree.

All of this was the result of Lt. Tom Boyhan's aggressive and imaginative operational planning. He was above all else a professional warrior and the finest officer I ever served with in my twenty years of naval service.

We shoved off from CG 36 and headed for Saigon. When we arrived bad news was waiting for us and it set everyone back on his heels. Rich Solano, our teammate, had just been killed during an administrative helicopter flight from Seafloat to Binh Thuy. He was enroute to Saigon to come home with us the very next day. Four other SEALs were also killed in the same accident. It is said to be the most tragic loss of life the SEALs suffered in Vietnam in a single incident.

The helicopter crashed for some unknown reason at the time. Years later at a SEAL reunion I learned from a SEAL then stationed at Seafloat that the crew had just returned from a hot landing zone where they'd taken fire. There had been an explosion and the slick had lost altitude, but then recovered. When the helo landed at Seafloat its crew checked it out but didn't shut the engine down. The SEALs were ready to leave Seafloat and no other helicopter would be available until the next day. So, they climbed aboard regardless of possible problems. Their decision cost them their lives. It was no fault of their own, any of us would have done the same thing. You possessed the attitude that if the pilots and crew would fly it, you'd do the same.

I knew how close Rich and Tom Boyhan had become in the last six months. It is impossible to lead patrol after patrol working with the same pointman without developing a relationship between the two of you that is special. Tom had spoken to me about the quick reactions Rich had and how Tom depended upon Solano on point. When Tom was told Rich was dead, his face betrayed no expression. We were all in a state of disbelief.

Mr. Boyhan asked if I would go to the morgue with him to identify the bodies. It was one of those requests you don't think to refuse, however, you certainly don't look forward to it. I recall four of us actually went. The only teammate I remember for sure was Hal Kuykendall and he was along because he knew all the SEALs on Seafloat. Tom borrowed a jeep and we left for the morgue at Tan Son Nhut.

After arriving we were told the bodies weren't ready for viewing. Tom informed the morgue personnel we were leaving the country and they let us come back. The morgue was the size of three large gymnasiums, with offices scattered throughout the huge structure. The work area itself had ten tables on one side of the room and six others opposite. There were body bags on the tables, and the bodies of our teammates were still in them.

At one point in our tour I'd asked Rich about the nasty scar he had on one of his wrists. He told me he'd been drilling a hole in a tin can with an electric drill when a young boy. The lid had slipped and cut his wrist. I asked the sergeant with us to see if such a scar was present and it was. There wasn't anything else I needed to see to know this was Rich Solano.

Hal called me over to where he was with the other body bags. "That's Toby Thomas, and that's Gore," he said, while pointing at their contents. Hal zipped open another bag and identified Durlin and Donnelly, as well. They were all wearing tan UDT swim trunks. Their skin had been burnished bronze by Vietnam's powerful sun and this made them stand out from other bodies also in the morgue. Tom came over to pay his respects, and then offered it was time to leave. We thanked the sergeant and made our way out.

It was time for the platoon to leave but I didn't want to leave Lieutenant Boyhan in Vietnam by himself. He was going to stay behind to break in the new SEAL platoon replacing us. I wanted to go home to be with my family more than anything. Still, the responsibility of helping Tom finish the job had my guts churning. Lieutenant Boyhan refused my offer to stay. Something about my seeing the platoon got back to the States all right. I knew there were others who could handle this job but I believe he wanted all of us out of Vietnam before something else happened.

Onboard the airplane I found my seat and fastened its belt around my lap. We were on our way. Most of the men were quiet and when they were talking it was to the man next to them. I'm sure their thoughts were on Rich. I still had Tom on my mind and maybe the platoon did too. If only he would just take the new platoon on a Sunday walk through the nipa palm and come home. Not Tom, not his style. Before coming back to the States he would go on another Brightlight operation with the new platoon.

It was a long flight home. There was an abundance of time to just sit and think. After about an hour of staring at white caps on the ocean far below I turned back to watch the men. Some of us would be returning to Vietnam. I've been asked many times why we went back again and again. I haven't been able until now to come up with an answer for this question, at least not a good one.

Was it for our country, or for freedom, or for the folks back home? Or was it just for the Navy? I don't think any of these fueled our true motivation. Sitting there watching Tom's and my men it hit me and I couldn't figure out why I hadn't seen it before now. We went back for each other. We go to war for each other. It is what being a teammate is all about, being there for each other.

The plane was quiet now and the only ones awake other than myself were Hal and Thornton. I don't think Mike knew how to be quiet. Hal was on Mike's case about something and Mike kept saying, "Ah, Cuz, you don't mean that." It was the normal banter between those two men and what made them inseparable. More than likely Hal was trying to convince Mike of how close he'd come to going to the brig just before we left the country.

It seemed Mike had gotten into a little contest with two Army MPs. He'd ended up lifting both men off the ground by their shirtfronts, slamming them into a nearby wall. The wide-eyed MPs could only grab Thornton by his arms as their feet were dangling eighteen inches off the floor of wherever it was they were on. In a very calm voice Lieutenant Boyhan had said, "Mike, put them down." Thornton did just that and Tom got him out of there as fast as he could. The MPs didn't push the matter. They were either shaken by the SEAL's matchless strength or just glad to be saved by our lieutenant. Maybe it was a little of both. Mr. Boyhan told me years later he'd never known a man as strong as Mike Thornton, and I had to agree.

It came to me that perhaps our platoon commander had sent me along with the platoon so I, its chief, could keep Thornton out of trouble . . . at least until we got back to the Silver Strand.

To say I was looking forward to seeing my wife and three children would be an understatement. I wondered if they would be at the North Island Naval Air Station when we landed? How would my wife know what plane we were coming in on? Or on what day, for that matter? Well, she'd always been there before and I was sure she'd find out one way or another. Who else would be there? Hal's, Thornton's, and LaCaze's wives would certainly be present. Maybe Mike Sands's wife too, if she was back from Montana by now. How about the single men? Would there be no one to meet them on the tarmac, no one to go home to or with? No one to give them a hug, to congratulate them for coming home alive and in one piece? Or would they still be there for each other? Was leave planned, leave going back to a home and family somewhere in the United States where they would be welcome and safe?

Hal and Mike were probably right about me. Maybe I was a "Mama Knock Knock." But these teammates had been my family for the last six months. Heck, I could worry over them a little, couldn't I?

I was happy we were returning to a military town like San Diego. We'd heard so much talk in Vietnam about veterans of the war who returned home and were made to feel unwelcome, and even unwanted. It was said some were even spat upon by their fellow Americans. I'd never heard of this happening to a SEAL, and if it had I'm sure someone would have gotten hurt and someone else would have gone to jail. I hoped our men would find the image they'd held of home the same as when they'd left. As for themselves, well, we'd all changed in one way or another.

Many would take offense to "longhairs" or "hippies," maybe even to college students in general for all the antiwar protesting and flag burning we'd heard and seen while in Vietnam. Did I really believe one of my men, or any SEAL, would just stand by and allow himself to be spat on by a hippie? No, not a SEAL fresh from facing enemy troops deep in the jungles and waterways of Vietnam. Certainly not a member of CHARLIE platoon, whose every member now had a huge hole in his heart from the loss of Rich Solano the day before we were all to fly to safety. Such an irrational and stupid action would deserve its just reward if anyone even thought of issuing such a "protest" in our direction.

My thoughts went back to the men and what was coming. Would the folks back home perhaps meet them with kindness? Would the families try to understand? Would the sweethearts and wives have the compassion necessary to bring their men back to a world they'd had to set aside in order to survive? I said a little prayer: "Lord, you have kept them safe. Now, let them feel warmth in returning, let them have a Homecoming."

As long as I live I will never get used to returning home. I always tremble inside before I step off the plane. When we touched down that time I was trembling. But to this day I still remember, still feel, little arms around my legs, two larger arms around my waist, and two very wonderful arms around my neck. As for me, I was afraid—really afraid—to hug back as hard as I wanted to and knew I could for fear I'd break something.

I was home again.

My work wouldn't be complete if I didn't report what happens to a burly SEAL commando once he stops being a jungle fighter. What happens to teammates who have become family to each other? How do they fit in when they return to civilian life? This may be the hardest part to put into words that I have written.

One of our teammates is a United States Senator and one is a minister of the Gospel. Some are firefighters and some are police officers. Others are farmers and still others the CEOs of major companies. Some went on to own their own businesses while other work for their teammates today. Some became naval officers and others stayed in the Navy, making it their life's career. Some went into sales and some became consultants. I know teammates who work offshore and teammates who work underwater. Some are teachers in our schools and some are students pursuing their education. Some of us retired. The list goes on and on and on.

What they do professionally doesn't really matter. What does is this. They are the next-door neighbor and members of the communities in which they live. They are Scout Masters, 4-H leaders, and they even coach Little League. You will find them to be family men who love and honor their wives, and they are fathers and some even grandfathers.

Once at a SEAL reunion for Vietnam Veterans held in Colorado I found myself talking with John Ware's wife, Jimmie. I asked her how John was doing and her answer was not what I was ready for. She didn't tell me what a good provider John was, or what a good husband. Rather, she looked me right in the eye and gave my teammate the greatest compliment a wife can give a husband. "He's a good daddy," Jimmie said. Then, as if she wanted to make sure I understood her she repeated herself. "He's a *good* daddy." I have never forgotten what Mrs. Ware told me or what John Ware, former jungle fighter, had become.

I have often been asked about drugs and drug use in Vietnam. You hear about it everywhere, in the movies and on television, and even in a variety of reading material, some about SEALs. In all my time in Vietnam I never knew of a SEAL involved with drugs. Not even experimentation. In my platoons I wouldn't tolerate it, and those who served with me knew this. In fact, I never knew of any military men who even used or talked about drugs. Maybe this was because of the work we did and the isolated, terribly remote areas we worked in.

For sure, we weren't Saigon warriors. That's not meant as

an excuse, it's just that drugs were not a part of my teammates' lives. They, like myself, wouldn't have put up with a drug user.

And I feel strongly about that statement.

When the war was over SEALs went in different directions, settling down in every state of the Union. Yet we stay in contact with each other, one way or another. I have one teammate in West Virginia who calls me about every other month. It's always after I've gone to bed. I'm delighted to hear his voice, however, regardless of the time. He is still that kind of friend. We have some help keeping up with each other and it's provided by the Fraternal Order of UDT/SEAL. If you have a lost teammate they will lend a hand in finding him.

The teams themselves host a reunion every summer and some smaller reunions are held from time to time, from state to state. Then there's the unexpected knock on the door and you find a teammate on your porch, just stopping by to say "hi." Twenty-five years or more and there's still something special in how we feel about each other. We will always be family.

This level of friendship and brotherhood may be hard for some to understand. For those who have missed it I am truly sorry. Men need friends who are men. A former Army ranger, Stu Weber, wrote a book titled *Tender Warrior*. He said the following:

> *Yes, beyond question, our wives are to be our most intimate companions. We're to be willing to die for our wives and children instantly, and many of us are ready to do just that. But within the willingness to die for family and home, something inside us longs for someone to die with . . . someone to die beside . . . someone to lock step with. Another man with a heart like our own.*

In this single paragraph Ranger Weber captures the heart of a SEAL. When I read his words I understand why I locked step with Bill Machen. I understand why he was willing to give up his life for his teammates instantly, without question or reservation. I understand fully why thirty-three other men from SEAL Team One followed Bill into the "dark waters" where they, as one, wait for us.

For they are our TEAMMATES.

Bibliography

BOOKS

Bosiljevac, T.L. *SEALs.* New York: Ivy Books, 1987.

Dockery, Kevin. *SEALs in Action.* New York: Avon, 1991.

Hoyt, Edwin P. *SEALs at War.* New York: Dell, 1993.

Kelly, Orr. *Brave Men—Dark Waters.* New York: Pocket Books, 1993.

Mills, Nick. *Combat Photographer.* Boston: Boston Publishing Co., 1983.

Walker, Greg. *At the Hurricane's Eye.* New York: Ivy Books, 1994.

Weber, Stu. *Tender Warrior.* Sisters, OR: Questar, 1993.

PERIODICALS

Couch, Richard. "My First Firefight." *Shipmate,* 1987.

Edwards, Steve. "Nasty Boats & Nasty Boys." *Fighting Knives,* 1991.

Bibliography

Edwards, Steve. "POWs, MIAs, and SEALs." *Fighting Knives,* 1991.

James, Frank. "Stoner 63." *Firepower,* 1986.

Jenkins, Lynn. "Sea, Air and Land." *All Hands,* 1987.

Kokalis, Peter. "Stoner Super 63." *Soldier of Fortune,* 1991.

Tarble, Jerry. "The Stoner Machine Guns." *Machine Gun News,* 1990.

Walker, Greg. "Elite SEAL Units." *International Combat Arms,* 1989.